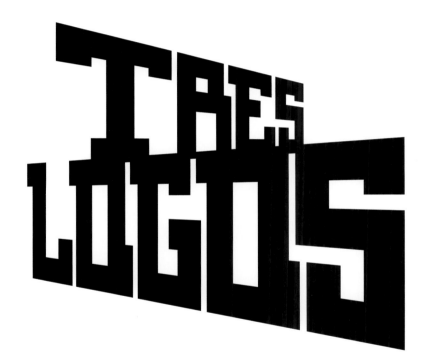

Table of contents   Inhaltsverzeichnis   3

Foreword   4

Vorwort   10

Corporate   Corporate   16

Culture   Kultur   84

Design   Design   132

Fashion   Mode   214

Motion/Games/Media   Motion/Games/Media   288

Music   Musik   316

Other/Art/Unclassifiable   Andere/Kunst/Unklassifizierbar   376

Political   Politik   416

Sports   Sport   432

Address Index   460

Work Index   475

Imprint   508

SOMETHING WANTS TO SEE THE LIGHT!

by Robert Klanten and Nicolas Bourquin

It germinates, proliferates, and explodes.
Everywhere are plants, animals, skulls, and thunderbolts.
All in all, these are very good signs.

The third installment of our "Logos" series again features a conspicuous number of animals. Lions, elephants, mice, cats, eagles, rabbits, zebras, giraffes, hamsters, hummingbirds and horses. Heavenly horses, winged horses, galloping horses and unicorns. Not to mention ducks, quails, flamingos, bulls, hyenas, dragons, trout and chickens. Each animal form undergoes all manner of transformations, probably a consequence of the fact that both designers and animals have been nibbling at overripe fruit. We find elephants with bags under their eyes, demonically glowering panda bears and lions with poodle manes.

This year, transformation, fertility, and the organic are central themes. Branches shoot out from names and titles, there are rampant ornaments and madly overloaded coats of arms. Illustrations sprawling around letters like viruses. Scratched messages, layered scrawls. The logos are proliferating. But what does it mean?

THE FERTILITY OF CHARACTERS

In line with the world's increasing diversity, signs and written characters are multiplying. Increasingly, commodity groups, brands, and enterprises, but our own interests and biographies as well, become differentiated, ramified. According to a study performed by Mercer Management Consulting, the number of products available for purchase has increased fivefold in the past 20 years. Every week, 600 new products vie for space on the shelves of German supermarkets. The average individual makes 100,000 decisions daily, the majority of them without conscious awareness. An average of 3,000 marketing messages assault us daily – and assuming eight hours of sleep, that means one every 30 seconds.

Given this fragmentation, the impact of each message is necessarily diminished. Brand names lose their lustre. Formerly they used to be reservoirs of our collective desires. But this ocean has become a sea of droplets. "Today, brand names embody the values attributed to them by the individual user," writes the Hamburg-based trend agency in their "Simplexity" study.

We join forces in mini-communities and publish weblogs. Thousands of new aesthetic concepts emerge from the soil. Things are faster, more creative, more anarchic than ever before. The proprietors of the most celebrated logos are beginning to observe all of this with curiosity. Every individual today is a potential target group and potential logo material.

The great challenge for every brand name today, then, is to be just like any other individual, while still representing a larger entity. To stay in the game, they need to cover both bases.

Complex, proliferating, weighed down with baubles and embellishments like a Christmas tree, overloaded and fragmented: these are the new logos. But none strive to conceal the contrast between simple and complex, between large and small, between strong and weak. For that is exactly where we are today.

The world is a madhouse. And the logos, too, are running riot. They celebrate the simultaneity of complexity and simplicity. They mix contradictions without resolving them. They say what they need to say concisely, directly and emotionally. In most cases, they are both engaging and entertaining. Small wonder: given the sheer quantity of messages, modesty and restraint will hardly serve.

THE END OF SOBRIETY

Logos used to be the identifiying mark of an organisational unit: enterprise, utility, political party, association. In those days, enterprises consisted of physical entities such as factories, conveyor belts and factory gates. The logo was an academic, simplified variant of core industrial activities, or else represented a firm's history like a coat of arms.

The four rings of the Audi logo, for example, stand for the founding enterprises of the Auto Union: the Audi, Horch, DKW automotive works and the automotive department of the Wanderer firm. The BMW logo represents an airplane propeller seen from the front. The three-part Mercedes star stands for the elements earth, water and air, since this mixed concern originally wanted to build motors capable of conquering all three natural forces. "Mitsu" "bishi" means "three" "diamonds", which in turn symbolises the ship propellers that once earned its revenues. The stacked chevrons of the Citroën logo stand for a specific type of cogwheel that made founder Andre Citroën famous even before he began building automobiles.

Today there are ideas, networks and services. No enterprise would dare to face the world armed with such an academic abstraction. First of all, because the elements expressed as signs in the logos of the old economy are today simply purchased from industrial suppliers. Secondly, brands, and not engineers, play a central role in today's enterprises. And thirdly, nowadays no one would understand these reductions as in the absence of their historical background, they appear cold and hollow.

Increasingly, global players are gearing their insignia toward the emotional. Years ago, the ice cream maker Langnese, for example, known in nearly every country of the world under a different name (Walls, Holanda, Miko, Frisko, Eskimo, Ola and Kibo, to name just a few) discarded its trademark marquee and replaced it with the globally recognised heart logo. In the age of globalisation, logos must be both emotionally appealing and readily comprehensible.

Emotion has become the commercial language of global marketing. Small or unknown firms strive to devise symbols that will trigger the same associations everywhere in the world. For a simple, emotional symbol can convey the allure of a brand via the narrowest channels and on the smallest display formats.

THE NEW LOQUACIOUSNESS

That was yesterday. But simple and emotional is no longer enough. Amid the sheer diversity of communication, the tried and tested quickly wears out. And just as this drive toward economic unification known as globalisation has incited a countertrend of rationalisation, the fact that we can be everything and everywhere simultaneously has allowed the world of signs to sprout and bloom like after a tropical rainstorm.

In former times, there was neon lighting, rubber stamps and the factory gates. Instead of reducing everything to a single statement, the new logo ornaments are complex and eventful, as though they could hardly wait to relate their entire histories.

Logos used to be signs of the first order. They stated: "I am." The new logos communicate: "I encounter you. I tell you about myself."

THE NEW ROMANTICISM

As late as the 1990s, business themes were illustrated with brisk individuals wearing ties who would listen to one another admiringly and shake hands. At some point, text and image façades became so perfect and that designers began to incorporate interference. It began with digital fuzz, fluff and scratches to endow the design with something handmade. By incorporating doodles, Apple, for example, endowed its iLife package with a touch of the analogue. Nowadays, we have arrived at the organic ornament, at the plant level. Coca-Cola makes its appearance as a youth movement, composing collages of people, floral patterns and birds for its global campaign "The March", an unfettered mixture of punk, hippie culture and Xerox art.

With these floral themes, scratch marks and ornaments, nature reaches directly into the world of digital objects – which remain intangible in the truest sense of the word. The ornament fills this comprehension gap. In the age of the MP3 player and digital exchange networks, the live concert is currently enjoying a glorious renaissance. The campaigns for the new generation of MP3 player mobile phones by Nokia and Sony Ericsson are bursting with floral energy. Nokia even features tendrils on one of its mobile phone ranges.

Every technical revolution gives rise to its own romantic countermovement. So it should not come as a surprise that these new flourishes are so reminiscent of earlier attempts at effecting aesthetic upheavals: the Renaissance, Art Nouveau and Psychedelic Pop.

Wild nature wants to return. The primeval forest emerges from the concrete.

SELL-OUT REVOLUTION

Ten years ago, "never touch the logo" was still an overriding law of design that only a few brands (like Burton, for example) dared to break. Stated differently: particularly with seasonal articles such as designer clothing and electronics, it is regarded as good form to develop ac-

tion logos which allow global brands to break into local scenes. Things are redesigned, sprayed on, reinterpreted and revolutionized – all on commission from marketing departments. Texts are translated into the lingo of target groups. The more fragmented the product portfolio, the more diverse the differing versions of the logo. Adidas, for example, developed its own spray-painted logo for its +10 Campaign, which was then applied by so-called "guerrilla teams" to public surfaces. Naturally, these concrete surfaces were leased in advance for advertising purposes. The triple-blade logo pops up in other locations as well, and young artists are hired to revive its paint-your-own shoe "Adicolor". The Y-3 label, too, a collaboration between fashion designer Yohji Yamamoto and Adidas, manifests itself in fractions: here the hero cult of the Chinese Cultural Revolution is cited; there cranes take flight from the logo.

In a now familiar strategy of appropriation, global brands usurp the codes used by activists such as Adbusters or by the political left: spontaneous poster-style silkscreen collages, East Coast campus look. In the case of Coca-Cola, the new look is even designed by protagonists of the movements or people from the art scene. But the big challenge facing businesses is to genuinely achieve the sense of closeness affected in their design and the messages they convey. For increasingly, they will be judged by the degree of consistency between reality and design.

And where the large brands start to fragment and seek out even the smallest target groups by tuning their action logos accordingly, smaller labels hit back by inflating themselves, getting rowdy and going up against the big players with brass knuckle logos. Many streetwear labels are emphatically martial in character. Thick lines, marker pen designs – one part sprayed tag, one part anti-capitalist barricade.

Of course, there are always hand-drawn tags, which are then scanned and converted into vectors. But it appears that the classic street or hip-hop logo is on the way out. Many sprayers who earlier graced entire urban districts with their work have lately discovered a fondness for architecture. Instead of drawing, their activities now revolve around

spaces and bodies. When they go to work at their computers or drawing boards or in their workshops, the results are massive, three-dimensional designs and collaborations with new partners and techniques.

PANDORA'S BOX

But of course, the bastardisation of drawing was not really concocted by marketing departments – large companies are too sluggish for that. This creative revolution – like every one before it – has its origins in technology. And it is only able to spread so quickly because it reflects social reality.

Just as the digitised Internet has been a driving force behind globalisation (the all-connecting movement of commodities, brands and manufacturers), digital vector graphics techniques have sparked a massive crossover of images and symbols. Just as the boundaries between branches of the industry are dissolving, for example when Apple penetrated the entertainment electronics market with its iPod or turned the music industry inside out with its iTunes, vector graphics have dismantled taboos, borders between scenes and inhibitions.

Vector graphics, the digitally-defined, filled-in surface, offer the perfect platform for all kinds of layerings, mixtures and bastardisations. Many designers, who have been exclusively occupied in this area for years, have accumulated gigantic data bases containing thousands of forms, structures and images.

And so missiles acquire legs, antlers grow out of letters, serif fonts form branches, Marx grows roots, chimpanzees nibble on a brain while sitting in an egg and grow dendrites. Texts, patterns and images sprawl into collages and coats of arms harbouring an undergrowth of strange characters. These proliferations are excessive and explosive, as though some maniac had opened Pandora's box. Dartboards on which everything tossed up in the process of brainstorming has simply stuck – it is precisely this absence of restraint that makes the new logo so entertaining.

By means of this inconsistency, they also embody the delights and the schizophrenia of the present – fortunately, without commentary. What could you say anyway? A single persistent theme: irony. Taboos are dissolved. It is this simultaneity of contradictions that comes closest to reality. Hip Hop meets Kiss meets Britney Spears meets Nazi Surfer.

These hyper-crests make up the wrought iron gates around enchanted gardens in which we lose ourselves in contemplation even before we enter – take for example the logo of the French restaurant/bar Omnia. Or the Kultivator logo: the central cow's head is surrounded by a star formation composed of a rake, a goose, tractors, vegetables, screw nuts, brushes, dowels, ducks and ears. The solution to this picture puzzle could only be some kind of artistic commune. Precisely so, for we are dealing with a hybrid of organic farm, workshop and arts project on the island of Öland in southern Sweden with its affiliated "Agri-Cultural Shop".

By contradicting our expectations of the traditional logo, such images are not always immediately legible. But that is not the point. It is a question of spatial scope, depth of content and the decoding of riddles. Such hybrid insignia often perform better than plain writing when it comes to holding the attention of the beholder.

The hyper-logos tell stories. Which is why they are more successful than others. To be sure, they are not immediately intelligible – but by way of compensation, they are all the more worth deciphering. Occasionally, the beholder's imagination assumes the role of the narrator, allowing these new crests and portals to emerge from the world of the image into that of language. They make up new hybrids mixing image and language. New grammars, new metaphors. Word. Image. Idea. Logo.

CORPORATE INNOCENCE

Small, young enterprises use story-telling logos to control their dimensions and identities – inventing their own instant histories. Larger enterprises use the same mechanisms, adopting the language of

small-scale symbols to appear naïve and approachable. Now they play at being revolutionary, now quaint. But the message remains the same: the world is complex, and so are we. More is the new more.

One corporation that has achieved a consistent translation of this harmony of contradictions is Unilever, a manufacturer of consumer products. Above the company name, seemingly executed with a paintbrush, we find a "U" consisting of smaller units. These include a bee, a pullover, a wave, a molecule, a sun, a recycling logo, ice cream, a dove and a number of other elements. Each symbol stands for a specific product, branch of operations or value.

Where the crests of smaller enterprises represent an anarchic commentary on the present, global businesses, of course, use theirs to convey fairy tales – not unlike Microsoft, for example, disguising its tentacular aggressiveness behind a butterfly logo. It wasn't long before a couple of graphic designers put a new Flash variant of the Unilever logo on the Internet, where it offers commentary on the rosy "Unilever Land" from a left-wing perspective.

But this activism-based critique mainly serves to confirm the effectiveness of the Unilever logo. It is perceived, taken seriously, elicits commentary. In design terms, it shifts the company into the realm of the avant-garde. The controversial whistle logo of the last soccer World Cup also pursued this new approach. The viewer's knowledge of the event's content, namely "football", is assumed. The logo transports purely emotional messages that were actually fulfilled by the subsequent event: fun, masquerade, party. The logo as mascot – something more suitable for a children's brand or a leisure park.

LOST WORLDS

Products, channels, devices, communication, visual languages, logo languages: the world proliferates, and the logos multiply accordingly. Noticeably, this growth follows acquired rules. Either the various signs organise themselves on shield-like surfaces like contemporary coats of arms, or else they expand organically, like artificial creepers, their empty surfaces crammed with metaphors. And nature is constantly cited. Coat of arms and ornament: both forms rely conspicuously on symbols related to flora and fauna.

With saucer eyes, flowers, rabbits, hummingbirds and winged bear cubs, childish traits invade the logos – even in the corporate world. The innocence exuded by these little darlings points directly towards descriptions of worlds we can never re-enter: paradisiacal landscapes, shapes and nests that can only be soiled by contact with us.

But this Bambi syndrome reveres a nature no one has ever encountered in reality. Logo nature remains sterile. They are idealised, fantasy archetypes that embody justice, authenticity and a mild yearning for order. These nature symbols and ornaments comment on digital reality in a voice that is both kitschy and romantic. Not unlike earlier renaissances, it is a question of spirituality, ant-rationalism and sensuality. Just like photography, where the hyperrealism of flash-startled eyes made way for an artificial, almost religious hyper-romanticism, the encompassing metaphor of nature symbolises our search for the roots that simply cannot take hold in a circuit board.

EXPECTO PATRONUM!

Where there is flora, there is fauna. The incredible throng of animals – whether Bambi or fantasy dragons – can no longer be explained solely by the fact that designers need to discover emotional references for their messages. Instead, we find new legions of heraldic animals. The old ones are still with us. Eagle, lion, unicorn, dragon. There are the construction kits for coats of arms, such as Logikwear's Crestbuilder, as well as droves of marvellous new totemic animals, spiritual escorts, guardian angels and Harry Potteresque spiritual guardians summoned by new enterprises, law firms, art galleries, design offices, cultural agencies, NGOs, global players, and one-man businesses in order to guard their wearers, especially in these troubled times.

Against this background, we can also interpret the non-symbolic/figurative ornaments, these colourful, layered kaleidoscopes composed of magical amulets. All of these create and shape identities. But crests, signet rings, gems and logos have also always served as protectors.

The numerous other natural symbols as well – thunderbolts, clouds, sunrises – are all anchored in a pre-digital era. All are aesthetic, material extensions designed to glorify the era of brands, ecstasy and the Internet. The grandchildren of the '68 generation cheerfully remix Woodstock, the Grateful Dead and everything else psychedelic. Which is why skulls and lightning bolts are popping up all over the place. Lightning strikes from the most unlikely places, and there are skulls in all imaginable variations. Skulls with crossed chopsticks, skulls concealed in audio cassettes, Mickey Mouse skulls, skulls with cigars, with spikes, with quills, skulls with roots.

These frequently baroque arrangements, this taboo-breaking mix and match of transient elements, is, of course, pure heavy metal. "Memento mori", they call out to us when they build their logo still lifes, reminding us of our own mortality. All of our creations are dedicated to Vanitas, to futile vanity. But to interpret these baroque logos as admonitions would be a mistake. For the downfall is part of change.

LET THERE BE LIGHT!

The new logos, the ornaments, the filled spaces, the wallpaper patterns and molecules, the anarchic still lifes, the freely associative, piled up, megalomaniac mountains of images, the enchanted portals and entwined letters: all of it mirrors the complexity of our times. Their prototypes are signets. They are reflections of a time characterised by creativity and insecurity.

But the palpable symbols in these patterns can be read as symbols of collective dreams. They provide hints about where things are headed.

It is common knowledge that we live in times of upheaval. The hordes of totemic beasts watch over us in our quest for the transcen-tental. Lightning bolts have always stood for energy, intuition and release. Clarity, strength, liberation and radicality. But also for steadfastness, for a bolt of lightning is not something half-hearted, not revocable. And many people seem to yearn for inspirational bolts from the sky to hurl us into states of rational confusion while clearing away old, decaying material.

The proliferation of skulls by no means indicates that designers worldwide are yearning for death. On the contrary. The skulls also stand for change, for the new and even for communication. In many folk festivals, from Mexico to Italy, skulls, often painted in garish colours, play a part in dramatising life. The hoisted skull-and-crossbones flag on a raiding pirate ship signalled a willingness to negotiate. It said: "You can talk to us." Only when the attackers raised a red flag it was clear: now it is a question of life and death.

A logo is always half yearning, half oracle. It is up to us which of the two prevails. The latest new signs are already visible on the horizon of the US-American West Coast: still more patterns, still more psychedelic art, resulting in correspondingly headache-inducing logos, tribalism, and eco-organic systems.

The prevailing mood is one of romanticism. What we see is complex. What we need: strength. What arrives is spiritual. Or psychedelic. All in all, the prospects look good.

ETWAS WILL ANS LICHT!

von Robert Klanten und Nicolas Bourquin

Es sprießt, wuchert und explodiert.
Überall Pflanzen, Tiere, Totenköpfe und Blitze.
Alles in allem sind das sehr gute Zeichen.

Auch in der dritten Ausgabe von unserer „Logos"-Reihe sind wieder auffällig viele Tiere dabei. Löwen, Elefanten, Mäuse, Katzen, Adler, Kaninchen, Zebras, Giraffen, Hamster, Kolibris und Pferde. Feuerpferde, geflügelte Pferde, galoppierende Pferde und Einhörner. Außerdem: Enten, Wachteln, Flamingos, Bullen, Hyänen, Drachen, Gänse, Forellen und Hühner. Die Tiergestalten machen allerhand Verwandlungen durch, die wohl daher stammen, dass Gestalter oder Tier vergorene Früchte genascht hat. So kommen Elefanten mit Augenringen zu Stande, teuflisch grollende Pandabären und Löwen mit Pudelmähne.

Verwandlung, Fruchtbarkeit und Organik, das sind die großen Themen dieses Jahr. Aus Namen und Schriftzügen schießen Knospen und Äste, es gibt wuchernde Ornamente und irrwitzig überladene Wappen. Illustrationen, die wie Geschwüre um Schrift wuchern. Geritzte Botschaften, geschichtetes Gekrakel. Die Logos wuchern. Aber was bedeutet das?

DIE FRUCHTBARKEIT DER ZEICHEN

Mit der Vielfalt der Welt vermehren sich natürlich auch die Zeichen. Warengruppen, Marken und Unternehmen, aber auch unsere eigenen Interessen und Lebensläufe nehmen immer feinere Verästelungen. Allein die Zahl der Produkte, die es zu kaufen gibt, hat sich laut einer Studie der Unternehmensberatung Mercer Management Consulting in den letzten zwanzig Jahren verfünffacht. Sechshundert neue Produkte drängen jede Woche neu in die Regale der deutschen Supermärkte. An die 100.000 verschiedene Entscheidungen treffen wir durchschnittlich jeden Tag, die meisten davon unbewusst. Durchschnittlich 3.000 Markenbotschaften prasseln täglich auf uns, bei acht Stunden Schlaf macht das alle dreißig Sekunden eine.

Mit dieser Fragmentierung nimmt die Wirkung jeder Botschaft zwangsläufig ab. Marken verlieren ihre Leuchtkraft. Früher waren sie Sammelbecken für unsere kollektiven Wünsche. Aus dem Ozean ist ein Meer der Tropfen geworden. „Marken verkörpern heute die Werte, die ihnen jeder einzelne Verbraucher zuschreibt", schreibt das Hamburger Trendbüro in seiner Studie ‚Simplexity'.

Wir schließen uns zu Mini-Communities zusammen und veröffentlichen Weblogs. Tausendfach schießen neue ästhetische Konzepte aus dem Boden. Schneller, kreativer und anarchischer als je zuvor. Die Großlogobesitzer gucken da erst einmal neugierig zu. Jeder Einzelne ist heute potenzielle Zielgruppe und er ist potenzielles Logo.

Die große Herausforderung für jede Marke ist es heute also, so zu sein wie jeder einzelne Mensch und gleichzeitig noch ein großes Ganzes darzustellen. Wer mitmachen will, der muss alles auf einmal sein.

Komplex, wuchernd, vollgehängt wie Weihnachtsbäume, überladen und fragmentiert sind die neuen Logos. Aber keines von ihnen versucht den Gegensatz zwischen einfach und komplex, zwischen groß und klein, zwischen stark und schwach zu kaschieren. Denn das ist genau der Ort, an dem wir heute stehen.

Die Welt ist ein Tollhaus. Und auch die Logos spielen verrückt. Sie feiern die Gleichzeitigkeit von Komplexität und Einfachheit. Sie vereinen Gegensätze, ohne sie aufzulösen. Was sie zu sagen haben, das sagen sie konkret, direkt und emotional. In den meisten Fällen ist das anziehend und unterhaltsam. Kein Wunder: Bei der Menge an Botschaften führt Bescheidenheit nicht weit.

DAS ENDE DER NÜCHTERNHEIT

Früher war das Logo ein Erkennungszeichen einer Organisationseinheit: Firma, Werk, Partei, Verein. Früher bestanden Unternehmen aus realen Dingen wie Fabriken, Förderbändern und Werkstoren. Das Logo war eine akademische, vereinfachte Variante der industriellen Kerntätigkeit oder es stellte wappenartig die eigene Historie dar.

Die vier Ringe des Audi-Logos zum Beispiel stehen für die Gründungsunternehmen der Auto-Union: Audi-Werke, Horchwerke, Zschopauer Motorenwerke und die Autoabteilung der Wanderer Werke. Das BMW-Logo zeigt einen Flugzeugrotor von vorne gesehen. Der dreiteilige Mercedes-Stern steht für die Elemente Erde, Wasser und Luft, für deren Überwindung der Mischkonzern einst Motoren bauen wollte. „Mitsu" „bishi" bedeutet „drei" „Diamanten", die wiederum die Schiffsschrauben symbolisieren, mit denen der Konzern früher Geld verdiente. Die übereinander stehenden, nach oben gerichteten Zacken im Citroën-Logo stehen für eine bestimmte Sorte Zahnräder, die den Gründer Andre Citroën berühmt machten, bevor er anfing Autos zu bauen.

Heute gibt es Ideen, Netzwerke und Dienstleistungen. Mit akademischen Abstraktionen würde sich kein Unternehmen mehr ans Licht der Welt trauen. Erstens werden heute die Komponenten, die in den Logos der alten Wirtschaft zeichenhaft umgesetzt sind, bei Zulieferbetrieben eingekauft. Zweitens stehen keine Ingenieure, sondern Marken im Kern der Unternehmen. Drittens würde keiner die Reduktionen verstehen, denn ohne die Markengeschichte, die wir mit ihnen verbinden, würden sie uns kalt und hohl erscheinen.

Die Global Player stellen ihre Zeichen und Bildsprachen daher nach und nach auf Gefühl um. Die Speiseeismarke Langnese zum Beispiel, die in fast jedem Land der Welt unter einem anderen Namen bekannt ist (Walls, Holanda, Miko, Frisko, Eskimo, Ola oder Kibo, um nur ein paar zu nennen) hat vor Jahren die Markise abgeschafft und durch das globale, emotional eindeutige Herzlogo ersetzt, denn mit der Globalisierung müssen Logos emotional und eindeutig lesbar sein.

Das Gefühl ist zur Geschäftssprache des Weltmarketings geworden. Wer heute nicht schon groß ist und bekannt, der sehnt sich nach einem Symbol, das überall gleich gelesen wird. Denn ein emotionales, einfaches Symbol distribuiert den Markenreiz noch durch die schmalsten Kanäle auf die kleinsten Displays.

DIE NEUE GESCHWÄTZIGKEIT

Das war gestern. Aber simpel und emotional ist nicht mehr genug. In der Vielfalt der Kommunikation nutzt sich das ewig Gleiche viel zu schnell ab. Und so wie dieses wirtschaftliche Einheitsformat namens Globalisierung den Gegentrend der Regionalisierung entfachte, so hat die Tatsache, dass wir alles und jedes gleichzeitig und überall sein können, die Welt der Zeichen sprießen lassen wie nach einem tropischen Regenschauer.

Früher gab es Leuchtschriften, Stempel und Werkstore. Statt alles auf eine Aussage zu reduzieren, sind die neuen Logo-Ornamente so komplex und ereignisreich, als wollten sie uns ihre ganze Geschichte jetzt und sofort erzählen.

Früher waren Logos Zeichen erster Ordnung. Sie sagten „Ich bin". Die neuen Logos sagen: „Ich begegne dir. Ich erzähle dir von mir."

DIE NEUE ROMANTIK

Noch in den Neunzigern wurden Businessthemen mit aufgeweckten, beschlipsten Menschen dargestellt, die sich gegenseitig zuhören, bewundern oder die Hände schütteln. Irgendwann waren die Zeichen- und Bildfassaden aber nur noch perfekt und glatt, so dass die Gestalter begannen, Störungen einzubauen. Es fing an mit digitalen Fusseln, Flusen und Kratzern, die dem Design etwas Handgemachtes gaben. Apple zum Beispiel verlieh seinen iLife-Paketen mit etwas Gekrakel einen Touch des Analogen. Heute sind wir beim organischen Ornament, beim Gewächs angelangt. Die Getränkemarke Coca-Cola tritt als Jugendbewegung auf, für ihre globale Kampagne „The March" baut sie Collagen aus Menschen, Blumenmustern und Vögeln, freizügig wird da Punk, Hippiekultur und Xerox-Art vermischt.

Mit den floralen Themen, den Kratzern und Ornamenten, greift die Natur nach der Welt der digitalen Dinge, die ja im wahrsten Sinne des Wortes nicht zu be-greifen ist. Das Ornament füllt diese Verständnislücke. Im Zeitalter der MP3-Player und digitalen Tauschbörsen erleben Livekonzerte eine glorreiche Renaissance. Die Kampagnen für die neue Generation von MP3-Player-Handys von Nokia und Sony Ericsson bersten vor floraler Energie. Bei Nokia finden sich Ranken sogar auf einer Handyreihe wieder.

Jede technische Revolution erfuhr immer ihre eigene, romantische Gegenbewegung. Kein Wunder, dass die neuen Schnörkel an frühere ästhetische Umsturzversuche erinnern: Renaissance, Jugendstil und Psychedelic Pop. Das Wilde will zurück. Der Urwald kriecht aus dem Beton.

SELLOUT REVOLUTION

„Never touch the logo" war noch vor zehn Jahren ein Topgebot des Designs, aus dem nur wenige Marken (wie zum Beispiel Burton) auszubrechen wagten. Anders heute: Es gehört zum guten Ton, gerade bei Saisonartikeln wie Mode und Elektronik, Aktionslogos entwickeln zu lassen, die das Auftreten der Global Brands auf lokale Szenen herunterbrechen. Da wird re-designt, gesprüht, interpretiert und revolutioniert – alles im Auftrag der Marketingabteilung. Der Kommunikationstext der Marke wird in den Slang der Zielgruppe übersetzt. Je fragmentierter das Produktportfolio, umso vielfältiger die Versionen der Logos. Adidas zum Beispiel hat für seine +10 Kampagne ein eigenes Spraypaint-Logo entwickelt, das von so genannten Guerilla-Teams an öffentlichen Plätzen gesprüht wurde. Die Betonflächen waren natürlich vorher brav als Werbeflächen gebucht. An anderer Stelle lässt man das Dreiblattlogo aufblitzen oder engagiert junge Künstler für eine Wiederbelebung des Anmalschuhs Adicolor. Auch das Y-3-Label, eine Zusammenarbeit des Modedesigners Yohi Yamamoto mit Adidas, gibt sich fraktal: Mal wird der Heldenkult der chinesischen Kulturrevolution zitiert, mal flüchten Krähen aus dem Logo.

In bekannter Vereinnahmungsstrategie übernehmen die Weltmarken Codes, die sie bei Aktivisten wie Adbusters oder der politischen Linken abgucken: Siebdruck, Sponti-Collage und posterartiger East-Coast-Campus-Look. Im Fall von Coca-Cola wird der neue Look sogar von Protagonisten der Bewegung oder von Leuten aus der Kunstszene entworfen. Die große Herausforderung für die Konzerne aber wird sein, die Nähe, die ihr Design und ihre Botschaften vorspielen, tatsächlich einzulösen. Denn an der Passgenauigkeit zwischen Sein und Design, werden sie verstärkt gemessen.

Wo die großen Marken sich also fragmentieren und ihre getunten Aktionslogos selbst in die kleinsten Zielgrüppchen einführen, da blasen sich die kleinen Labels reflexartig auf, machen auf halbstark und halten den Big Playern Schlagringlogos entgegen. Viele Streetwear Labels betonen noch das Martialische. Fette Linien, Edding-eskes Design – halb gesprühter Tag, halb antikapitalistischer Schutzwall.

Natürlich gibt es noch immer von Hand gemachte Tags, die anschließend eingescannt und in Vektoren umgerechnet werden. Aber es scheint, das klassische Street- und HipHop-Logo ist auf dem Weg nach draußen. Viele Sprayer, die früher ganze Stadtviertel veredelten,

haben mittlerweile ihre Liebe zur Architektur entdeckt. Statt um Zeichen dreht sich ihre Arbeit heute um Räume und Körper. Wenn sie an ihre Rechner, Zeichenbretter oder in ihre Werkstätten gehen, entstehen wuchtige, dreidimensionale Entwürfe – und neue Kooperationen mit neuen Partnern und Techniken.

PANDORAS BÜCHSE

Die Bastardisierung der Zeichen ist natürlich nicht wirklich in den Marketingabteilungen ausgeheckt worden, dafür sind Konzerne viel zu träge. Diese kreative Revolution hat, wie jede andere vor ihr auch, technische Ursachen. Und sie kann sich nur so schnell verbreiten, weil sie gesellschaftliche Realität spiegelt.

Ähnlich wie das digitale Internet die Globalisierung angeschoben hat – diese alles verbindende Bewegung der Waren, Marken und Fabriken – genauso hat die digitale Technik der Vektor-Grafik das große Crossover der Bilder und Symbole entfacht. So wie sich heute Branchengrenzen auflösen, wenn zum Beispiel Apple mit seinem iPod in den Unterhaltungselektronikmarkt eindringt oder mit iTunes die Musikbranche umkrempelt, so hat die Vektorgrafik Tabus, Szenegrenzen und Berührungsängste abgebaut.

Vektorgrafik, die digital definierte gefüllte Fläche, bietet sich als perfekte Plattform an für Überlagerungen, Mischungen und Bastarde aller Art. Viele Designer, die sich seit Jahren mit nichts anderem beschäftigen, sitzen heute auf riesigen Datenbanken mit abertausenden Formen, Strukturen und Bildern.

Und so bekommen Raketen Beine, Hirschgeweihe wachsen aus Buchstaben, Serifenschriften bilden Äste, Marx schlägt Wurzeln, Schimpansen knabbern in einem Ei sitzend Gehirn und treiben Dendriten. Schriften, Muster und Bilder wuchern zu Collagen und Wappen, in deren Gestrüpp seltsame Gestalten hausen. Diese Wucherungen sind übervoll und explosiv, als hätte ein Spaßvogel Pandoras Büchse geöffnet. Dartscheiben, an denen einfach mal alles haften blieb, was man beim Brainstorming so drauf los geworfen hat, und es ist dieses Fehlen von Beschränkung, das die neuen Logos so unterhaltsam macht.

Mit dieser Widersprüchlichkeit bilden sie die Reize und Schizophrenie der Gegenwart ab – zum Glück kommentarlos. Was will man auch sagen? Einzig durchgehendes Statement: Ironie. Tabus sind aufgelöst. Es ist die Gleichzeitigkeit der Gegensätze, die der Wahrheit am nächsten kommt. HipHop meets Kiss meets Britney Spears meets Nazi Surfer.

Die Hyperwappen sind wie schmiedeeiserne Pforten zu Zaubergärten, in deren Betrachtung wir uns verlieren, noch bevor wir eintreten – wie zum Beispiel im Logo der französischen Restaurantbar Omnia. Oder das Logowappen von Kultivator: In der Mitte ein Kuhkopf, sternförmig darum angeordnet sind ein Rechen, eine Gans, Traktoren, Gemüse, Schraubmuttern, Pinsel, Dübel, Enten und Ohren. Ein Bilderrätsel, dessen Auflösung nur auf eine Art Kunstkommune hinauslaufen kann. Und richtig, es handelt sich um eine Mischung aus Biobauernhof, Seminar- und Kunstprojekt auf der südschwedischen Insel Öland, mit angeschlossenem „Agri-Cultural Shop".

Solche Schaubilder sind nicht immer sofort lesbar, wie man das von einem Logo klassischerweise erwartet. Aber darum geht es nicht. Es geht um räumliche Breite, inhaltliche Tiefe und die Dechiffrierung von Rätseln. Es sind oft diese hybriden Plaketten, die gegen die flachen Schriftzüge gewinnen, wenn es darum geht die Aufmerksamkeit des Betrachters zu halten.

Die Hyperlogos sind Geschichtenerzähler. Und damit kommen sie weiter als andere. Sie sind zwar nicht unmittelbar lesbar, aber dafür umso lesenswerter. Manchmal übernimmt auch die Fantasie des Betrachters die Rolle des Geschichtenerzählers, und damit betreten die neuen Wappen und Portale, aus der Welt der Bilder kommend, die Welt der Sprache. Sie bilden neue Mischformen aus Bild und Sprache. Neue Grammatiken, neue Metaphern. Wort. Bild. Idee. Logos.

CORPORATE INNOCENCE

Kleine, junge Unternehmen steuern mit ihren Erzähllogos ihre Größe und Identität – und erfinden ihre eigene Instantgeschichte. Große Konzerne nutzen dieselbe Mechanik, wenn sie die Sprache der vielen kleinen Symbole einsetzen, um sich naiv und nahbar zu geben. Sie geben sich mal revolutionär, mal blümerant. Auch hier bleibt die Botschaft dieselbe: Die Welt ist komplex. Wir sind es auch. Mehr ist das neue mehr.

Wer diese Harmonie des Widerspruchs konsequent als Logo umgesetzt hat, ist der Konsumgüterkonzern Unilever. Über dem wie gepinselten Namen Unilever steht ein U, das aus kleineren Einheiten besteht. Da gibt es Biene, Pullover, Welle, Molekül, Sonne, Welle, Recyclinglogo, Eiskrem, Taube und noch so einiges mehr. Jedes Symbol steht für bestimmte Produkte, Unternehmensbereiche oder Werte.

Wo die Wappen der Kleinunternehmer noch einen anarchischen Kommentar auf die Gegenwart abgeben, erzählt der Weltkonzern natürlich Märchen – ähnlich wie Microsoft zum Beispiel, der seine krakenhafte Aggressivität mit einem Schmetterlingslogo tarnt. Und so hat es nicht lange gedauert, bis ein paar Grafikdesigner eine neue Flash-Variante des Unilever-Logos ins Netz stellten, das die Elemente des lila Unileverlands aus einer linken Perspektive kommentiert.

Aber die aktivistische Kritik zeigt doch vor allem eins: Das Unilever-Logo funktioniert. Denn es wird gelesen, ernst genommen und kommentiert. Gestalterisch rückt der Konzern damit zur Avantgarde auf. Auch das umstrittene Trillerpfeifenlogo der letzten Fußballweltmeisterschaft folgte bereits dieser neuen Linie. Der Inhalt des Events, nämlich „Fußball", wurde beim Betrachter vorausgesetzt. Das Logo transportierte rein emotionale Botschaften, die von der Veranstaltung Jahre später sogar komplett eingelöst wurden: Spaß, Verkleiden, Party. Das Logo als Maskottchen – noch besser hätte das zu einer Kindermarke gepasst, oder einem Freizeitpark.

VERLORENE WELTEN

Produkte, Kanäle, Geräte, Kommunikation, Bildsprachen, Logosprachen – die Welt wuchert. Die Logos wachsen mit. Dabei fällt auf, dass dieses Wachstum gelernten Regeln folgt. Entweder ordnen sich die Zeichen auf schildartigen Flächen an, zu modernen Wappen. Oder sie breiten sich organisch aus, gestalterische Schlingpflanzen, die Freiflächen mit Metaphern füllen. Und immer wird Natur zitiert. Beide Formen, Wappen und Ornamente, verarbeiten auffällig oft Symbole der Flora und Fauna.

Mit Kulleraugen, Blumen, Hasen, Kolibris und geflügelten Bärchen nistet sich das Kindchenschema ins Logo ein – sogar in der Corporate-Welt. Die Unschuld, die von diesen Knupperschnupperfiguren ausgeht, mündet fast anschlusslos in Beschreibungen von Welten, in die wir ebenfalls nie wieder zurück können: paradiesische Szenerien, Formen und Nester, die wir mit unserer Berührung nur verschmutzen würden.

Mit diesem Bambi-Syndrom wird aber eine Natur verehrt, in der wir uns nie bewegt haben. Die Logo-Natur bleibt steril. Idealisierte, Fantasy-Archetypen sind das, die für Gerechtigkeit, Authentizität und dann doch ein wenig Sehnsucht nach Ordnung stehen.

Die Natursymbole und Ornamente kommentieren unsere digitale Wirklichkeit mit einer kitschig/romantischen Stimme. Ähnlich wie in früheren Renaissancen geht es inhaltlich um Spiritualität, Antirationalismus und Sinn. So wie in der Fotografie der Hyperrealismus angeblitzter Augen einer künstlichen, fast religiösen Hyperromantik Platz macht, so steht die Übermetapher Natur für die Suche nach Wurzeln, die wir auf Platinen eben nicht schlagen können.

EXPECTO PATRONUM!

Wo Flora ist, ist Fauna. Die unglaubliche Menge an Tieren, ob Bambi oder Fantasydrachen, ist allein dadurch, dass die Gestalter emotionale Referenzen für ihre Botschaften finden mussten, nicht mehr zu erklären. Viel eher begegnen wir hier einer neuen Heerschar an Wappentieren. Die alten sind noch alle da. Adler, Löwe, Einhorn, Drache.

Es gibt Wappenbaukästen, wie den Crestbuilder von Logikwear und es gibt Herden an neuen, wunderschönen Totemtieren, Schutzengeln, spirituellen Begleitern und Harry-Potterschen Schutzgeistern, die von Jungunternehmern, Anwaltskanzleien, Galerien, Designbüros, Kulturreferaten, NGOs, Global Playern und Ich-AGs gerufen werden, damit der Wappenträger geschützt werde und gestärkt bei seiner Überfahrt durch diese bewegten Zeiten.

Vor diesem Hintergrund können auch die nicht-symbolisch/bildlichen Ornamente, diese bunt überlagerten Kaleidoskope, als magische Amulette gedeutet werden. Identität stiften sie ja alle. Aber Wappen, Siegelringe, Gemmen und Logos waren immer auch Beschützer.

Auch die vielen anderen Natursymbole – Blitze, Wolken, Bäume, Sonnenaufgänge – sie alle verankern sich in der vordigitalen Zeit. Ästhetische Materialerweiterungen sind das, die die Zeit vor Marken, Ecstasy und Internet verherrlichen. Die Enkel der Achtundsechziger zitieren und remixen munter Woodstock, Grateful Dead und alles, was psychedelisch ist. Folgerichtig tauchen überall Totenköpfe und Blitze auf. Aus den sonderbarsten Ecken schießen Blitze, und auch die Totenköpfe gibt es in allen Variationen. Totenköpfe mit gekreuzten Essstäbchen, in Audiokassetten versteckte Totenköpfe, Mickymaus-Totenköpfe, Totenköpfe mit Zigarren, mit Stiften, Federkielen und Totenköpfe mit Wurzeln.

Die oft barocke Anordnung, das tabulose Kombinieren des Vergänglichen ist natürlich Heavy Metal pur. „Memento mori" rufen sie uns zu, wenn sie ihre Logostillleben bauen, und erinnern uns daran, dass wir sterblich sind. All unser Schaffen sei der Vanitas geweiht, der vergeblichen Eitelkeit. Aber diese barocken Logos als Mahnungen zu deuten wäre ein Fehler. Denn der Untergang gehört zum Wandel.

ES WERDE LICHT!

Die neuen Logos, die Ornamente, die ausgefüllten Freiflächen, die Tapeten und Moleküle, die anarchischen Stillleben, die frei assoziierend aufgetürmten, größenwahnsinnigen Bilderberge, die Zauberportale und Wortranken, sie alle spiegeln die Komplexität der Gegenwart. Die Muster sind Siegel. Und sie sind Spiegelbilder einer Zeit, die geprägt ist von Kreativität und Unsicherheit.

Die konkreten Symbole aber, die in diesen Mustern immer wieder auftauchen, lassen sich lesen wie kollektive Traumsymbole. Sie zeigen ein wenig, wohin die Reise geht.

Dass wir uns im Umbruch befinden, weiß ohnehin jeder. Die Herden an Totemtieren beschützen uns bei unserer Übersinnsuche. Blitze standen schon immer für Energie, Intuition und Entladung. Klarheit, Kraft, Befreiung und Radikalität. Aber auch für Konsequenz, denn ein Blitzeinschlag ist keine halbe Sache, die man rückgängig machen kann. Da scheinen sich viele Menschen Geistesblitze zu wünschen, die ins rationale Wirrwarr einschlagen und das alte, morsche Material zerstören.

Die vielen Totenköpfe bedeuten jedoch mitnichten, dass sich die Gestalter weltweit nach dem Tode sehnen. Im Gegenteil. Der Totenkopf steht ebenfalls für Veränderung, für das Neue und sogar für Kommunikation. In vielen Festen von Mexiko bis Italien sind Totenköpfe, teilweise in grellen Farben bemalt, Teil von lauten Inszenierungen des Lebens. Die gehisste Totenkopfflagge auf einem angreifenden Piratenschiff signalisierte Verhandlungsbereitschaft. Sie sagte: „Mit uns könnt ihr reden." Erst wenn die Angegriffenen die rote Fahne sahen, wussten sie: Es geht um Leben und Tod.

Logos sind immer halb Sehnsucht, halb Orakel. Was von beiden am Ende überwiegt, liegt an uns. Die nächsten neuen Zeichen ziehen bereits vor der US-amerikanischen Westküste am Horizont auf: noch mehr Muster, noch mehr Psychedelic-Art, folglich ein paar komplizierte Kopfschmerzlogos, Tribals und ökoorganische Systeme.

Wo wir heute stehen, ist Romantik. Was wir sehen, ist komplex. Was wir brauchen: Kraft. Was kommt, ist spirituell. Oder psychedelisch. Alles in allem sind das doch schöne Aussichten.

CORPORATE

PRAGMATIC, NOT TRENDY

As the representatives of the corporate world need to communicate a huge range of offers and strategic objectives, it is impossible
to make general assertions about this discipline of present-day logo
design. The strategies of a financial institution are simply too different from those of a restaurant chain, for example. Despite this, one
tendency is clearly observable: the innovative impulses unleashed by
designers two years ago have now arrived in the corporate world.

THE SHATTERED TABOO

With the inflation of the symbol, the designer is confronted by
increasing demands for symbols characterised by originality, dis-
tinctiveness and forcefulness, symbols capable of working as logos.
Consequently, he must constantly seek out new sources, and to an
increasing degree older ones: mythology, esotericism, religion.

The - deliberate or naïve - probing of taboos is conspicuous
among contemporary strategies, whose results are socially accept-
able only as long as certain boundaries are not transgressed. But to
what does the word "taboo" (with its origins in the Polynesian Tonka
language) actually refer? A prohibition to engage in certain activities,
to come into contact with, to look at, or to name forbidden objects.
"A shattered taboo is a taboo no longer," asserted French author Jean
Genet. A pithy proverb, but one that does not necessarily do justice
to (contemporary) reality, and one which, accordingly, should be filed
alongside 20th century ideological utopias.

FRANKFURT AM MAIN, GERMANY

SIMON & GOETZ

Design follows strategy.

What must a trademark actually accomplish? What tasks must it fulfil in the strategic framework of the enterprise for which it stands? Reduced to its core function, it serves mainly to earn profits. For it is primarily an instrument of marketing. This direct, pragmatic interpretation reflects the laws of the market and is closely linked to the interests of shareholders and stakeholders. At the same time, it is a realistic interpretation, and one which defines a specific strategic approach to the task of corporate visualisation, namely that of the design agency Simon & Goetz.

Here superior strategic competency is joined to creative design that capably positions a firm within the marketplace: these complementary functions are united at the highest level by this agency, which was founded in Frankfurt am Main in 1991. They are its credo. An ideal combination, and one embodied by its two founders: Matthias Simon, a marketing strategist by training, and Rüdiger Goetz, a designer.

The development of strategies for branding and market positioning and their respective visual realisations as logo and corporate design: the activities of Simon & Goetz Design revolve around these concerns. With a staff of 30, the agency supervises various well-known brands and enterprises. Their customer portfolio is multifaceted and ranges from bank to bike, from fashion to furniture.

According to Simon & Goetz, corporate design conveys the brand's core, the soul of an enterprise. The creation of a corporate trademark represents the greatest challenge: it visualises the firm's message and communicates its positioning concept in its most compressed form. The task is to create an independent, timeless, easily identifiable symbol that can be deployed functionally. A brand without a powerful trademark is doomed to remain weak. And weakness is the worst possible precondition for prevailing in an environment characterised, by sceptical consumers and omnipresent rival companies.

But how does the Frankfurt-based design agency Simon & Goetz define a powerful trademark? In their own words: "If corporate design constitutes the public face of a brand, then the trademark is roughly equi-valent to its DNA. Unmistakable and immutable, even when the design world changes. This stable visual core at the heart of a brand provides confidence, security, and orientation in the face of a never-ending flood of novel visual stimuli."

CORPORATE

PRAGMATISCH STATT TRENDY

Weil die Vertreter der Corporate World die unterschiedlichsten Angebote und strategischen Ziele kommunizieren, lässt sich keine generelle Aussage über das aktuelle Logodesign für diese Disziplin treffen. Zu verschieden sind die Strategien etwa eines Finanzinstitutes von denjenigen einer Restaurantkette. Trotzdem wird eine Tendenz klar sichtbar: Was Designer vor zwei Jahren an Innovationsschüben ausgelöst haben, ist jetzt in der Corporate World angekommen.

DAS ZERSCHLAGENE TABU

Mit der Inflation der Zeichen wachsen die Ansprüche an den Gestalter nach Originalität, Eigenständigkeit und Kraft der Zeichen als Logos. Deshalb versucht er ständig, neue Quellen zu erschließen die in zunehmendem Maße auch „alte Quellen" sind: Mythologie, Esoterik, Religion. Das - bewusste oder naive? - Antasten von Tabus gehört zu den aktuellen Strategien, deren Resultate von der Gesellschaft akzeptiert werden, solange gewisse Grenzen nicht überschritten werden. Doch was bezeichnet eigentlich das ursprünglich aus dem polynesischen Tonga kommende Wort Tabu? Ein Verbot, bestimmte Handlungen auszuführen, Gegenstände zu berühren, anzublicken, zu nennen. „Ein zerschlagenes Tabu ist kein Tabu mehr", behauptete der französische Autor Jean Genet. Ein schöner Satz, der allerdings der Realität (auch der heutigen) nicht immer standhält und folglich in die ideologische Utopienkiste des 20. Jahrhunderts gehört.

FRANKFURT AM MAIN, DEUTSCHLAND
SIMON & GOETZ

Design follows strategy.

Was muss eigentlich eine Marke leisten? Welche Aufgaben hat sie im Kontext der Strategie des Unternehmens zu erfüllen, für das sie steht? Auf ihre eigentliche Kernfunktion reduziert, muss sie vor allem Geld verdienen. Denn sie ist primär ein kaufmännisches Instrument. Das ist eine sehr direkte, pragmatische, die Gesetze des Marktes reflektierende, eng an den Shareholder und Stakeholder Values orientierte Interpretation. Aber es ist eine realistische Interpretation, die gleichzeitig eine strategische Herangehensweise an die Aufgabe ihrer Visualisierung definiert: diejenige der Designagentur Simon & Goetz.

Hohe strategische Kompetenz und positionierungsadäquates, kreatives Design zu einem eigenständigen Dienstleistungsangebot auf hohem Niveau verbinden. So lautet das Credo der 1991 in Frankfurt am Main gegründeten Agentur. Eine ideale Verbindung, die von den beiden Agenturgründern gleich selbst personifiziert wird: Matthias Simon ist von Haus aus Marketingstratege Rüdiger Goetz Designer.

Die Entwicklung von Marken- und Positionierungsstrategien und deren visuelle Umsetzung in Logo und Corporate Design bilden die Schwerpunkte der Tätigkeit von Simon & Goetz Design. Mit dreißig MitarbeiterInnen betreut die Agentur bekannte Marken und Unternehmen. Das Kundenportfolio ist vielseitig und reicht von der Bank und dem Bike bis zu Mode und Möbeln.

Das Corporate Design transportiert nach Simon & Goetz den Markenkern, die Seele des Unternehmens. Dabei stellt die Entwicklung des Markenzeichens die größte Herausforderung dar: Sie ist das Ins-Bild-setzen der Unternehmenskommunikation und der Kommuni-

kation der Positionierungsidee in ihrer komprimiertesten Form. Sie ist die Schaffung eines eigenständigen, zeitlosen, leicht identifizierbaren, funktional einsetzbaren Zeichens. Eine Marke ohne starkes Markenzeichen kann keine starke Marke sein, bleiben oder werden. Ganz einfach deshalb nicht, weil Schwäche die schlechtmöglichste Voraussetzung ist, sich in einem Umfeld durchzusetzen, das von kritischen Konsumenten und omnipräsenten Mitbewerbern geprägt ist.

Und wie definiert die Frankfurter Designagentur Simon & Goetz ein starkes Markenzeichen? So: „Wenn das Corporate Design das Gesicht einer Marke ist, dann ist das Markenzeichen so etwas wie ihre DNS. Unverwechselbar und unveränderlich, auch wenn die Gestaltungswelt variiert. Diese visualisierte Konstanz im Kern der Marke gibt Vertrauen, Sicherheit und Orientierung in der Flut ständig neuer visueller Reize."

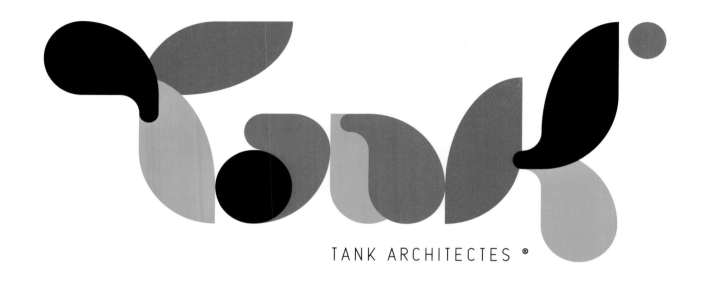

TANK ARCHITECTES ©

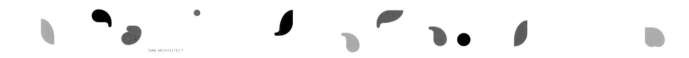

01 Atelier Télescopique

01 Insect Design

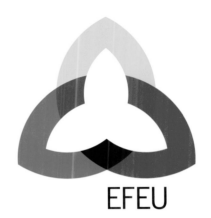

02 Discodoener

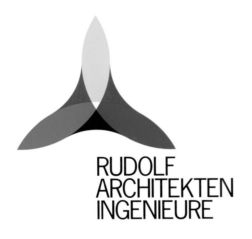

03 Discodoener

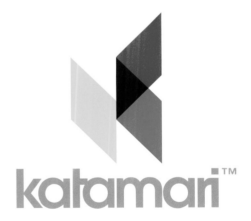

04 Zion Graphics

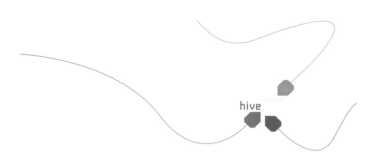

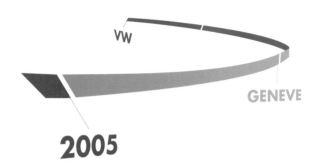

01 Fupete Studio

02 Rocholl Selected Designs

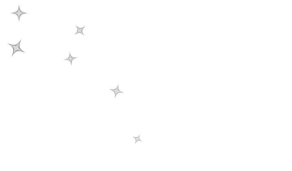

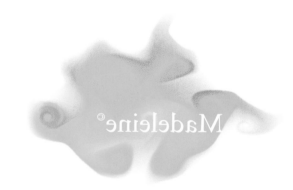

03 David Maloney

04 Kontrapunkt

BYGTEQ A/S

01 Emil Hartvig

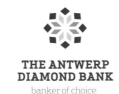

THE ANTWERP DIAMOND BANK
banker of choice

02 Flink

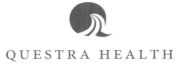

QUESTRA HEALTH

03 strange//attraktor:

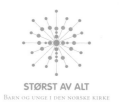

STØRST AV ALT
BARN OG UNGE I DEN NORSKE KIRKE

04 bleed

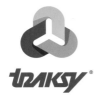

05 Bionic Systems

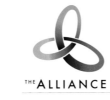

06 Futro

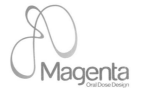

07 JDK

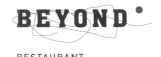
RESTAURANT
LOUNGE
TAKE AWAY

08 Borsellino & Co.

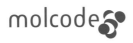

09 Velvet

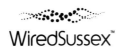

10 Crush Design

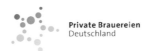

11 KMS Team

12 Alexander Fuchs

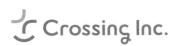

13 Raredrop

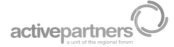

14 Rob Chiu

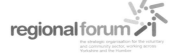

15 Rob Chiu

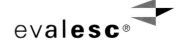

16 Annabelle Mehraein

01 Martha Stutteregger

 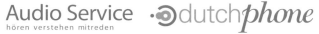

02 kw43

03 310k

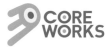

04 Raredrop

05 Axel Raidt

06 Jon Ari Helgason

07 WGD

08 Systm

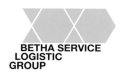

09 sunrise studios

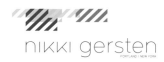

10 makelike

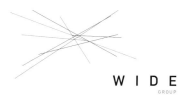

11 eduhirama

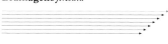

12 Georg Schatz

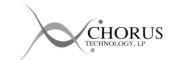

13 J6Studios

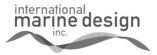

14 William Morrisey

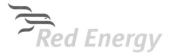

15 David Maloney

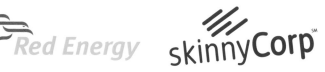

16 Jeffrey Kalmikoff

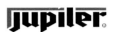 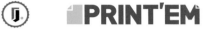 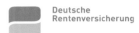 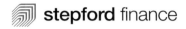

01 Pfadfinderei   02 Raredrop   03 KMS Team   04 Velvet

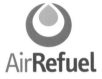 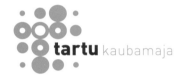 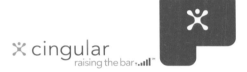

05 Sesame Studio   06 Velvet   07 Mattisimo

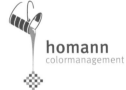 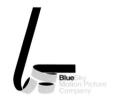 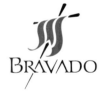 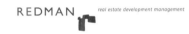

08 Rosendahl Grafikdesign   09 Insect Design   10 Kimera   11 Velvet

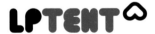 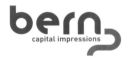 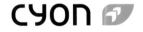 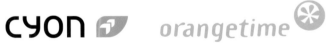

12 Trafik   13 Balsi Grafik   14 nothing from outer space   15 Velvet

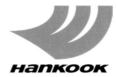

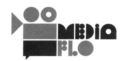

01 archetype : interactive   02 archetype : interactive   03 Research Studios Berlin   04 Stolen Inc.

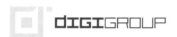

05 Borsellino & Co.   06 Research Studios Berlin   07 Norwegian Ink   08 Futro

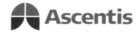

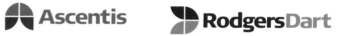

09 Sesame Studio   10 Sesame Studio   11 Sesame Studio   12 Sesame Studio

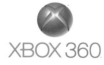

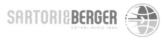

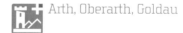

13 JDK   14 Stolen Inc.   15 Axel Domke   16 Carsten Raffel

FEDERATION OF
**BELGIAN
DIAMOND
BOURSES**

01 Flink

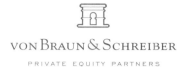

TIMEDON

02 Fluid Creativity

VON BRAUN & SCHREIBER
PRIVATE EQUITY PARTNERS

03 Simon & Goetz Design

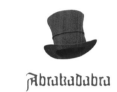

zineKING

04 nothing from outer space

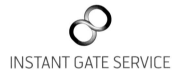

HERKULES

05 Felix Braden

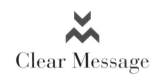

MADHIMA GULGAN
TOURS

06 GillespieFox

ROYAL MEDIA
Hotels & Resorts

07 Toxic design

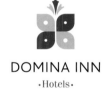

Abrakadabra

08 Sensus Design Factory

INSTANT GATE SERVICE

09 Systm

Clear Message

10 Toxic design

Union Bank

11 mateuniverse

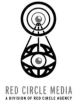

DOMINA INN
·Hotels·

12 Toxic design

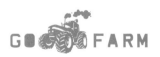

GO FARM

13 Stolen Inc.

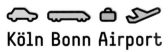

Köln Bonn Airport

15 Intégral Ruedi Baur

MART
SHIPPING LTD.
ISTANBUL

15 Cape Arcona Typefoundry

RED CIRCLE MEDIA
A DIVISION OF RED CIRCLE AGENCY

16 David Maloney

01 Chapter3

02 Fluid Creativity

03 Attak

04 Emil Hartvig

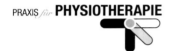

05 Strukt Visual Network

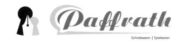

06 Mutabor Design

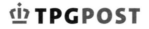

07 friederike preuschen

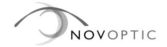

08 Mathilde Quartier

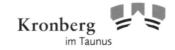

09 Miha Artnak

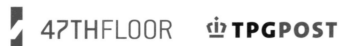

10 Toxic design

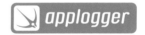

11 Studio Dumbar

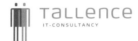

12 nothing from outer space

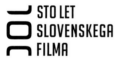

13 Felix Braden

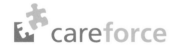

14 Labor f. visuelles Wachstum

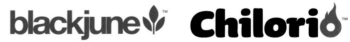

15 blackjune

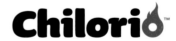

16 AmorfoDesignlab™

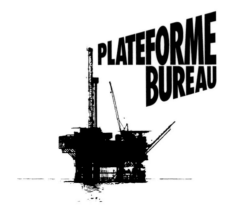

01 Paul Snowden

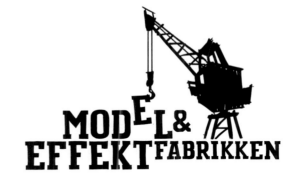

02 Spild af Tid ApS

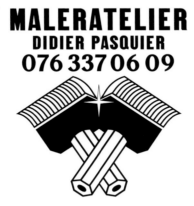

03 The Remingtons

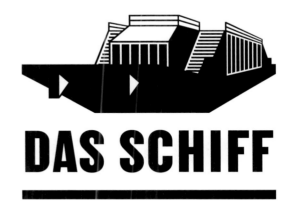

04 Ludovic Balland

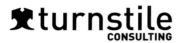 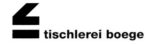 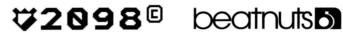 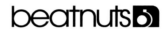

01 Crush Design   02 Carsten Giese   03 2098   04 Christian Rothenhagen

 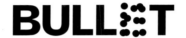 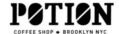 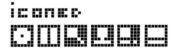

05 Keep Left Studio   06 Double Standards   07 I-Manifest   08 Loic Sattler

 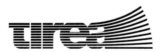 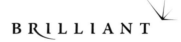 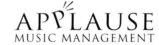

09 Atomic Attack   10 Alexander Wise   11 Velvet   12 Velvet

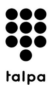 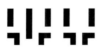

13 Niels Shoe Meulman   14 Emil Hartvig   15 310k   16 less rain

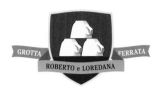

01 Jakob Straub

02 XYZ.CH

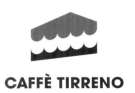

03 Georg Schatz

04 DigitalPlayground Studio

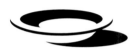

05 donat raetzo union

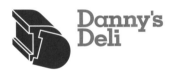

06 morphor

07 Visual Mind Rockets

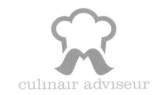

08 Attak

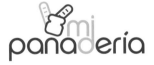

09 Nohemi Dicuru

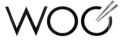
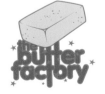

10 Emmi Salonen

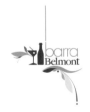

11 La Superagencia ®

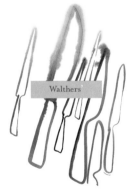

Kebap da Demir
autentico döner kebap turco

12 Dimomedia Lab

13 :phunk studio

WOO

14 onrushdesign / front

15 granit di Lioba Wackernell

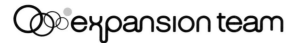

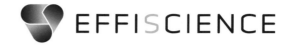

01 Studio Five

02 AmorfoDesignlab™

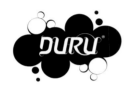

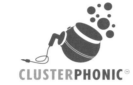

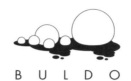

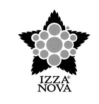

03 29 degres

04 Kanardo

05 Kanardo

06 Martin Kvamme

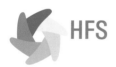

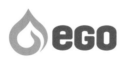

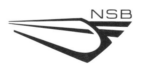

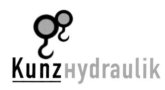

07 Moving Brands

08 Jon Ari Helgason

09 WGD

10 Felix Braden

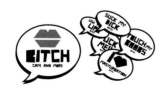

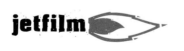

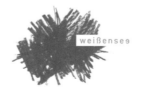

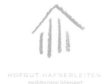

11 the red is love

12 Rosendahl Grafikdesign

13 Alexander Fuchs

14 Strada

THE
RESTORE CREATION
PROJECT

 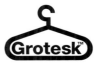 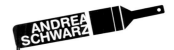

01 asmallpercent

02 the red is love

03 Cuartopiso

04 Martin Kvamme

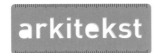

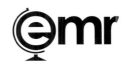

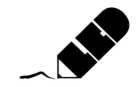

05 Studio 3

06 Luka Mancini, Katarina

07 Grotesk aka Kimou Meyer

08 seventysix

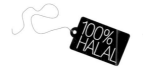

09 feurer network

10 Resin[sistem] design

11 Sanjai Bhana Illustration

12 onrushdesign / Front

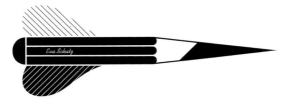

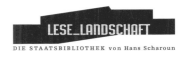

13 Georg Schatz

14 News

15 Thomas Beyer Design

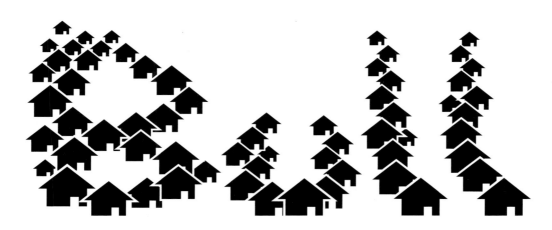

01 GUAK

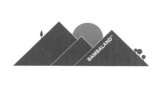

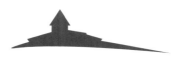

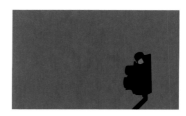

02 Muller

03 Thomas Nolfi

04 Marc Atlan

05 Mattisimo

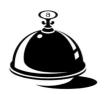

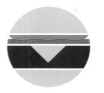

06 morphor

07 Mattisimo

08 Mattisimo

09 Mattisimo

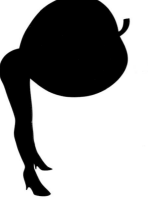

01 Mattisimo

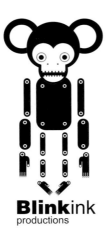

Blinkink
productions

02 Katharina Leuzinger

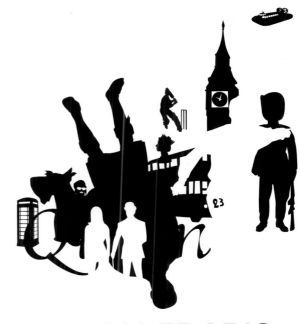

HARRAP'S

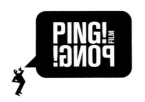

03 Büro Destruct

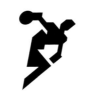

04 Felix Braden

05 june

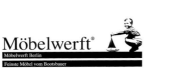

06 sunrise studios

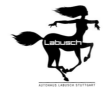

07 Discodoener

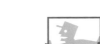

08 Formikula

09 Carsten Raffel

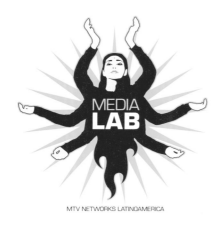

MTV NETWORKS LATINOAMERICA

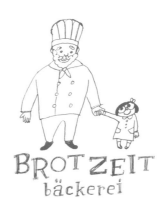

01 NeoDG

02 Naho Ogawa

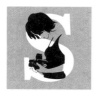

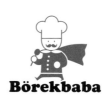

03 bandage

04 Atelier Télescopique

05 Atelier Télescopique

06 Flexn

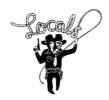

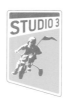

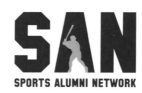

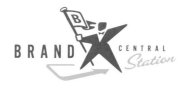

07 Miki Amano

08 Studio 3

09 Jeffrey Kalmikoff

10 Axel Domke

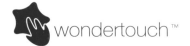

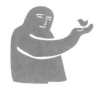

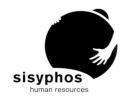

01 zookeeper

02 fatbob

03 Paco Aguayo

04 Paco Aguayo

05 Simian

06 Hayato Kamono

07 Formikula

08 Raredrop

A LIFE ONCE LOST

09 Jeffrey Kalmikoff

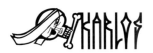

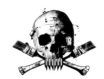

10 Zion Graphics

11 44 flavours

12 Insect Design

13 Lorenzo Geiger

02 Thomas Nolfi

03 Simon & Goetz Design

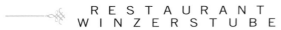

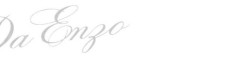

01 Labor fuer visuelles Wachstum™

04 derek johnson

05 Engine

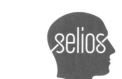

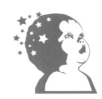

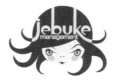

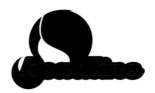

06 Superfamous

07 I Am Human

08 Balsi Grafik

09 Catalina Estrada Uribe

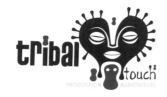

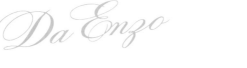

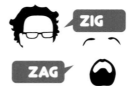

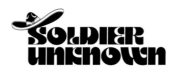

10 zookeeper

11 Mikkel Grafixico Westrup

12 the red is love

13 Nathan Jobe

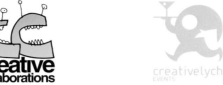

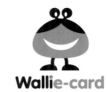

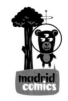

01 Jon Burgerman

02 Rinzen

03 KesselsKramer

04 Dr. Alderete

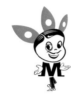

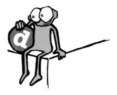

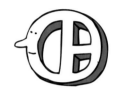

05 Studio 3

06 FireGirl

07 Christian Rothenhagen

08 Lousy Livincompany

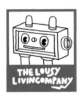

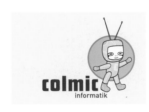

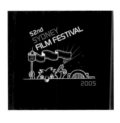

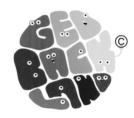

09 Lousy Livincompany

10 Judith Zaugg

11 jeremyville

12 Creative Pride

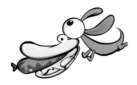

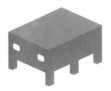

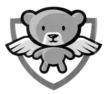

13 austrianilllustration.com

14 Alexander Fuchs

15 Formikula

16 IDolls GrafikModeDialog

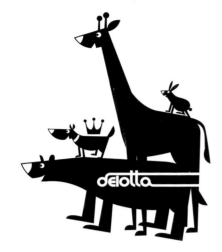

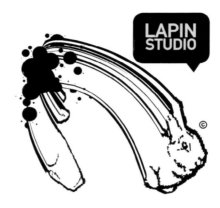

01 Yuu Imokawa

02 Lapin

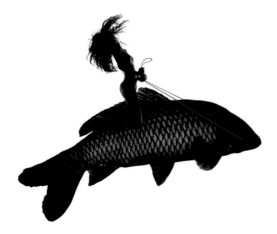

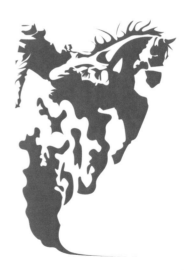

03 eduhirama

04 Attak

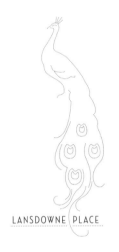

01 red design

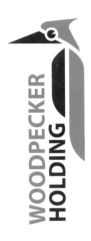

02 Joe A. Scerri

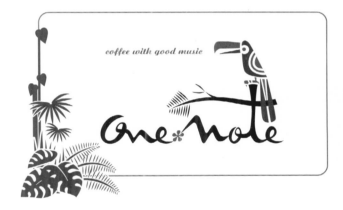

03 Amore Hirosuke

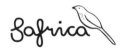

04 Alphabetical Order®

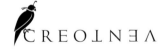

05 Mark Sloan

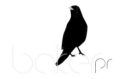

06 Jawa and Midwich

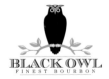

07 jl-prozess

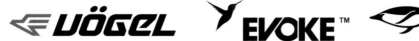

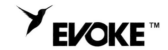

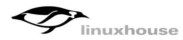

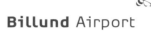

01 Power Graphixx

02 Chapter3

03 Axel Raidt

04 Kontrapunkt

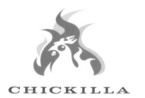

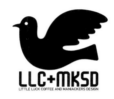

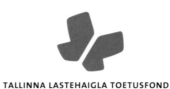

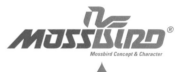

05 Axel Domke

06 Maniackers Design

07 Velvet

08 Bionic Systems

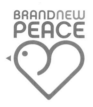

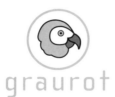

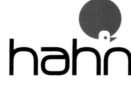

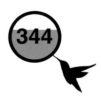

09 Hayato Kamono

10 Cape Arcona Typefoundry

11 tapetentiere

12 344 Design, LLC

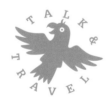

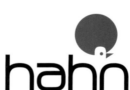

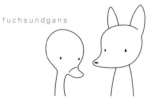

13 milchhof : atelier

14 Extraverage Productions

15 Labooo

16 Juju's Delivery

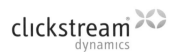

01 Superfamous

02 Attak

03 milchhof : atelier

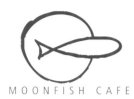

04 GrafficTraffic

05 Miha Artnak

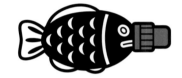

06 jum

07 Oscar Salinas Losada

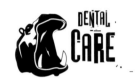

08 Maria Elena Velasco Rojas

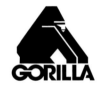

09 the wilderness

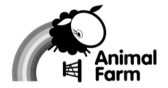

10 DED Associates

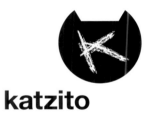

11 Georg Schatz

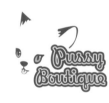

12 Studio Output

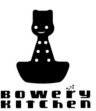

13 Positron

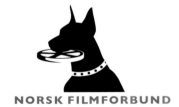

14 Studio 3

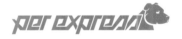

15 Attak

16 Mattisimo

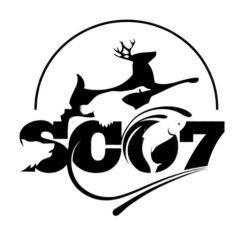

01 Seth Rementer

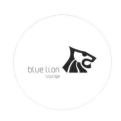

02 domenico catapano

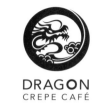

03 artless Inc

04 Karoly Kiralyfalvi

05 Rosendahl Grafikdesign

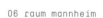
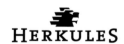

06 raum mannheim

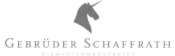
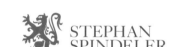

07 Stylepatrol.com

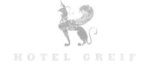

08 weissraum.de(sign)

09 chemicalbox

HERKULES

10 Felix Braden

GEBRÜDER SCHAFFRATH
DIAMANTENMANUFAKTUR

11 Simon & Goetz Design

HOTEL GREIF

VERY PERSONAL

12 granit Di Lioba Wackernell

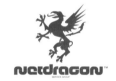

13 Karoly Kiralyfalvi

01 bleed

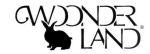

02 Kingsize

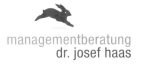

03 Felix Braden

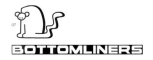

04 Ottograph

05 bleed

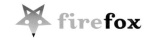

06 Miha Artnak

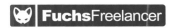

07 DigitalPlayground Studio

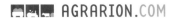

08 Labor f. visuelles Wachstum

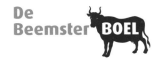

09 DTM_INC

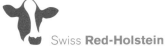

10 kong. funktion gestaltung

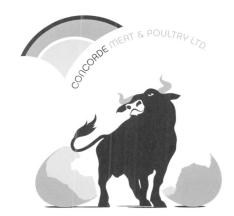

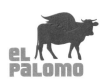

11 Oscar Salinas Losada

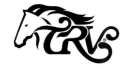

12 Keep Left Studio

13 Lunatiq

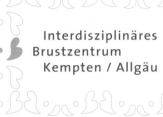

**Interdisziplinäres
Brustzentrum
Kempten / Allgäu**

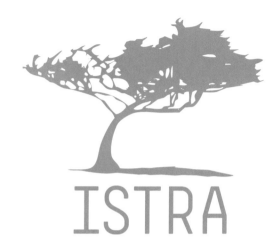

02 Amen

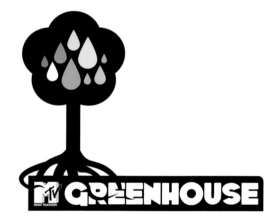

01 Juli Gudehus   03 Tado

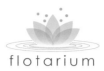

01 Catalina Estrada Uribe

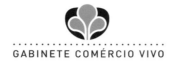

02 FireGirl

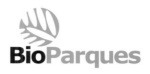

03 Annella Armas

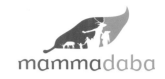

04 Gints Apsits

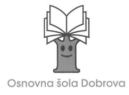

05 Luka Mancini, Katarina

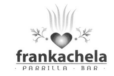

06 Catalina Estrada Uribe

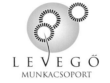

07 Extraverage Productions

08 spin

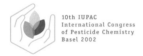

09 AND

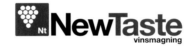

10 Mikkel Grafixico Westrup

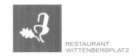

11 selanra grafikdesign

12 DTM_INC

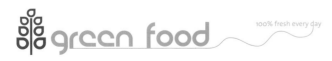

13 sunrise studios

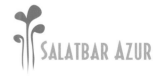

14 Cyklon

15 29 degres

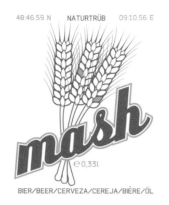

BIER/BEER/CERVEZA/CEREJA/BIÈRE/ÖL

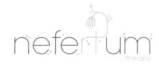

02 Nohemi Dicuru

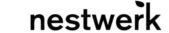

03 29 degres

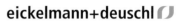

04 Karoly Kiralyfalvi

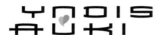

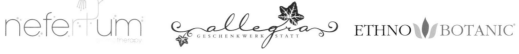

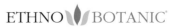

01 Discodoener

05 Jon Ari Helgason

06 büro uebele

07 jl-prozess

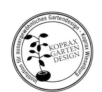

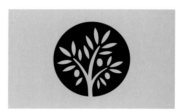

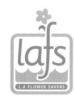

08 Mattisimo

09 Designkitchen

10 Simon & Goetz Design

11 Semisans

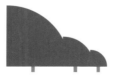

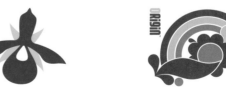

12 austrianilllustration.com

13 Mattisimo

14 David Maloney

15 A-Side Studio

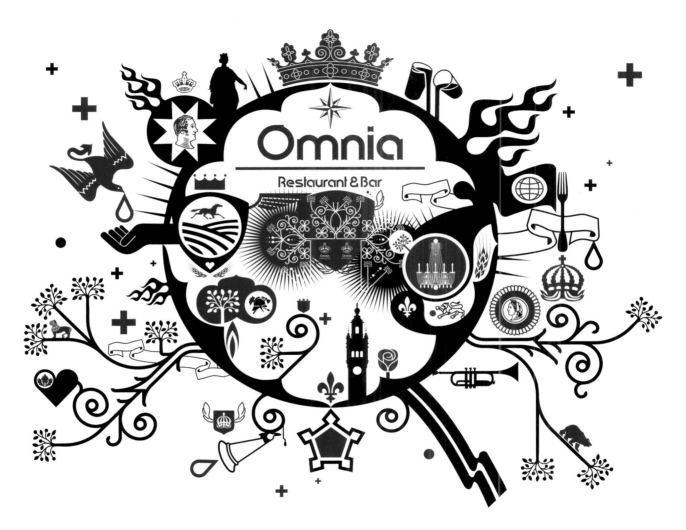

01 Atelier Télescopique

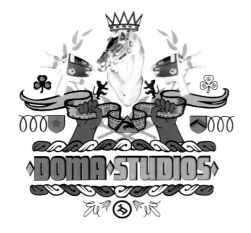

01 Doma

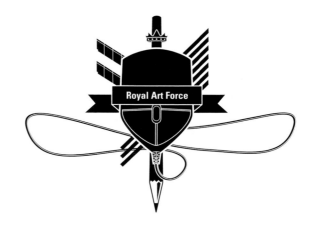

02 backyard 10

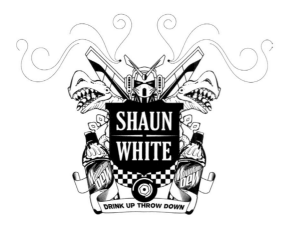

03 Colletivo Design

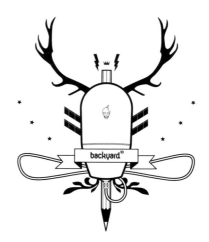

04 backyard 10

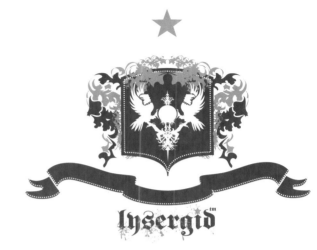

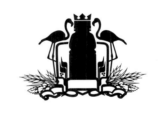

02 Loic Sattler

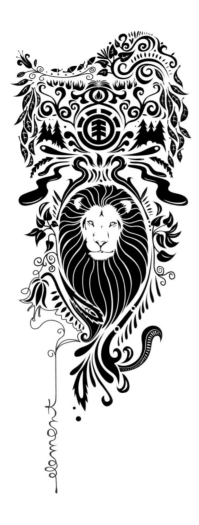

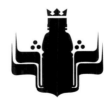

01 National Forest

03 Keep Left Studio

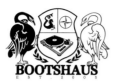

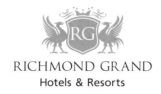

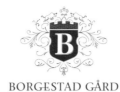

01 Discodoener

02 Toxic Design

03 Skin Design AS

04 Karoly Kiralyfalvi

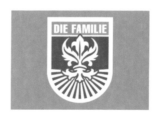

05 Klaus Wilhardt

06 blackjune

07 Adhemas

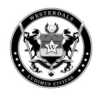

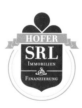

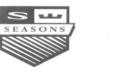

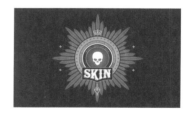

08 Studio 3

09 Karoly Kiralyfalvi

10 Le_Palmier Design

11 Skin Design

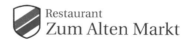

12 Alëxone

13 Axel Domke

14 raum mannheim

15 Designunion

1/33 productions.

5 Rue Marcel Monge   92150 Suresnes   Tél. 0141389138
fax. 0141380133   email   info @ 1-33. com

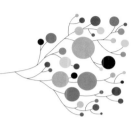

1/33 productions.

5 Rue Marcel Monge   92150 Suresnes   Tél. 0141389138
fax. 0141380133   email   info @ 1-33. com

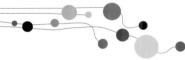

1/33 productions.

5 Rue Marcel Monge   92150 Suresnes   Tél. 0141389138
fax. 0141380133   email   info @ 1-33. com

01 Katharina Leuzinger

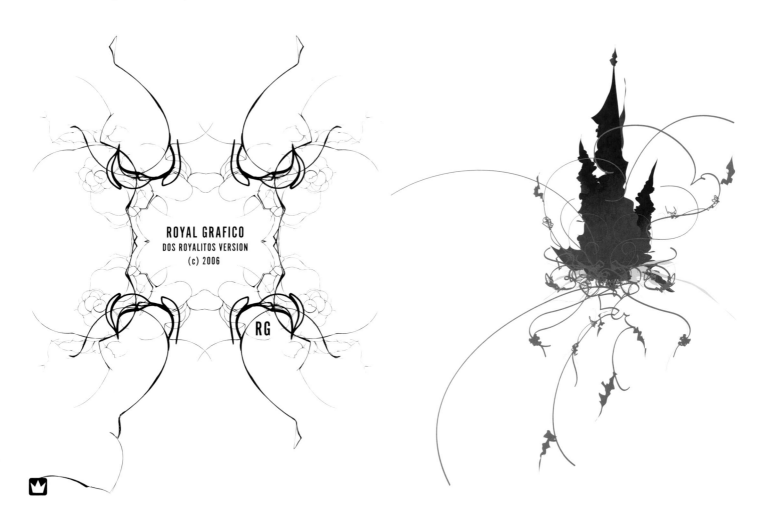

ROYAL GRAFICO
DOS ROYALITOS VERSION
(c) 2006

RG

01 Accident Grotesk!   02 Loic Sattler

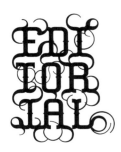

01 Magma

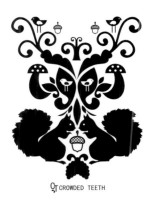

02 Cassie Leedham

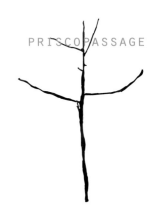

03 YellowToothpick

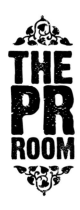

04 Amen

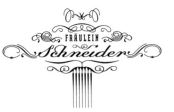

05 Rosendahl Grafikdesign

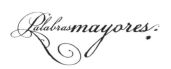

06 anna-OM-line.com

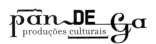

07 Caótica

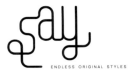

08 Thomas Nolfi

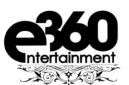

09 Hydro74

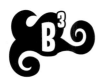

10 Magma

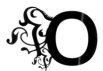

11 ROM studio

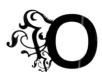

12 Power Graphixx

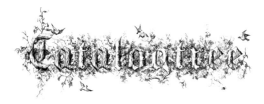

01 Catalogtree

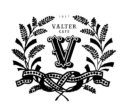

02 Hula Hula

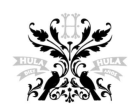

03 Sueellen

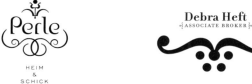

04 Thomas Beyer Design

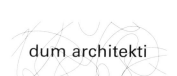

05 Tender

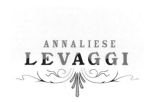

06 William Morrisey

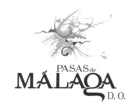

07 FÓSFORO

08 MvM

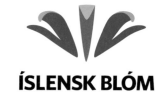

09 Petr Babák, Laborator

10 Jon Ari Helgason

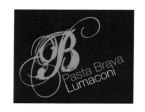

11 Norwegian Ink

12 Miha Artnak

13 Holzschuherstrasse

14 Gazelle Communication

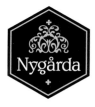

15 Zion Graphics

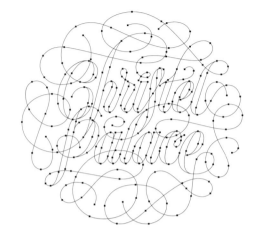

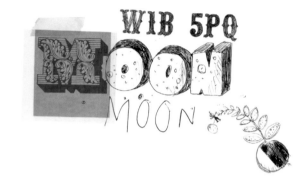

01 Niels Shoe Meulman

02 Katharina Leuzinger

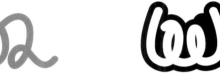

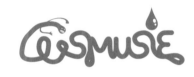

03 Pietari Posti

04 BankerWessel

05 Jun Watanabe

06 Flexn

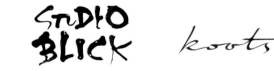

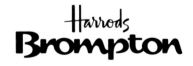

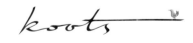

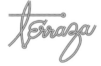

07 Positron

08 Nonstop

09 Resin[sistem] design

10 Dr. Alderete

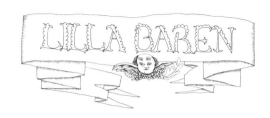

02 Vår

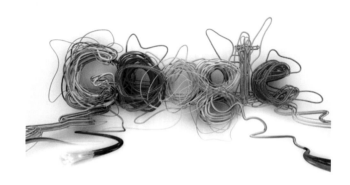

01 Laundry

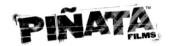

03 AmorfoDesignlab™

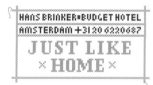

04 Jeffrey Kalmikoff

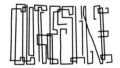

05 44 flavours

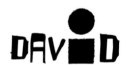

06 Miha Artnak

07 Velvet

08 KesselsKramer

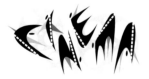

09 Escobas

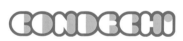

10 Hula Hula

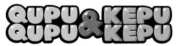

11 Furi Furi Company

12 Freaklüb

AMIRA

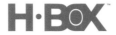

sɔsɹɔʌıɒ ıɒɔɔs

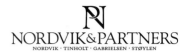
NORDVIK&PARTNERS
NORDVIK · TINHOLT · GABRIELSEN · STØYLEN

01 MWK

02 Mattisimo

03 Lorenzo Geiger

04 Martin Kvamme

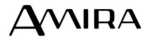

you are here

a|sterdorf

ZÆFFERÆNO

05 Brighten the corners

06 bleed

07 büro uebele

08 viagrafik

Lydia &
Töchter

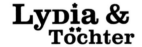Liguria living
SECOND HOMES IN ITALY

ENTRY2006

BYGGERIETS/NNOVATION
BUILDING LAB DK

09 Designunion

10 Tim Bjørn

11 KMS Team

12 1508 A/S

 ALBDRUCK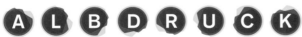

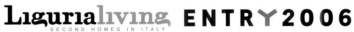CORPORATE COOL

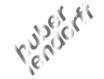

13 Neeser & Müller

14 44 flavours

15 unfolded

eraser

GASAG

ANORAK ^{agency}

TOPTRENDS PUBLISHING

01 stylodesign

02 Läufer + Keichel

03 Nonstop

04 DTM_INC

argon SUPPORT

MAIK ROBERTS FOTOGRAPHIE

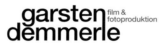

garsten demmerle film & fotoproduktion

lau photos

05 Maik Brummundt

06 123buero

07 seventysix

08 :phunk studio

I amsterdam.

BLUEF**ANT** .DE

Mu||er ©

dag°

09 KesselsKramer

10 Georg Schatz

11 Muller

12 Sensus Design Factory

BUSINESS unusual ™

eight studios

HILLSIDE VENEERS Fine Veneer Design

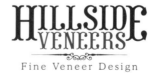

OFFICE Greminger EST JULY2005

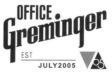

13 radargraphics

14 urbn;

15 Three Negative

16 Ashi & office Greminger

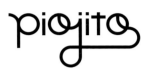

01 Laura Varsky

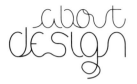

02 Accident Grotesk!

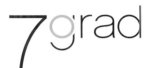

03 Etienne Heinrich

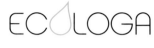

04 Glauco Diogenes

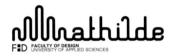

05 Salon Vektoria

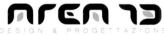

06 Rinzen

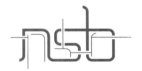

07 actiondesigner

08 XYZ.CH

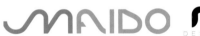

09 DTM_INC

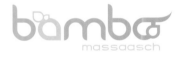

10 Dimomedia Lab

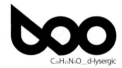

11 propella, konzept + design

12 Loic Sattler

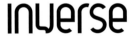

13 Emil Kozak

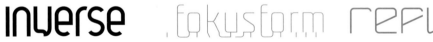

14 Bringolf Irion Vögeli

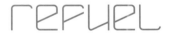

15 Hayato Kamono

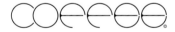

16 Maniackers Design

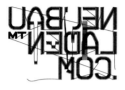

01 Neubau.

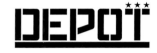

02 Büro Destruct

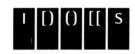

03 IDolls

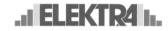

04 Carsten Giese

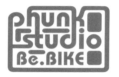

05 :phunk studio

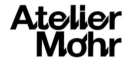

06 Neubau.

07 Neubau.

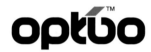

08 Emmi Salonen

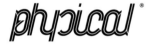

09 Pfadfinderei

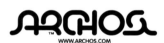

10 viagrafik

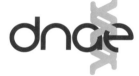

11 Jawa and Midwich

12 Mattisimo

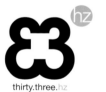

13 Extraverage Productions

14 Systm

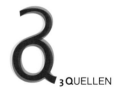

15 IDolls

16 44 flavours

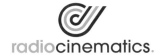

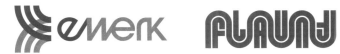

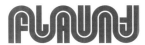

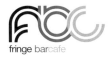

01 blackjune

02 blackjune

03 Rinzen

04 red design

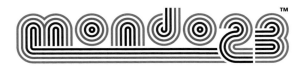

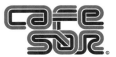

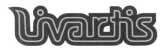

05 Rob Meek

06 Kallegraphics

07 Luka Mancini, K. Mrvar

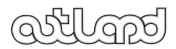

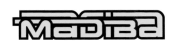

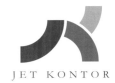

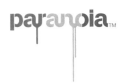

08 Norwegian Ink

09 Ottograph

10 I&EYE

11 Urs Lehni

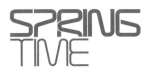

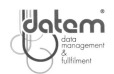

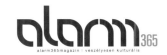

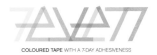

12 Keep Left Studio

13 june

14 Karoly Kiralyfalvi

15 Lunatiq

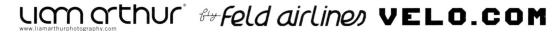 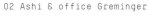 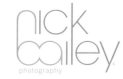

01 A-Side Studio   02 Ashi & office Greminger   03 Ludovic Balland   04 A-Side Studio

05 A-Side Studio   06 Joe A. Scerri   07 unfolded   08 Omochi

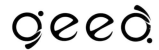 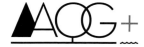

09 Semitransparent Design   10 SAT ONE   11 Omochi   12 Carsten Raffel

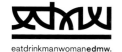 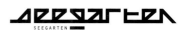 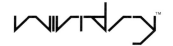 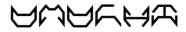

13 Borsellino & Co.   14 Borsellino & Co.   15 Omochi   16 Omochi

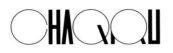

01 Omochi

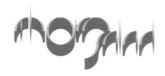

02 Omochi

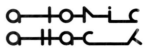

03 Atomic Attack

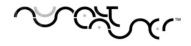

04 AmorfoDesignlab™

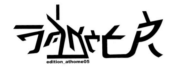

05 44 flavours

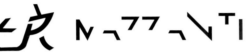

06 Cuartopiso

07 Paco Aguayo

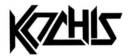

08 Jason Kochis

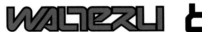

09 Büro Destruct

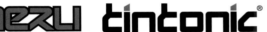

10 viagrafik

11 Omochi

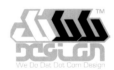

12 Koadzn

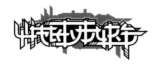

13 44 flavours

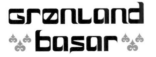

14 bleed

15 44 flavours

16 44 flavours

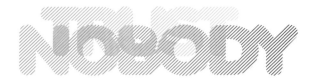

01 Freaklüb

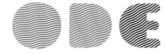

02 Floor Wesseling Ix Opus

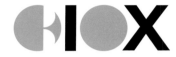

03 Karoly Kiralyfalvi

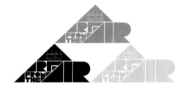

04 Keep Left Studio

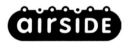

05 Airside

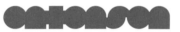

06 Akira Sasaki

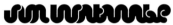

07 Jun Watanabe

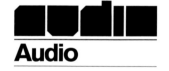

08 red design

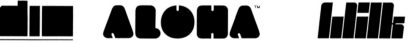

09 AmorfoDesignlab™

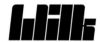

10 raum mannheim

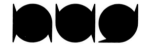

11 Omochi

12 Karoly Kiralyfalvi

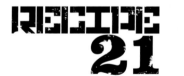

13 Crush Design

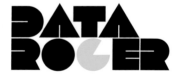

14 Kallegraphics

15 Tohyto

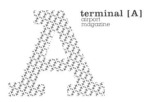 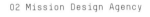

01 cabina

02 Mission Design Agency

03 Superfamous

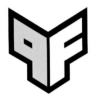

04 Die Gestalten

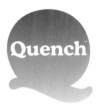

05 stylodesign

06 Axel Domke

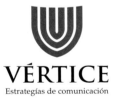

07 Paco Aguayo

08 Trafik

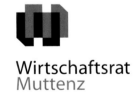

09 Joe A. Scerri

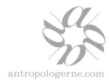

01 Flink

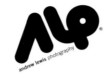

02 A-Side Studio

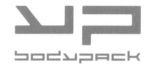

03 martinaigner.com

04 clandrei

05 sidsel stubbe

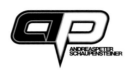

06 Georg Schatz

07 kw43

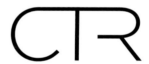

08 Trafik

09 radargraphics

10 Emil Hartvig

11 Mwmcreative

12 Mattisimo

13 Bo Lundberg Illustration

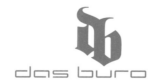

14 Klaus Wilhardt

15 Paco Aguayo

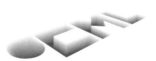

16 Thonik

01 archetype : interactive

02 makelike

03 Annabelle Mehraein

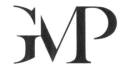

04 chris bolton

05 Kjetil Vatne

06 Toko

07 Moving Brands

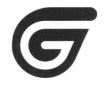

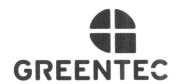

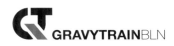

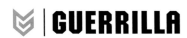

08 Mutabor Design

09 Velvet

10 blackjune

11 Out Of Order

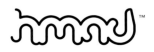

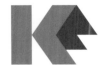

12 precursor

13 Mathilde Quartier

14 Toko

15 And

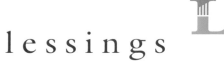
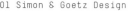

01 Simon & Goetz Design

02 Superlow

03 martinaigner.com

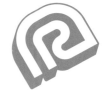

04 Muller

05 Rocholl Selected Designs

06 Sensus Design Factory

07 MaMadesign AB

08 Sesame Studio

09 A-Side Studio

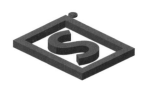

10 Attak

11 Le_Palmier Design

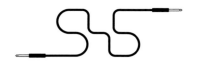

12 Tim Bjørn

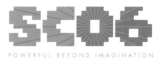

13 Out Of Order

14 Russ Yusupov

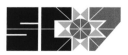

15 Russ Yusupov

01 Moving Brands

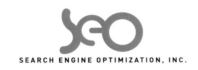

02 2Advanced Studios

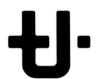

03 weissraum.de(sign)

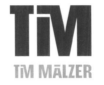

04 Power Graphixx

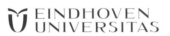

05 Attak

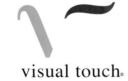

06 DTM_INC

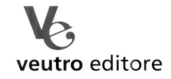

07 Sarah Grimaldi

08 Ketchup Arts

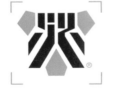

09 GWG

10 Fiftyeight3d

11 iaah

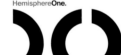

12 :g / studio-gpop

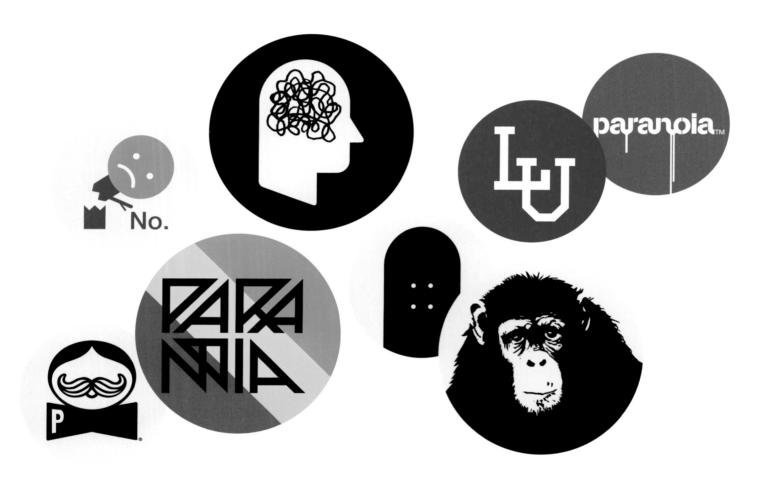

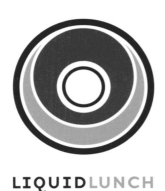

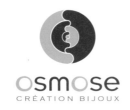

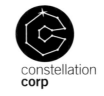

02 Mathilde Quartier

03 Alexander Wise

04 Karoly Kiralyfalvi

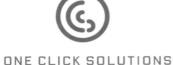

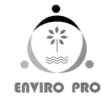

01 selanra grafikdesign

05 Moniteurs

06 Simon & Goetz Design

07 DTM_INC

08 Karoly Kiralyfalvi

09 Jeffrey Kalmikoff

10 a+morph

11 Pentagram

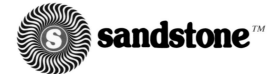

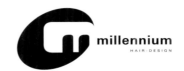

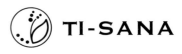

12 Extraverage Productions

13 flat

14 Mathilde Quartier

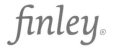

01 Tsuyoshi Hirooka

02 Superfamous

03 Tilt

04 Thomas Nolfi

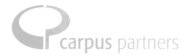
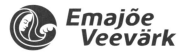
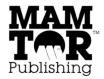

05 Katrin Acklin

06 Karoly Kiralyfalvi

07 Velvet

08 Muller

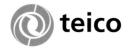
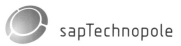

09 Escobas

10 flat

11 Ottograph

12 kw43

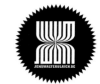

13 PMKFA

14 hijack graphics

15 Studio Output

16 Neeser & Müller

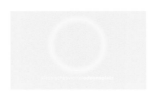

01 Amen

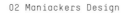

02 Maniackers Design

03 austrianilllustration.com

04 A-Side Studio

05 Katrin Acklin

06 jum

07 29 degres

08 Büro Destruct

09 Doma

10 Maniackers Design

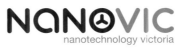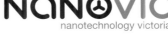

11 Resin[sistem] design

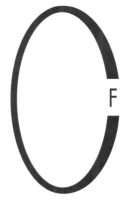

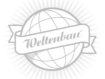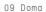

12 Tilt

13 the wilderness

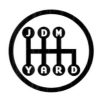

14 GillespieFox

15 Mattisimo

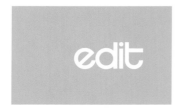

01 unfolded

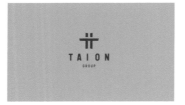

02 GWG

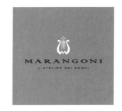

03 Simon & Goetz Design

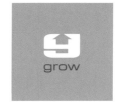

04 Simon & Goetz Design

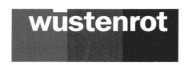

05 kw43

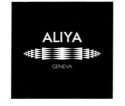

06 Sueellen

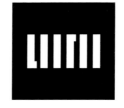

07 Accident Grotesk!

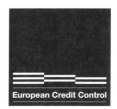

08 Engine

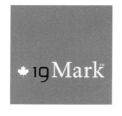

09 Ashi & office Greminger

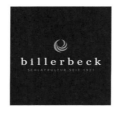

10 Simon & Goetz Design

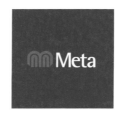

11 Sesame Studio

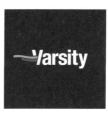

12 Sesame Studio

13 Jawa and Midwich

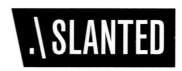

14 Magma

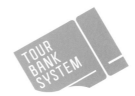

15 GWG

16 Sesame Studio

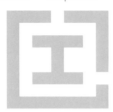

01 FoURPAcK ontwerpers

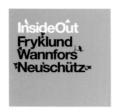

02 112 Ocean Drive

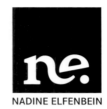

03 blackjune

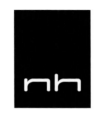

04 flat

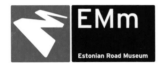

05 Velvet

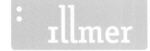
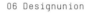

06 Designunion

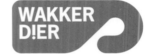

07 KesselsKramer

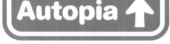

08 GillespieFox

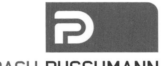

09 blackjune

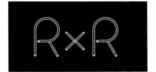

10 evaq studio

11 Laborator

12 Niels Shoe Meulman

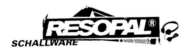

13 Resopal-Schallware

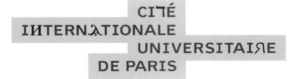

14 Intégral Ruedi Baur et associés

15 Sensus Design Factory

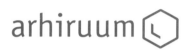 institute of visual culture

Cambridge

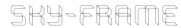 SKY-FRAME

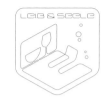

01 Martha Stutteregger

02 Bringolf Irion Vögeli

03 weissraum.de(sign)

arhiruum

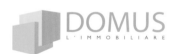 DD DESIGN

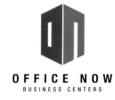 Escape Studios

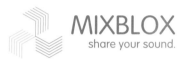 MIXBLOX
share your sound.

04 Velvet

05 DTM_INC

06 stylodesign

07 Jeffrey Kalmikoff

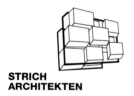 STRICH ARCHITEKTEN

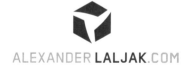 DOMUS
L'IMMOBILIARE

 OFFICE NOW
BUSINESS CENTERS

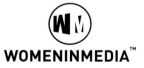 PEDANTEN.COM

08 Daniela Grundmann

09 Dimomedia Lab

10 Paco Aguayo

11 Axel Peemöller

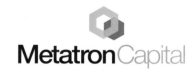 Metatron Capital

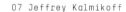 DITG
Digital Interactive Television Group

ALEXANDER LALJAK.COM

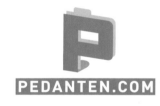 WOMENINMEDIA™

12 Sesame Studio

13 red design

14 blackjune

15 Crush

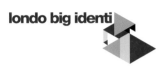 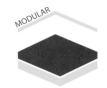 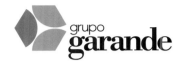 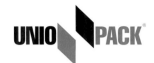

MODULAR

grupo **garande**

01 Labooo

02 raum mannheim

03 Luis E. Montenegro Lafont

04 Karoly Kiralyfalvi

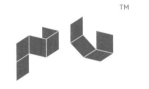

ports:united
streaming media systems.

FEDERATIE KOEPEL ORGANISATIES IN DE FINANCIËLE DIENSTVERLENING

05 yippieyeah cooperative

06 310k

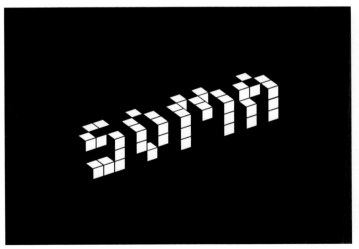 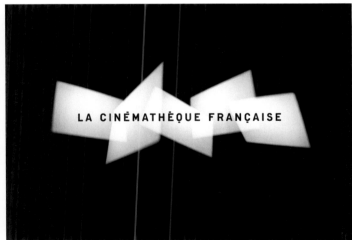

07 morphor

08 Intégral Ruedi Baur et associés

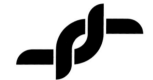

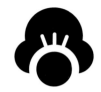

01 Labor f. visuelles Wachstum   02 Paco Aguayo   03 Sarah Grimaldi   04 Umeric

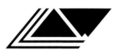

05 martinaigner.com   06 domenico catapano   07 the red is love   08 dextro.org

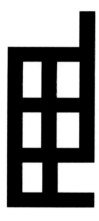

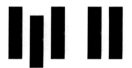

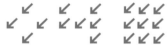

10 Emmi Salonen   11 Omochi   12 Sito

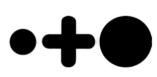

09 Euro RSCG Fuel Worldwide   13 Sito   14 büro uebele   15 nothing from outer space

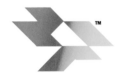

01 raum mannheim

02 Labor f. visuelles Wachstum

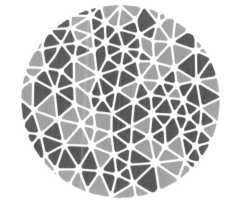

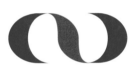

03 diamond

04 Pep Karsten

05 Katrin Acklin

06 makelike

07 Futro

08 makelike

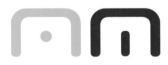

09 Jon Ari Helgason

01 Raredrop

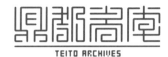

02 Zetuei Fonts

介護保険ナビ®

03 everyday icons

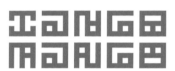

04 Omochi

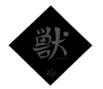

05 Coldwater Graphiix

06 kame design

07 Omochi

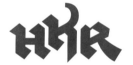

08 Velvet

09 Maniackers Design

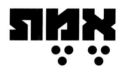

10 Power Graphixx

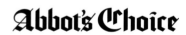

11 QuickHoney

HKR

12 Oscar Salinas Losada

Abbot's Choice

13 Raredrop

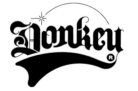

14 No-Domain

Maniackers Design

15 Maniackers Design

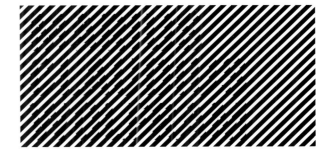

02 Axel Peemöller

Institut Fuer Musik Und Medien
Robert Schumann Hochschule Duesseldorf

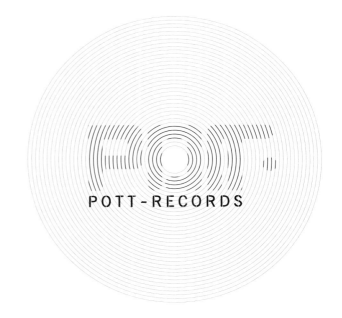

POTT-RECORDS

01 Double Standards   03 IDolls GrafikModeDialog

CULTURE

BALANCED

Things are not always easy for the inventor of symbols who is involved with culture. Many of the things offered in museums or found on the programs of theatres and concert halls fail to live up to their own aesthetic standards. And there exists a yawning gap between the tastes of the educated middle class and the consumers of events culture. Nonetheless, symbols are needed. Creative, even innovative, they must nonetheless renounce explosive outbreaks of colours or forms.

IRONY IS INNOVATION

The announcement, back then - in the wake of an unspeakable event habitually referred to with three numerals - that the "fun society" had come to an end, was not merely premature. It was perhaps also only intended ironically. Like so many things in our world. In the arts, irony has come to be regarded as a method for calling conventional aesthetic ordering principles into question, with the intention of unsettling beholders and their habitual patterns of perception. That was back in Classical Modernism. Which is now behind us. Adieu, Duchamp and Magritte. Ordering principles have taken their leave; patterns of perception have multiplied a million-fold. According to American philosopher Richard Rorty, the individual who relies on irony expresses a sense of doubt, and a sense of distance in relation to his or her own vocabulary in order to perpetually renew it. Should we not see the ironically intended codes contained in the logo – the smallest projection surface in the world – for what they really are: reflections of our society's patterns of communication?

AMSTERDAM, THE NETHERLANDS
FONS SCHIEDON

A good logo is an icon.

His logos often tell complex stories, ones that are a pleasure to read - always absorbing, never banal. Designer Fons Schiedon, who lives in Amsterdam, is an illustrator by training. But graphic design and film interested him right from the beginning. It seemed only logical to combine these disciplines and use them in his design work. Today, animation and motion design dominate his creative activities, with illustration and graphic design also playing important roles. And, of course, logo design.

Frans Schiedon has a special relationship to the logo. "I love logos. Even bad logos are fascinating because ultimately, every attempt to design one harbours the desire on the part of both designer and client to make something that is iconic and which communicates something 'essential' about an enterprise. A logo is the ultimate in identity design. Nothing else is as complex as this kind of composition, involving graphics or text or their combination. Given the pivotal importance ascribed to it, any logo design is pretentious. If a logo turns out well, it is a treat to admire its iconic value or intriguing way of capturing a complex matter. If it goes wrong, it often reveals how it fails to translate its intentions. In that case, it is great for speculating as to where the problem lies; is the logo a boardroom compromise, was the client indecisive, was the designer incompetent?"

But is a logo really a logo at all, in the textbook sense? With an ironic undertone, Fons Schiedon expresses concern about this object of his affections, which offers so many different facets for interpretation: "I have always believed that logos should capture the essence of whatever they are intended to represent in one clear, simple image. Almost like an illustration. If you have a salon for dogs, you show a dog and then some visual take on the idea of shaving, and you place the name of the company somewhere nearby. But the best logos don't do that."

Logos can be extremely minimal, says Fons, referring to the prime example of Big Blue IBM. But also extremely complex. And, in digital media, genuinely 'moving,' when slowly on a computer monitor. Good logo design - and this is the gist of this Dutch designer's deliberations - should start with a broader perspective: "You start by working 'around' it - creating shapes and colours, drawings and associative elements - avoiding obvious allusions to the logo. You assemble a collection of ingredients, adding and removing elements until you have something that captures a hint, an essence of the wider world you already worked in before. That's the hope, that a logo reflects some of where it came from."

KULTUR

AUSBALANCIERT

Für die in der Kultur involvierten Zeichenmacher ist es nicht immer einfach. Einiges, was in Museen geboten wird oder in Theatern und Konzertsälen auf dem Programm steht, entspricht nicht ihren eigenen ästhetischen Vorlieben. Und dann klafft auch ein Graben zwischen Bildungsbürgertum und Eventkulturkonsumenten. Zeichen werden trotzdem benötigt. Kreative, auch innovative, auf explosive Farben- und Formenausbrüche jedoch eher verzichtende.

IRONIE IST INNOVATION

Die Behauptung vom Ende der Spaßgesellschaft, damals, nach dem unaussprechlichen, nur in drei Zahlenchiffren nennbaren Ereignis, war nicht nur voreilig. Sie war vielleicht selbst nur ironisch gemeint. Wie vieles in dieser unserer Welt. In der Kunst galt die Ironie einmal als Methode, tradierte ästhetische Ordnungsprinzipien auf ironische Weise in Frage zu stellen, um den Betrachter und seine Wahrnehmungsmuster zu verunsichern. Das war in der klassischen Moderne. Vorbei. Adieu Duchamps und Magritte. Ordnungsprinzipien haben sich verabschiedet, Wahrnehmungsmuster millionenfach multipliziert. Nach dem amerikanischen Philosophen Richard Rorty drückt ein ironisch agierender Mensch damit den Zweifel und die Distanz gegenüber dem eigenen Vokabular aus, um es ständig erneuern zu können. Warum sollte man dann die ironischen Chiffren im Logo, der kleinsten Projektionsfläche der Welt, nicht als das nehmen, was sie sind: Reflexionen der Kommunikationsmuster unserer Gesellschaft?

AMSTERDAM, NIEDERLANDE

FONS SCHIEDON

Ein gutes Logo ist eine Ikone.

Seine Logos erzählen oft komplexe Geschichten, die man gerne liest, weil sie so spannend und nie banal sind. Der in Amsterdam lebende Designer Fons Schiedon ist von Haus aus Illustrator. Doch sein Interesse galt schon früh auch dem Graphic Design und dem Film. Die logische Konsequenz war, diese Disziplinen zu kombinieren und für seine gestalterische Arbeit zu nutzen. Animation und Motion Design bilden heute die Schwerpunkte seines Schaffens. Daneben Illustration und Graphic Design. Und eben auch Logos.

Frans Schiedon hat eine besondere Beziehung zu den Logos. „Ich liebe Logos. Selbst schlechte Logos sind faszinierend. Denn das Bestreben ein Logo zu entwickeln ist immer mit dem ultimativen Wunsch des Designers und seines Kunden verbunden, etwas zu kreieren, das ikonisch ist und etwas Essenzielles über das Unternehmen aussagt. Ein Logo, das ist die fundamentale Herausforderung des Identity Designs. Nichts ist so komplex wie diese Komposition aus Grafik und/oder Text. Weil ihm eine so zentrale Bedeutung zukommt, ist Logodesign immer prätentiös. Wenn ein Logo gelingt, dann ist es eine Freude seinen ikonischen Wert zu bewundern oder seine überzeugende Art, eine komplexe Botschaft auszudrücken. Wenn ein Logo misslingt, dann offenbart es oft, wie es seine Intentionen verfehlt hat. Das eröffnet Raum für Spekulationen: Wo lag das Problem? Ist es ein Konferenzzimmer-Kompromiss? War der Kunde zu wenig entscheidungsfreudig, der Designer unfähig ... ?“

Aber ist ein Logo überhaupt ein Logo, lehrbuchmäßig gesehen? Mit ironischem Unterton macht sich Fons Schiedon auch ‚Sorgen‘ über dieses, so viele Interpretationsflächen bietende Objekt seiner Liebe: „Ich habe immer geglaubt, Logos sollten das ausdrücken, für was sie stehen - in einem möglichst einfachen, klaren Bild. Wenn du einen Trimmsalon für Hunde hast, dann zeigst du einen Hund und irgendeine visuelle Idee über das Scheren von Hundehaaren, und dann arrangierst du den Namen des Salons darum herum. Doch die besten Logos tun dies eben gerade nicht.“

Logos können extrem reduziert sein, meint Fons, und verweist auf das Paradebeispiel Big Blue IBM. Aber auch extrem komplex. Und dazu, in Digitalmedien, echt ‚moving‘, indem sie sich am Bildschirm langsam aufbauen. Gutes Logodesign sollte, und das ist die Quintessenz der Überlegungen des holländischen Designers, von einer größeren Perspektive ausgehen: „Du arbeitest zu Beginn ‚darum herum‘, kreierst Formen, Farben, Zeichnungen, vermeidest konkrete Bezüge zum Logo. Du legst eine Sammlung von Bestandteilen an, fügst welche hinzu, nimmst welche weg, bis du einen Hauch, eine Spur, eine Essenz von der größeren Welt ‚eingefangen‘ hast, in der du schon vorher gearbeitet hast. Das ist die Hoffnung - ein Logo etwas davon reflektiert, wo es herkommt.“

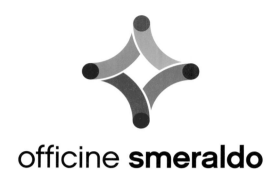

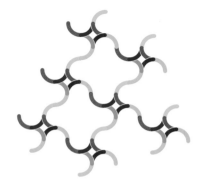

officine **smeraldo**

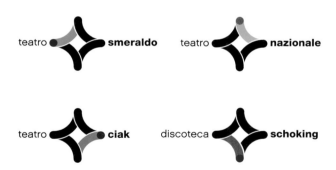

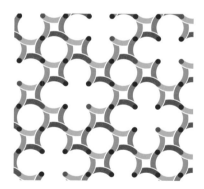

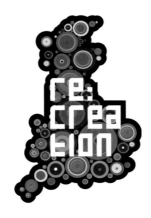

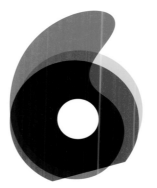

6th Biennial of
Towns and
Townplanners
in Europe

**City Living
Living City**

Copenhagen
2005

01 Form. Design and Art direction

02 Mai-Britt Amsler

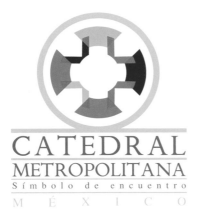

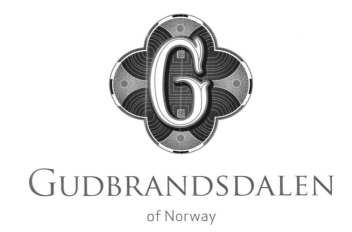

03 Pantiestudio

04 bleed

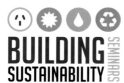

01 GillespieFox

02 Syrup Helsinki

03 Velvet

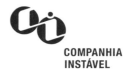

04 FireGirl

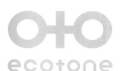

05 asmallpercent

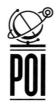

06 jum

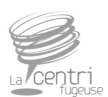

07 fireondesign / herborize

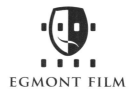

08 fireondesign / herborize

09 Fósforo

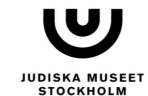

10 MaMadesign AB

11 zookeeper

12 Miha Artnak

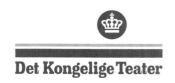

13 e-Types

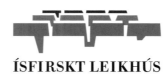

14 sidsel stubbe

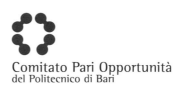

15 fireondesign / herborize

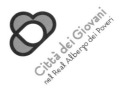

16 Perndl+Co

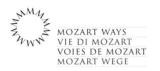

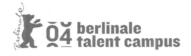

01 Pentagram

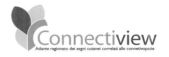

02 Rosendahl Grafikdesign

03 Dimomedia Lab

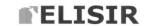

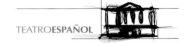

04 Dimomedia Lab

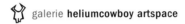

05 Laurent Fétis

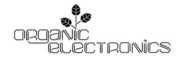

06 44 flavours

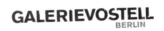

07 sidsel stubbe

08 Fósforo

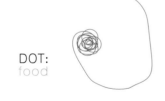

09 urbn;

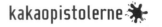

10 3 deluxe

11 Thomas Beyer Design

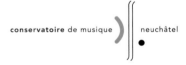

12 Mathilde Quartier

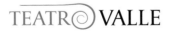

13 Jakob Straub

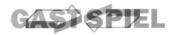

14 Neeser & Müller

15 3 deluxe

16 desres design group

confer, confide, contemplate, converse,

reflect,

discourse,

commune,

communicate,

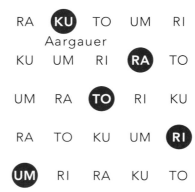

01 Magenta Creative Networks

02 Klauser Weibel Design

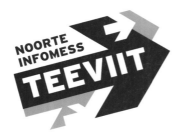

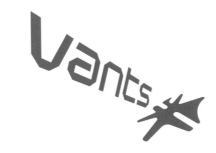

03 Velvet

04 Velvet

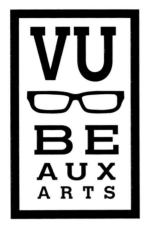

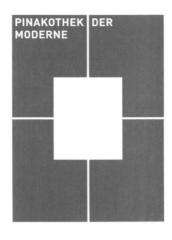

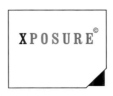

03 Matthias Gephart

04 raum mannheim

01 M!ch Welfringer

02 KMS Team

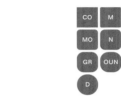

05 re-public

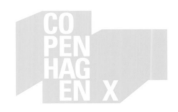

06 kummer & herrman

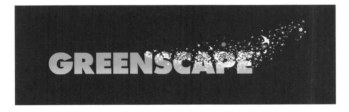

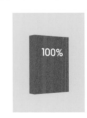

07 Engine

08 Mai-Britt Amsler

09 kummer & herrman

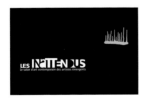

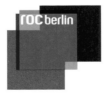

10 Alëxone

11 Fons Hickmann m23

12 Carsten Giese

13 Ariel Pintos

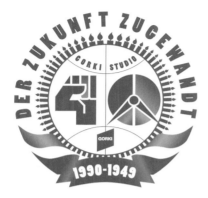

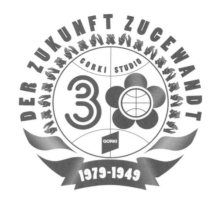

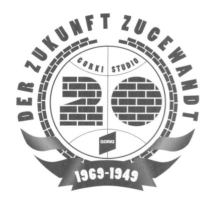

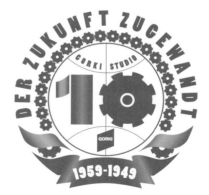

01 milchhof : atelier

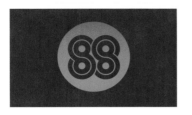

01 Sesame Studio

02 unfolded

03 unfolded

04 Supermundane

05 Raredrop

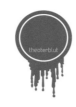

06 Cassie Leedham

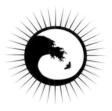

07 Cassie Leedham

08 Sensus Design Factory

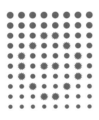

09 310k

10 Zucker und Pfeffer

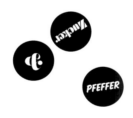

11 eduhirama

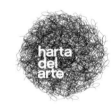

12 cabina

13 Grandpeople

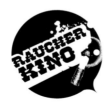

14 clandrei

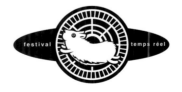

15 Benwar Home Design

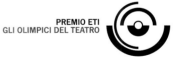

16 Jakob Straub

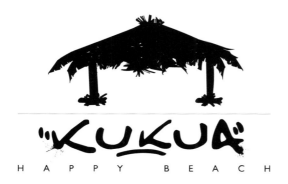

01 Dimomedia Lab

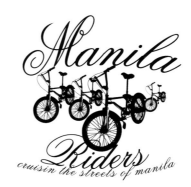

02 Team Manila

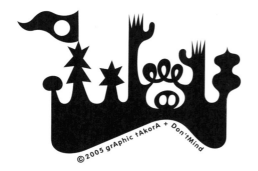

03 Takora

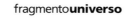

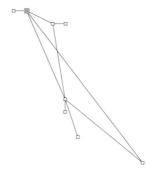

04 La Superagencia©

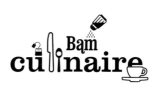

05 M!ch Welfringer

06 M!ch Welfringer

01 Team Manila

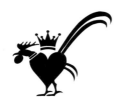

02 BEKO3

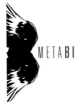

03 Alexandre Orion

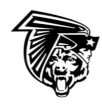

04 raum mannheim

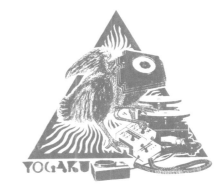

05 Hiroki Tsukuda

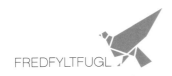

06 Kjetil Vatne

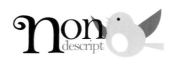

07 Cassie Leedham

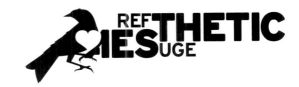

08 HandGun

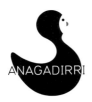

09 Kjetil Vatne

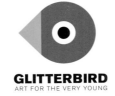

10 Rune Mortensen Design Studio

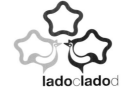

11 Dimaquina

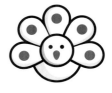

12 Kjetil Vatne

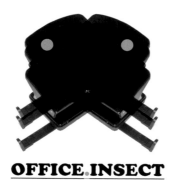

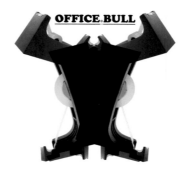

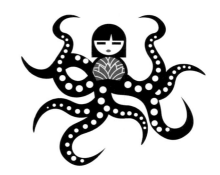

01 raum mannheim

02 raum mannheim

03 Keep Adding

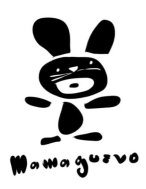

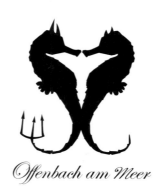

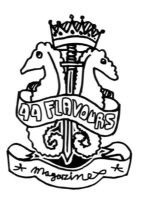

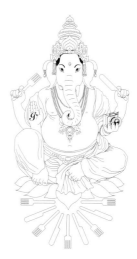

04 Magnetofonica

05 Salon Vektoria

06 44 flavours

07 Salon Vektoria

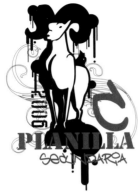

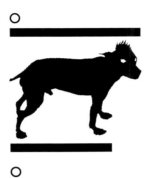

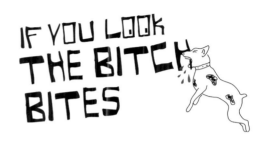

01 Escobas

02 The Remingtons

03 Transittus

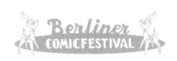

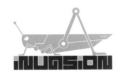

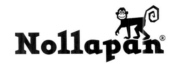

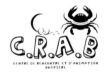

04 Judith Drews

05 Attak

06 Cyklon

07 Benwar Home Design

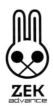

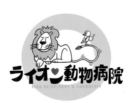

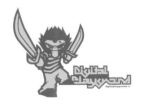

08 Miha Artnak

09 QuickHoney

10 Amore Hirosuke

11 DigitalPlayground Studio

02 Polygraph

03 News

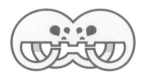

04 Toko

05 Sat One

06 310k

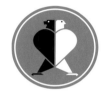

07 Attak

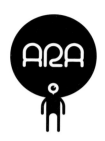

01 Atelier télescopique

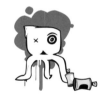

08 J. Tuominen, Jukka Pylväs

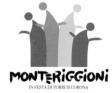

09 Fupete Studio

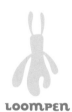

10 Oscar Salinas Losada

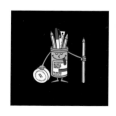

11 Grotesk

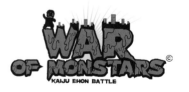

12 Koadzn

13 Canefantasma Studio

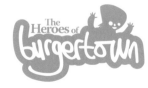

14 Jon Burgerman

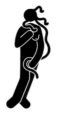

01 FireGirl

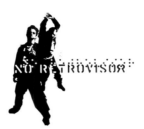

02 resistro®

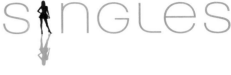

03 DTM_INC

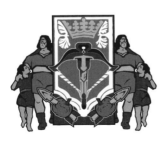

04 Jürgen und ich

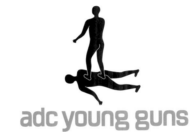

05 karlssonwilker inc.

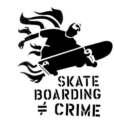

06 ROM studio

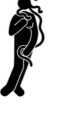

07 Sat One

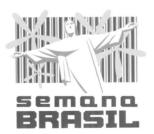

08 Mariana de Vasconcellos Lameiro da Costa

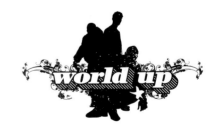

09 HandGun

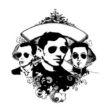

01 Team Manila

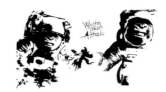

02 Norwegian Ink

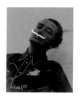

03 Norwegian Ink

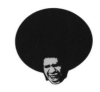

04 underson

05 Iván Solbes

06 Emil Hartvig

07 Jason Kochis

08 bisdixit

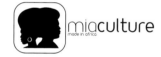

09 29 degres

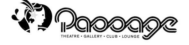

10 viagrafik

11 HardCase Design

12 Tohyto

13 Resin[sistem] design

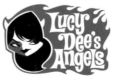

14 Sektie

15 Escobas

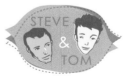

16 Miki Amano

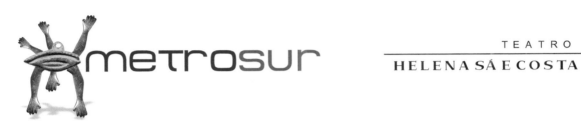

01 Escobas

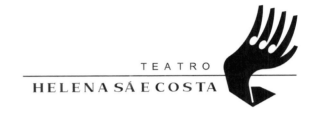

02 FireGirl

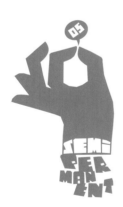

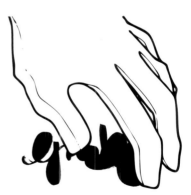

03 Adam Cruickshank

04 Pandarosa

05 Fupete Studio

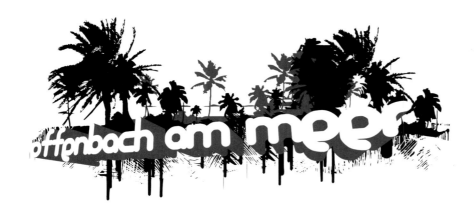

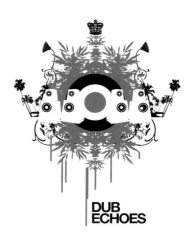

01 Salon Vektoria

02 Dimaquina

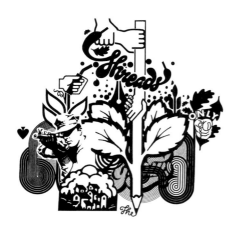

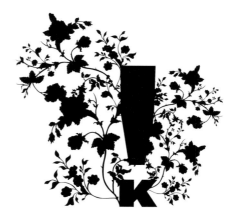

03 Keep Left Studio

04 Mutabor Design

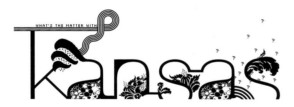

01 decoylab

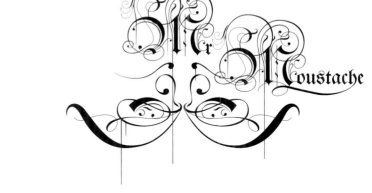

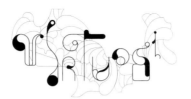

02 the Legalizer ApS

03 zinestesia

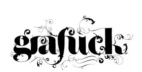

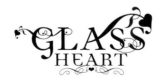

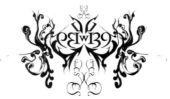

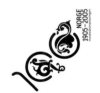

04 Me, Me

05 A-Side Studio

06 Superlow

07 Superlow

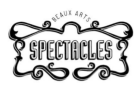

08 M!ch Welfringer

09 Molho

10 Toko

11 base

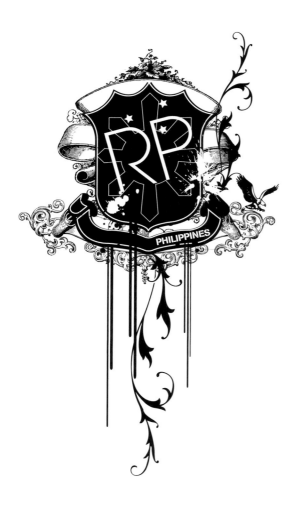

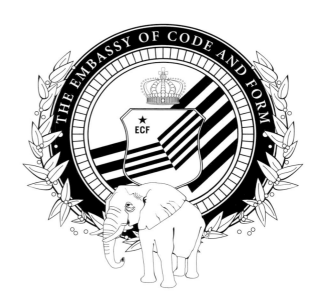

01 Team Manila

02 Supershapes

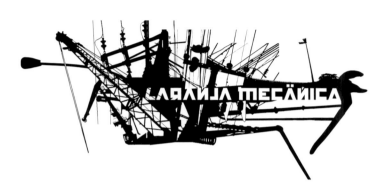

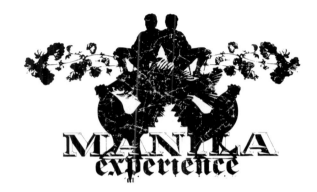

01 Caótica

02 Team Manila

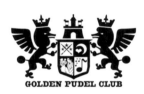

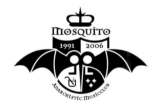

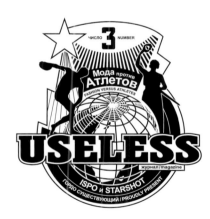

03 Typeholics

04 Strukt Visual Network

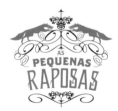

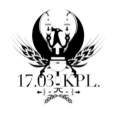

05 Caótica

06 raum mannheim

07 Magma

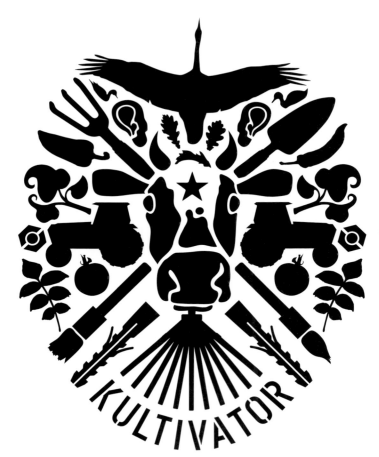

01 Floor Wesseling Ix Opus Ada

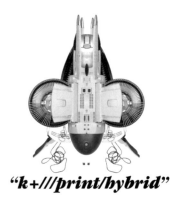

"k+///print/hybrid"

02 raum mannheim

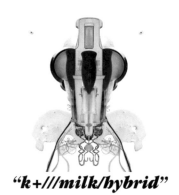

"k+///milk/hybrid"

03 raum mannheim

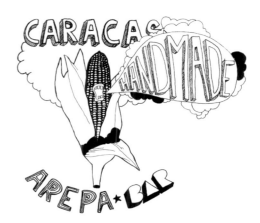

02 Tohyto

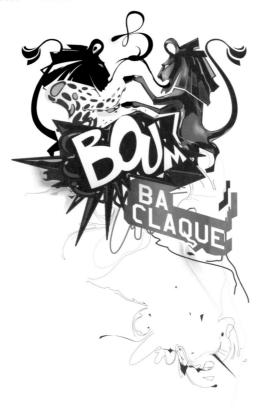

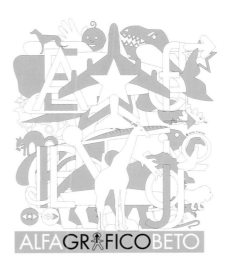

01 Fons Schiedon   03 Ariel Pintos

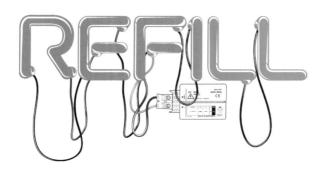

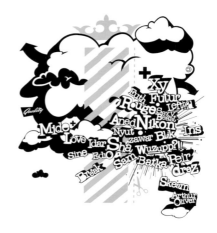

01 Keep Left Studio

02 Extraverage Productions

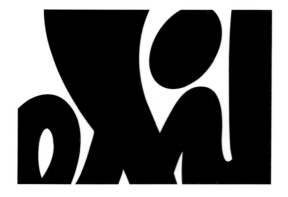

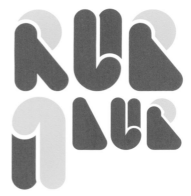

03 Keep Left Studio

04 Lucias Westrup

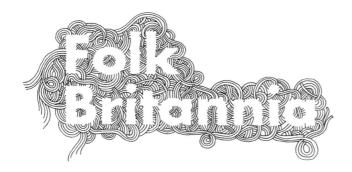

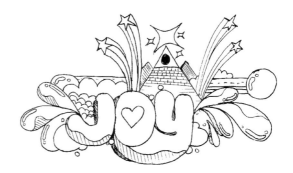

01 ZIP Design   02 Laundry

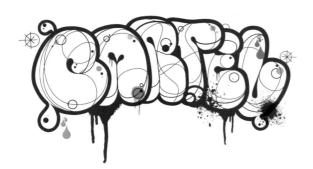

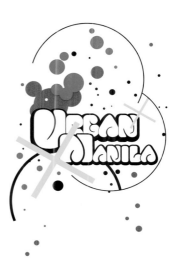

03 Masa   04 Team Manila

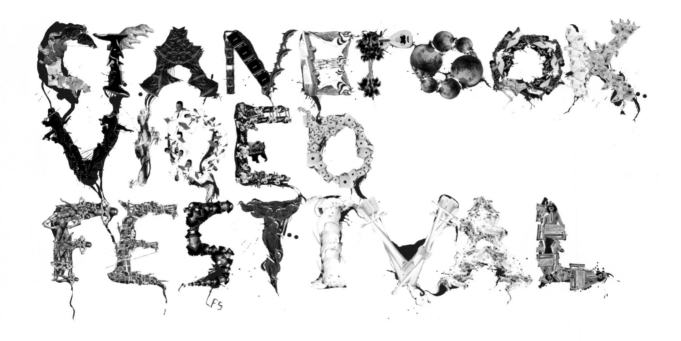

01 lifelong friendship society

WE ARE
GOING
UNDER
GROUND

01 bleed

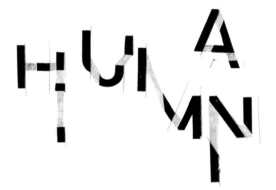

02 Molho

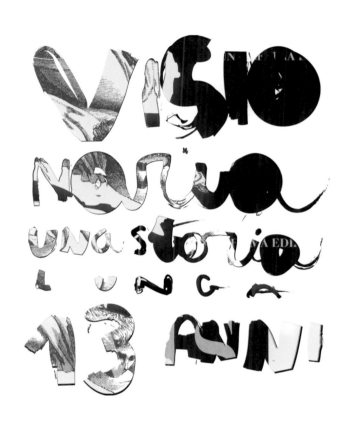

03 Canefantasma Studio

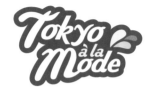

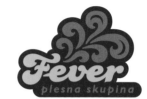

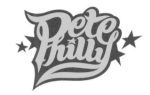

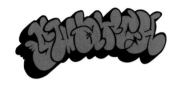

01 Meomi Design

02 Sektie

03 Lukatarina

04 Karoly Kiralyfalvi

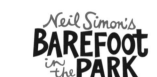

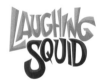

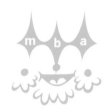

05 typotherapy+design inc.

06 BankerWessel

07 Stolen Inc.

08 Gastón Caba

Neil Simon's
BAREFOOT
in the PARK

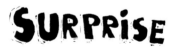

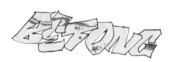

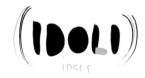

09 Bo Lundberg Illustration

10 Attaboy

11 Dennis Eriksson

12 Sektie

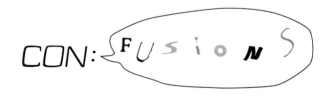

13 Spild af Tid

14 Martin Kvamme

15 Canefantasma Studio

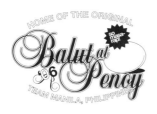

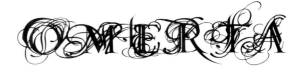

01 Team Manila

02 milchhof : atelier

03 The KDU

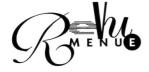

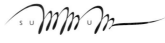

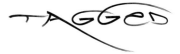

04 HardCase Design Dmitri

05 milchhof : atelier

06 Niels Shoe Meulman

07 MvM / Maarten van Maanen

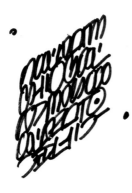

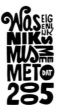

09 a+morph

10 raum mannheim

11 Fupete Studio

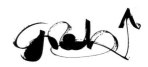

08 Michael Genovese

12 Parra

13 Catalogtree

14 Dennis Eriksson

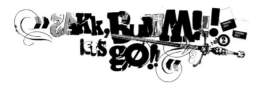

01 Zeek&Destroy

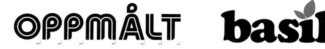

02 Underware

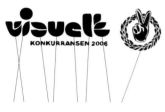
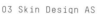

03 Skin Design AS

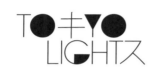
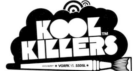

04 The KDU

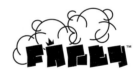

05 Skin Design AS

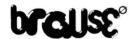

06 Luca Forlani

07 Zeek&Destroy

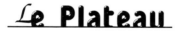

08 Laurent Fétis

09 viagrafik

10 viagrafik

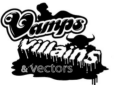

11 Digart Graphics

12 Alëxone

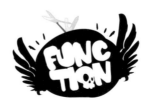

13 Clrqa

14 Luca Forlani

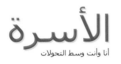 الأسرة
أنا وأنت وسط التحولات

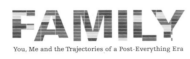 FAMILY
You, Me and the Trajectories of a Post-Everything Era

DISPLACED

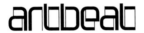

01 Canefantasma Studio   02 Alexander Fuchs   03 actiondesigner

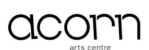 artbeat   stadtlicht   CAC BRETIGNY   KUNSTVERMITTLUNG

04 Norwegian Ink   05 Neeser & Müller   06 Vier5   07 Lorenzo Geiger

acorn
arts centre

TOTAL RECALL
INT. FESTIVAL DES NACHERZÄHLTEN FILMS

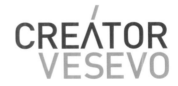 CREATOR
VESEVO

49 NORD
6 EST
FRAC
LORRAINE
FONDS RÉGIONAL D'ART CONTEMPORAIN DE LORRAINE
1ᴿᴱ RUE DES TRINITAIRES. F-57000 METZ
↘

08 A-Side Studio   09 Lollek und Bollek   10 fireondesign / herborize   11 re-p

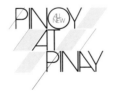 PINOY AT PINAY   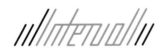   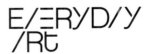 EVERYDAY /ART   BLINDSTADT
Labor für Reflexion

12 Team Manila   13 visomat inc.   14 automatic   15 substrat

Focustyle™   BABYgallery   ATELIFRANKFURT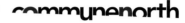

01 artless Inc   02 Julie Joliat   03 Fuenfwerken Design   04 Magenta Creative Networks

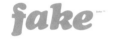   MANZPORTAL   portes ouvertes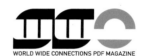

05 Brighten the corners   06 archetype : interactive   07 Neeser & Müller   08 Extraverage Productions

THE USE EXHIB AGAIN ITION   mumok slw   zuidelijk toneel   şimdi now

09 Flink   10 Martha Stutteregger   11 Toko   12 ständige vertretung

MUSEUM CHECKPOINT CHARLIE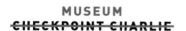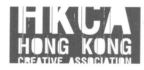

13 Fuenfwerken Design   14 Vier5   15 Double Standards   16 archetype : interactive

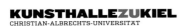 **KUNSTHALLEZUKIEL**
CHRISTIAN-ALBRECHTS-UNIVERSITÄT

aktive archive

rpotsdam

hansottotheate

01 Mutabor Design

02 Atelier Mühlberg

03 formdusche büro für gestaltung

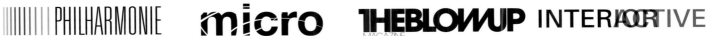 PHILHARMONIE

micro

1HEBLOWUP MAGAZINE

INTERAC**TI**VE

04 Pentagram

05 3 deluxe

06 Nish

07 Semitransparent Design

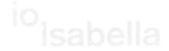 io Isabella

muthesius kunsthochschule

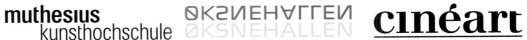 ØKSNEHALLEN
ØKSNEHALLEN

cinéart

08 Fons Schiedon

09 Tilt

10 Kontrapunkt

11 Jonas Ganz

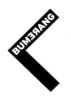 BUMƎRANG

 PIE NI TAI VAS
DEN LILLA HIMLEN
SMALL HEAVEN

 KUNST INDUSTRI MUSEET
DANISH MUSEUM OF ART & DESIGN

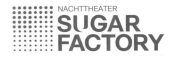 NACHTTHEATER **SUGAR FACTORY**

12 Futro

13 Syrup Helsinki

14 Kontrapunkt

15 310k

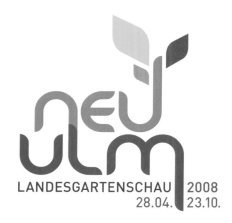

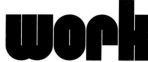
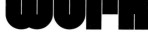

02 viagrafik

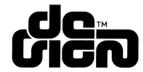

03 Intercity

01 propella, konzept + design

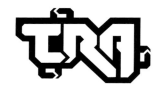

04 HelloBard.com

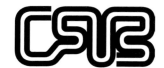

05 Sito

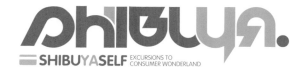

06 Axel Domke

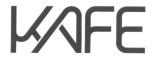

07 backyard 10

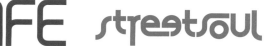

08 Karoly Kiralyfalvi

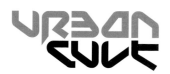

09 DTM_INC

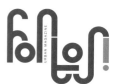

10 Karoly Kiralyfalvi

11 News

12 Superlow

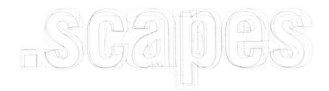

.scapes

01 granit di Lioba Wackernell

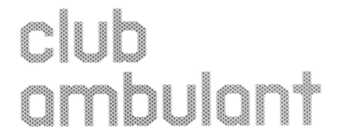

club
ambulant

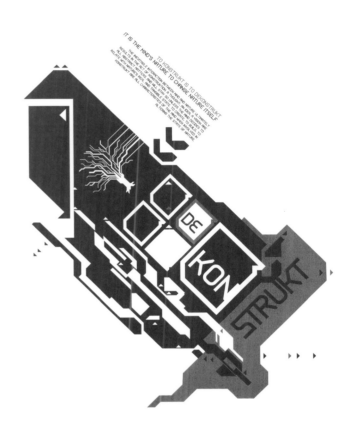

IT IS THE MIND'S NATURE TO KONSTRUKT IS TO DEKONSTRUKT

02 chris bolton   03 Lunatiq

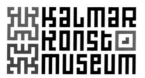

01 Floor Wesseling Ix Opus

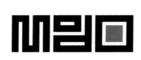

02 Paco Aguayo

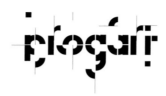

03 red design

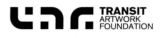

04 29 degres

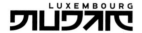

05 strange//attraktor:

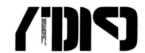

06 Superlow

07 artless Inc

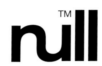

08 Caótica

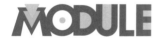

09 hirschindustries

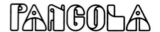

10 sophie toporkoff

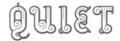

11 unfolded

12 Niels Shoe Meulman

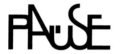

13 Laurent Fétis

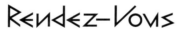

14 No-Domain

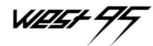

15 Jürgen und ich

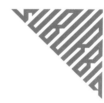

16 jewboy Corporation™

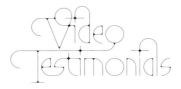

01 Niels Shoe Meulman

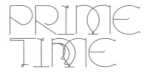

02 Superlow

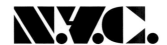

03 Superlow

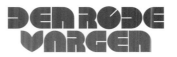

04 Tohyto

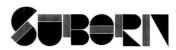

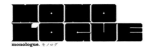

05 rtr

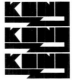

06 Nish

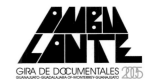

07 Plastic Kid

08 No-Domain

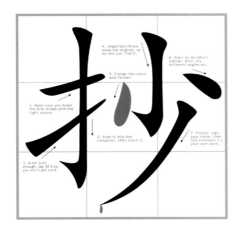

09 Atomic Attack

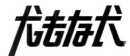

10 Raredrop

11 Martin Kvamme

12 archetype : interactive

13 Power Graphixx

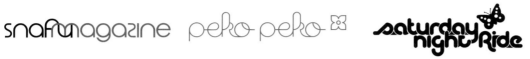 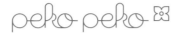 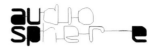 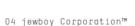

01 GrafficTraffic

02 3 deluxe

03 3 deluxe

04 jewboy Corporation™

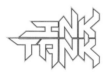 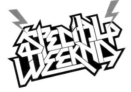 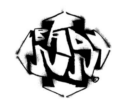

05 La Superagencia©

06 Superlow

07 Superlow

08 Caótica

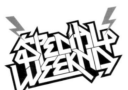

09 ruse76

10 Karoly Kiralyfalvi

11 Mikkel Grafixico Westrup

12 JAKe

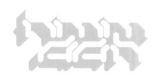 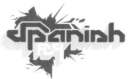 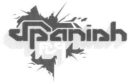 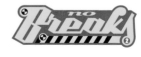

13 paulroberts.tv

14 44 flavours

15 44 flavours

16 Sektie

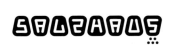

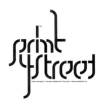

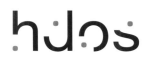

01 Hausgrafik

02 hirschindustries

03 Karoly Kiralyfalvi

04 Formgeber

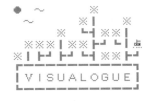

ZEPH4R C4.9

DESIGN GRAFICO BRASILEIRO

balcony le magazine

05 ten_do_ten

06 env-design

07 Molho

08 123Buero

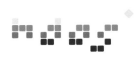

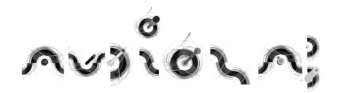

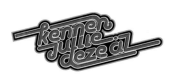

09 Formgeber

10 Laurent Fétis

11 Out Of Order

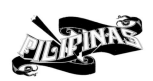

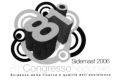

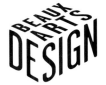

12 Team Manila

13 Dimomedia Lab

14 M!ch Welfringer

15 büro uebele

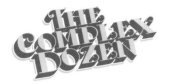

01 Razauno

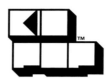

02 Konstantinos Gargaletsos

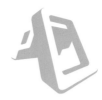

03 viagrafik

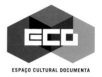

04 WGD

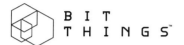

05 Semitransparent Design

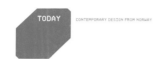

06 bleed

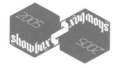

07 Superlow

08 William Morrisey

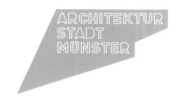

09 Brighten the corners

10 Fons Hickmann m23

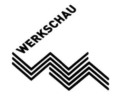

11 visomat inc.

12 Le_Palmier Design

13 Otherways 5th Floor Studio

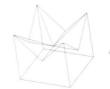

14 granit di Lioba Wackernell

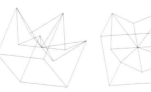

15 Floor Wesseling

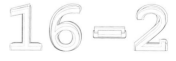

01 Attak

02 FireGirl

03 Thonik

04 visomat inc.

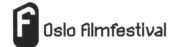

05 Simian

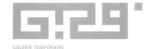

06 29 degres

07 Studio Dumbar

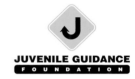

08 Semisans

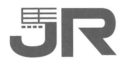

09 dainippon

10 ständige vertretung

11 raum mannheim

12 Jonas Ganz

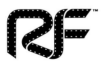

13 Keep Left Studio

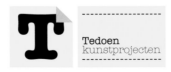

14 Toko

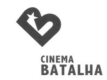

15 derek johnson

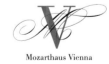

16 Pentagram

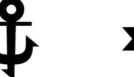

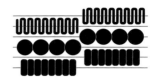

01 News

02 Ludovic Balland

03 Accident Grotesk!

04 Team Manila

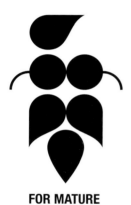

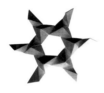

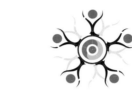

06 Catalogtree

07 Kjetil Vatne

08 Tender

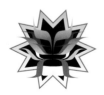

**FOR MATURE
READERS ONLY**

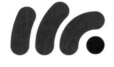

05 Flexn / BANK™

09 fireondesign / herborize

10 Annabelle Mehraein

11 makelike

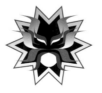

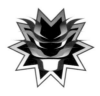

12 3volt Design

13 3volt Design

14 3volt Design

15 viagrafik

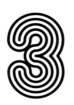

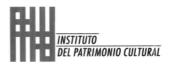

INSTITUTO
DEL PATRIMONIO CULTURAL

02 Balsi Grafik

03 Annella Armas

04 Annella Armas

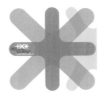

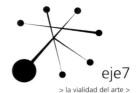

eje7
> la vialidad del arte >

05 Matthias Gephart

06 Annella Armas

07 Pantiestudio

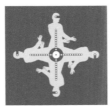

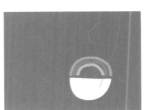

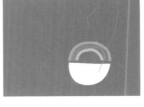

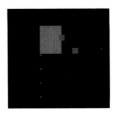

01 Atelier télescopique

08 FireGirl

09 Laundry

10 Loic Sattler

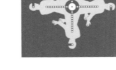

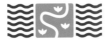

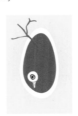

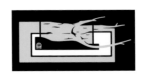

11 Lucias Westrup

12 Axel Raidt

13 Laundry

14 Sat One

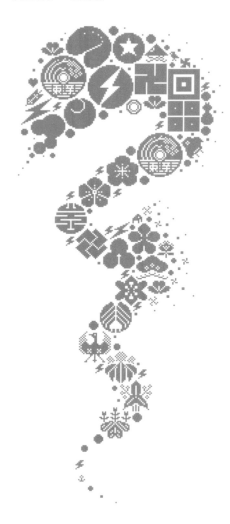

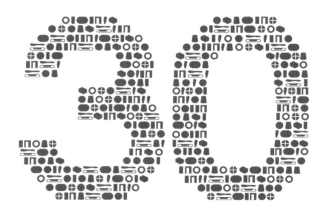

02 chris bolton

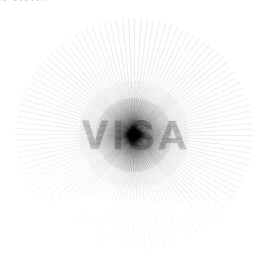

01 ten_do_ten

03 Fons Hickmann m23

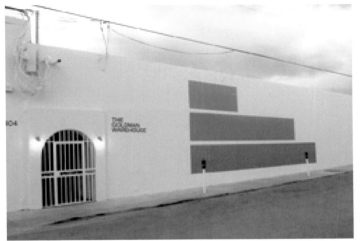

01 karlssonwilker

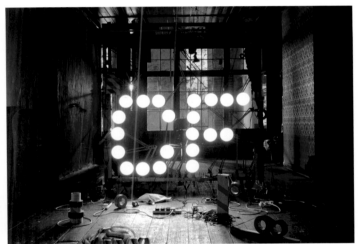

03 Tsuyoshi Kusano Design

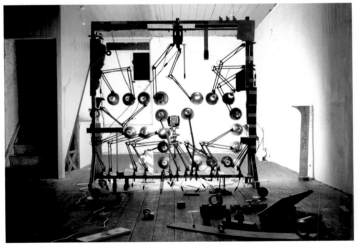

03 Creative Review

04 Creative Review

DESIGN

PROVOCATION IS AN ASPECT OF SELF-PORTRAYAL

A designer who respects prevailing CI rules when creating logos for commercial clients will make a 360° turn when it comes to his own trademark. This needs to be striking, abstract, absurd. Light years away from marketability. But aligned to the market nonetheless. Paradoxical? Not at all: the designer's own logo needs to function within his or her own scene and should ideally betray an affinity to experimental art.

MUCH LIGHTNING, LITTLE THUNDER

There is nothing new about cultural critics bemoaning the loss of social significance and relevance of traditional signs and symbols. Nor is there anything really new about designers helping themselves to this inventory of symbols without caring a straw about their original meanings. The main thing is to make them look cool. The lightning bolt, frequently represented in Tres Logos, is one such symbol. Does its shape not convey something fascinatingly aggressive? Its shape perhaps, but certainly not its original symbolic significance. Blitzkrieg and fascism were 20th century. The myths go back further. For the ancient Greeks, the lightning bolt signified the creative power of Zeus, father of the gods. In the Old Testament, it stood for spiritual enlightenment. One such myth remains alive and well to this day. And this example actually turns the symbol's supposed aggressiveness on its head: Blitzen (lightning) is the name of one of the reindeers pulling Santa's sleigh.

NEW YORK, UNITED STATES
DEANNE Y. CHEUK

"My mind is always ticking with too many ideas"

To the New York's Art Director's Club, she is one of the 34 top guns under the age of 30. A qualification that strikes one as rather ironic in light of her poetic creations, evocative of an entirely new Romanticism. There is no shooting where fantasy landscapes sprout with flowers of paradise. Time Magazine lists her among "The best people of 2004." Neomu, the smallest magazine in the world – no words, no advertising, no compromise – and refered to by herself as a "graphic zine of inspiration," has already achieved something like cult status. And 2005 saw the publication of her first book, Mushroom Girls Virus.

Designer Deanne Y. Cheuk, who grew up in Perth, Australia and now lives and works in New York City, is a pioneer when it comes to introducing illustrative typography to the magazine world. This much is clear from her work for contemporary cutting edge magazines since 1994, and as art director and designer for the likes of Big and Tokion. In the process, her style and her language have continued to evolve: her creations have become increasingly complex, organic, multi-faceted. Very few magazine art directors double as successful illustrators, and Deanne Y. Cheuk is one of them. And moreover in a decidedly innovative way that opens up new perspectives: Deanne Y. Cheuk has succeeded in blending her highly personal illustrative and painterly techniques with typography and editorial design. A perfect fusion and one that has yielded extraordinary results.

When it comes to current tendencies in design and her own work, this New York artist has definite opinions: "I think most graphic design today is derivative, but every now and then you see something that is so original, whether in the execution or in the design itself, maybe it's the typeface, the illustration, the photo, the colours, the printing, it can be any or all of those elements, or something else that creates something that is so inspired that it makes me really happy to be a designer. I love that feeling of wishing I had thought of it first, it's what drives me, it's that longing for inspiration - of finding it, and of giving it, it's an addiction."

Besides her numerous projects, many of them non-profit, Deanne Y. Cheuk is also commercially successful: Nike, Converse, Penguin Books, Target, Sprint, Urban Outfits, ESPN and MTV2 are among the companies that have commissioned this New York designer.

DESIGN

PROVOKATION GEHÖRT ZUR SELBSTDARSTELLUNG

Ein Designer, der beim Kreieren von Logos für kommerzielle Kunden bestehende CI-Regeln beachtet, vollführt eine Kehrtwendung um 360 Grad, wenn es um sein eigenes Zeichen geht. Krass, abstrakt, absurd muss es sein. Lichtjahre entfernt von der Marktfähigkeit. Trotzdem marktkonform. Paradox? Gar nicht: Das Logo des Designers soll in der eigenen Szene funktionieren und im Idealfall eine Affinität zur experimentellen Kunst haben.

VIEL BLITZ UND WENIG DONNER

Es ist nicht neu, dass Kulturkritiker das Vergessen von Bedeutung und Relevanz traditionsverbundener alter Symbole und Zeichen in unserer Gesellschaft beklagen. Und es ist ebenfalls kein wirklich neuer Trend, dass sich Gestalter aus diesem Fundus bedienen und sich keinen Deut darum scheren, was die ursprüngliche Bedeutung ist. Hauptsache, es sieht cool aus. Der Blitz, zahlreich vertreten in Tres Logos, ist eines dieser Zeichen. Hat seine Form nicht etwas faszinierend Aggressives? Seine Form vielleicht schon, seine ursprüngliche symbolische Bedeutung aber keineswegs. Blitzkrieg und Faschismus waren im 20. Jahrhundert. Die Mythen waren früher. Bei den alten Griechen galt der Blitz als Zeichen kreativer Kraft des Göttervaters Zeus. Im Alten Testament steht der Blitz als Zeichen spiritueller Erleuchtung. Ein Mythos ist sogar noch quicklebendig. Ausgerechnet einer, der die vorgebliche Aggressivität dieses Zeichens praktisch auf den Kopf stellt: Blitz heißt eines der Rentiere, die den Schlitten von Santa Claus ziehen.

NEW YORK, VEREINIGTE STAATEN

DEANNE Y. CHEUK

„In meinem Kopf ticken ständig viel zu viele neue Ideen."

Für den New Yorker Art Directors Club ist sie eine von 34 „Top Guns" unter 30. Ein Attribut, das ziemlich ironisch anmutet - angesichts der poetischen, eine ganz neue Romantik evozierenden Kreationen dieser Designerin. Denn: In imaginären Fantasielandschaften erblühende Paradiesblumen schießen nicht. Time Magazine reihte sie unter „The best people of 2004" ein. Das von ihr selbst als „graphic zine of inspiration" bezeichnete „neomu", kleinstes Magazin der Welt, ohne Worte, ohne Werbung, ohne Kompromisse, hat bereits so etwas wie Kultstatus erreicht. Und seit 2005 gibt es auch ein erstes Buch: „The Mushroom Girls Virus Book".

Die Designerin Deanne Y. Cheuk, im australischen Perth aufgewachsen, in New York City lebend und arbeitend, gilt als Pionierin beim Einsatz illustrativer Typografie im Magazinbereich. Das hat Deanne Y. Cheuk, die seit 1994 für moderne und zeitgeistige Magazine tätig ist, als Art Director und Designerin zum Beispiel für Big und Tokion eindrücklich bewiesen. Dabei hat sich ihr Stil, ihre Sprache kontinuierlich weiterentwickelt: Ihre Kreationen wurden immer komplexer, organischer, vielschichtiger. Es gibt wenige Art Directors für Magazine, die gleichzeitig erfolgreiche Illustratoren sind. Deanne Y. Cheuk ist eine der wenigen unter ihnen. Und sie ist es auf eine ausgesprochen innovative, neue Sichtweisen provozierende Art: Deanne Y. Cheuk hat es geschafft, ihre ureigenen illustrativen und Maltechniken mit der Typografie und dem Editorial Design zu verbinden. Eine perfekte Fusion, die außergewöhnliche Resultate zeitigt.

Was die aktuellen Tendenzen im Design und ihre eigene Arbeit angeht, so vertritt die New Yorker Künstlerin eine klare Meinung: „Grafikdesign ist heute derivativ, von irgendwoher abgeleitet. Doch ab und an entdeckst du etwas, das ist so echt, das wirkt so inspirierend, dass ich mich richtig glücklich fühle, Designerin zu sein. Dabei spielt es eigentlich gar keine Rolle, was es ist: Es kann die Ausführung oder das Design selbst sein. Vielleicht ist es das Schriftbild, die Illustration, das Foto, der Druck; es kann all das sein oder etwas ganz anderes. Ich liebe dieses Gefühl, dieses ‚Feeling of Wishing', das mich seit jeher begleitet. Es ist das, was mich antreibt. Es ist dieses Verlangen nach Inspiration, sie zu finden und weiterzugeben - es ist wie eine Sucht."

Neben ihren zahlreichen Projekten, die nicht selten Nonprofit-Projekte sind, ist Deanne Y. Cheuk auch kommerziell erfolgreich: Nike, Converse, Penguin Books, Target, Sprint, Urban Outfits, ESPN und MTV2 gehören zu den Unternehmen, die von der New Yorker Gestalterin bereits mit Designprojekten betraut worden sind.

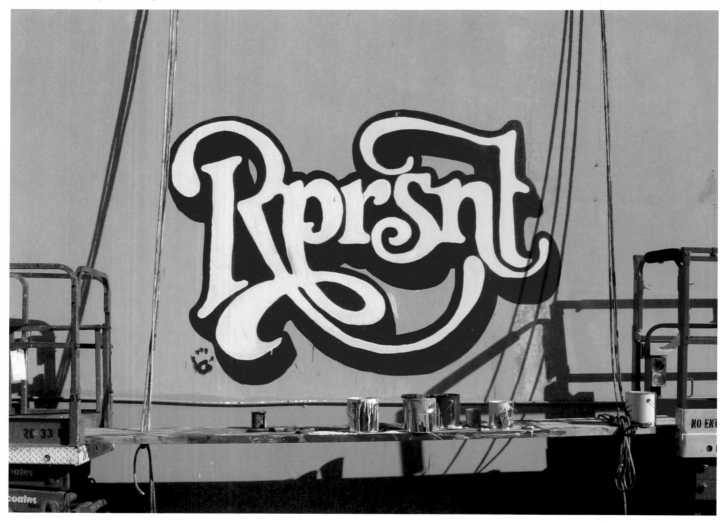

01 Keep Left Studio

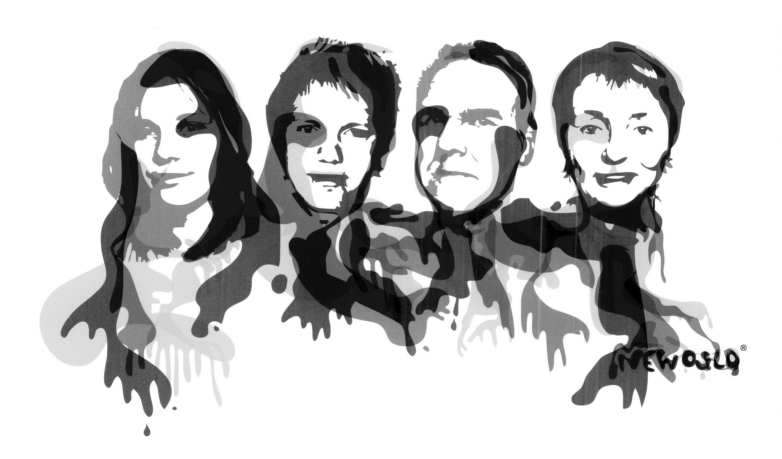

01 newoslo

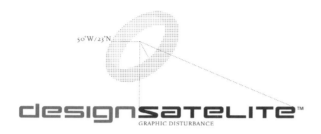

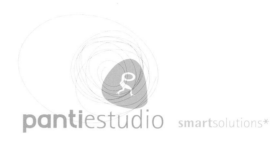

01 Labor für visuelles Wachstum™

02 Pantiestudio

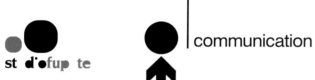

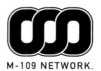

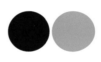

03 Fupete Studio

04 Kosta Lazarevski / rdy

05 Futro

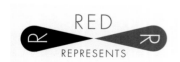

06 Insect

07 Borsellino & Co.

08 Intercity

09 Simian

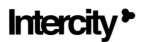

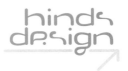

TOCA ME

pixelprinz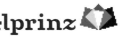

01 Intercity

02 brandigloo

03 Toca Me

04 donat raetzo union

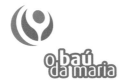
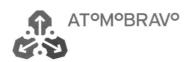

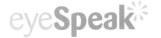

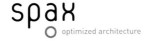

05 FireGirl

06 Toxic design

07 resistro®

08 Emil Hartvig

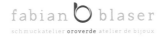

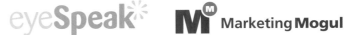

09 moxi

10 moxi

11 David Maloney

12 lindedesign

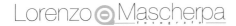

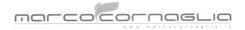

^ / Huippu / Design / Management

13 Dimomedia Lab

14 Dimomedia Lab

15 Syrup Helsinki

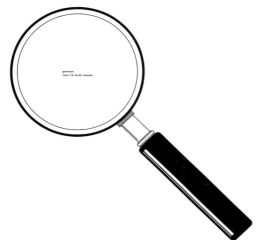

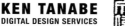

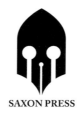

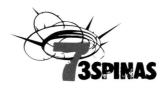

02 Cruz Creative

03 Keloide.net

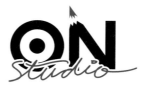

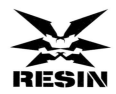

01 Amseldrossel

04 Resin[sistem] design

05 Resin[sistem] design

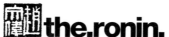

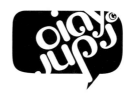

06 Ken Tanabe

07 Rob Chiu

08 Stolen Inc.

09 Karoly Kiralyfalvi

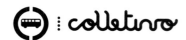

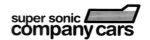

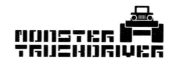

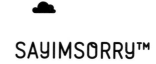

10 Colletivo Design

11 sunrise studios

12 DigitalPlayground Studio

13 123Buero

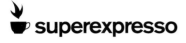
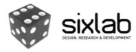

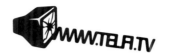

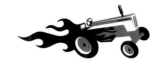

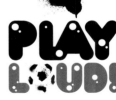

01 Superexpresso

02 cubegrafik - 100% Digital

03 Alexandre Orion

04 Norwegian Ink

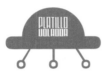

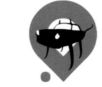

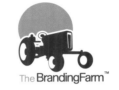

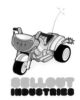

05 Dr. Alderete

06 Lapin

07 Ninjacruise

05 Sellout Industries

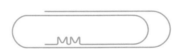
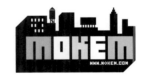

09 Chris Hutchinson

10 Mattisimo

11 jeremyville

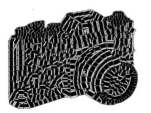

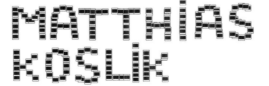

13 Frederique Daubal

14 Frederique Daubal

16 Masa

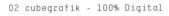

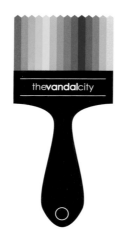

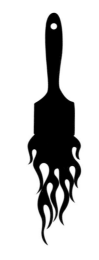

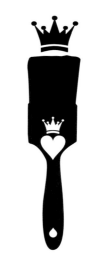

01 Karoly Kiralyfalvi

02 Karoly Kiralyfalvi

03 BEK03

04 BEK03

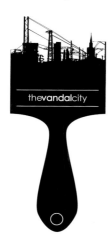

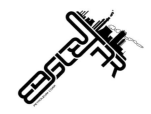

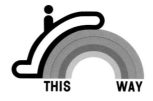

06 Carsten Raffel

07 Emmi Salonen

08 Lunatiq

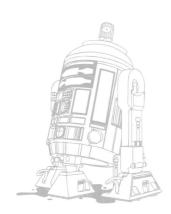

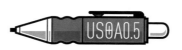

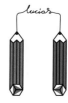

05 Keep Left Studio

09 jum

10 Felix Braden

11 Lucias Westrup

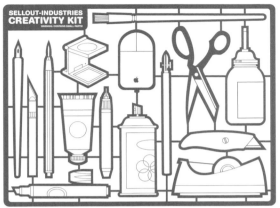

01 Sellout Industries

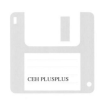

02 Amseldrossel

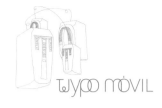

03 Blu Design

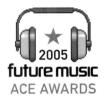

04 QuickHoney

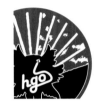

05 Heiko Hoos

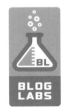

06 actiondesigner

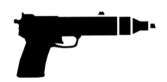

07 Matthias Gephart

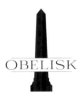

08 Nish

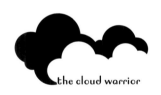

09 Karoly Kiralyfalvi

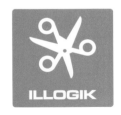

10 Draplin

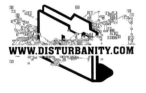

11 Karoly Kiralyfalvi

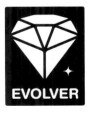

12 Emil Kozak

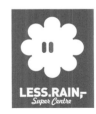

13 less rain

01 Karoly Kiralyfalvi

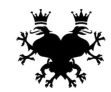

02 Robert Lindström

03 BEKO3

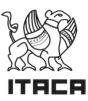

04 2Advanced Studios

05 BEKO3

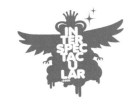

06 interspectacular

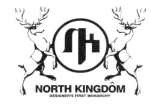

07 DesignChapel

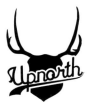

08 Canefantasma Studio

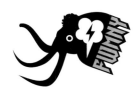

09 Cupco!

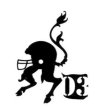

10 BEKO3

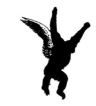

11 apishAngel

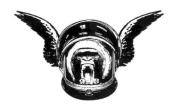

12 apishAngel

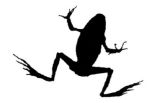

13 Georg Schatz

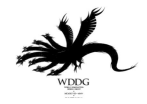

14 Nish

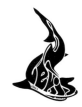

15 Studio Oscar

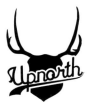

16 Upnorth

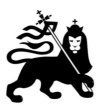

01 The Skull Dezain

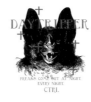

02 Microbot David Fuhrer

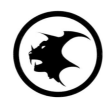

03 hijack graphics

04 hijack graphics

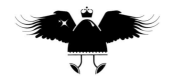

05 No-Domain

06 ROM studio

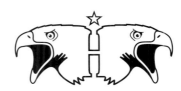

07 Yo Freeman

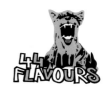

08 44 flavours

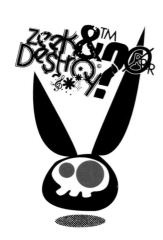
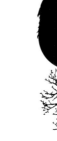

09 Zeek&Destroy

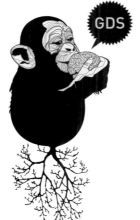

10 Glauco Diogenes

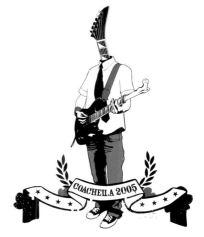

11 Tohyto

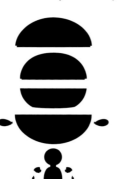

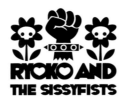

02 Tado

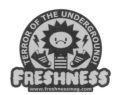

03 Tado

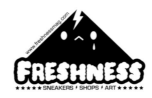

04 Tado

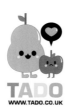

01 Rolitoland

05 Tado

06 Cupco!

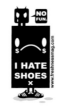

07 Tado

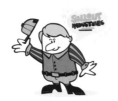

08 Tado

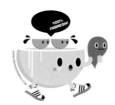

09 Tado

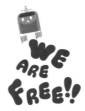

10 Takora

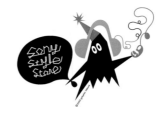

11 Takora

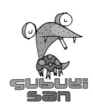

12 Sellout Industries

13 tapetentiere

14 redaktion »echtzeit«

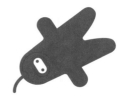

15 Alexander Fuchs

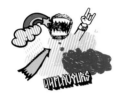

01 44 flavours

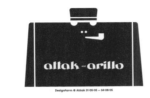

02 Attak

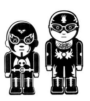

03 Cuartopiso

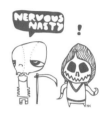

04 A-Side Studio

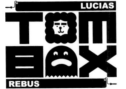

06 Lucias Westrup

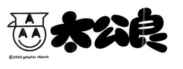

07 Takora

08 Lunatiq

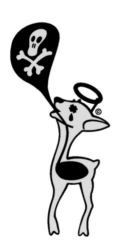

05 Lapin

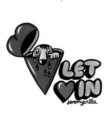

09 jeremyville

10 Rolitoland

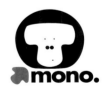

11 La Superagencia ®

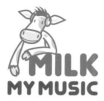

01 lindedesign

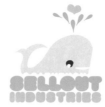

02 Tado

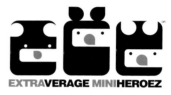

03 Sellout Industries

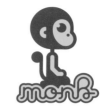

04 Lukatarina

05 Norwegian Ink

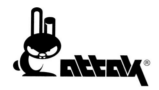

06 Attak

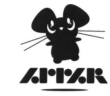

07 Attak

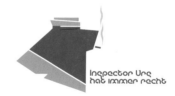

08 Karoly Kiralyfalvi

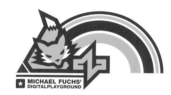

09 DigitalPlayground Studio

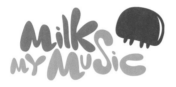

10 lindedesign

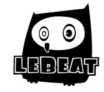

11 leBeat

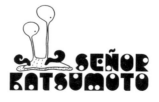

12 Attak

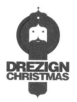

13 Karoly Kiralyfalvi

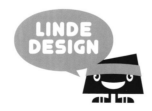

14 lindedesign

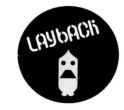

15 tapetentiere

16 Regina

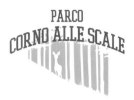

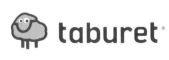

01 Axel Peemöller

02 AmorfoDesignlab™

03 Stockbridge International

04 Designbolaget

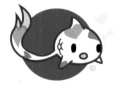

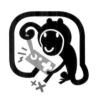

05 Tokidoki LLC

06 Fons Schiedon

07 Fons Schiedon

08 Fons Schiedon

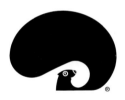

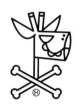

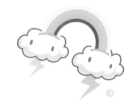

09 Tilt

10 Chris Hutchinson

11 Sellout Industries

12 Tokidoki LLC

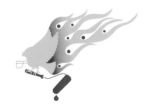

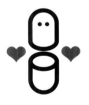

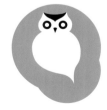

13 mateuniverse

14 BEK03

15 :g / studio-gpop

16 Chris Rubino

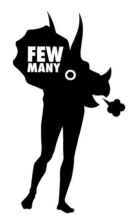

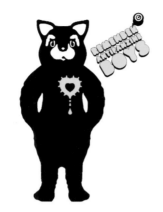

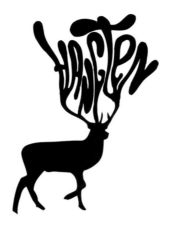

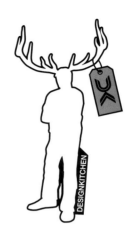

01 Cupco!   02 Lapin   03 Stockbridge International   04 Designkitchen

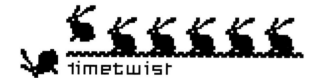

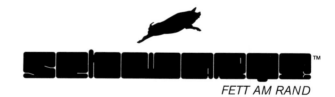

05 Felix Braden   06 Labor für visuelles Wachstum™

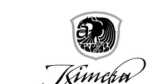

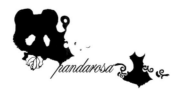

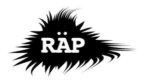

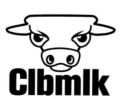

07 Kimera   08 Pandarosa   09 44 flavours   10 hijack graphics

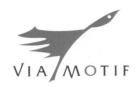

01 Vrontikis Design Office

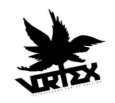

02 Karoly Kiralyfalvi

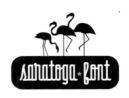

03 Dr. Alderete

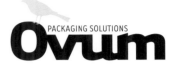

04 Cuartopiso

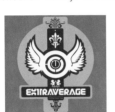

05 Karoly Kiralyfalvi

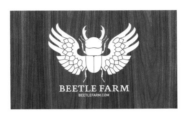

06 Cuban Council

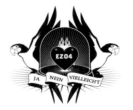

07 redaktion »echtzeit«

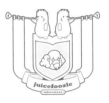

08 DigitalPlayground Studio

09 Cassie Leedham

10 Kanardo

11 bianca strauch

12 Nando Costa

13 Norwegian Ink

14 Fase

15 Karoly Kiralyfalvi

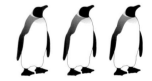

16 Shintaro Yarimizo

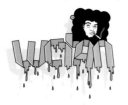

01 Lucias Westrup

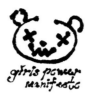

02 Furi Furi Company

03 Jon Burgerman

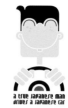

04 Attak

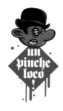

05 Escobas

06 Raffaele Primitivo

07 Gastón Caba

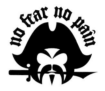

08 Attak

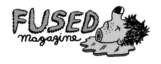

09 jeremyville

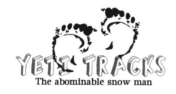

10 Gianni Rossi

11 Yo Freeman

12 Shivamat

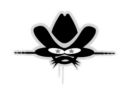

13 Fritz Torres

14 Dr. Morbito & 1000Changos

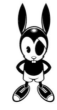

15 Carsten Raffel

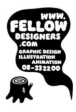

16 Fellow Designers

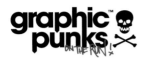

01 viagrafik

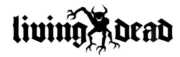

02 Jun Watanabe

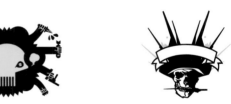

03 Cherrybox Studios

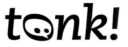

04 mateuniverse

05 Ashi & office Greminger

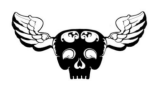

06 Atomic Attack

07 Norwegian Ink

08 Lapin

09 Jun Watanabe

10 No-Domain

11 Dr. Morbito & 1000Changos

12 DigitalPlayground Studio

13 Shivamat

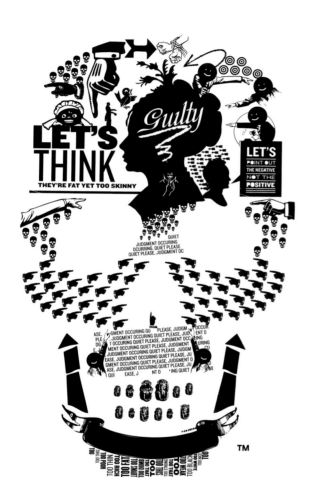

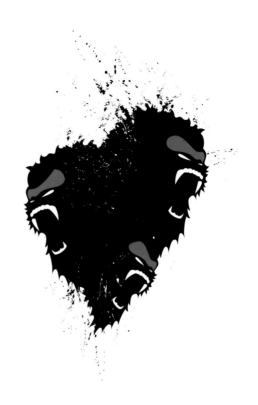

01 iaah

02 Attak

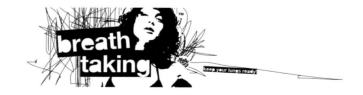

03 viagrafik

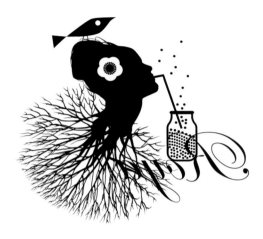

01 Roya Hamburger

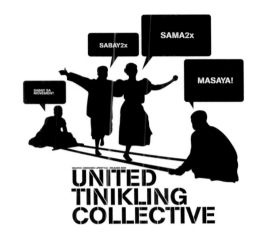

02 Team Manila

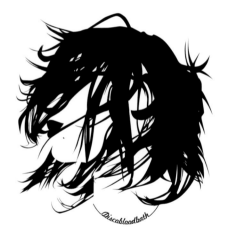

03 Nathan Jobe

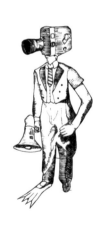

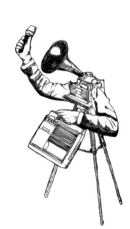

04 No-Domain   05 No-Domain

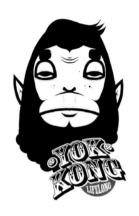

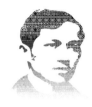

02 Team Manila

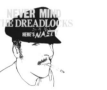

03 Yo Freeman

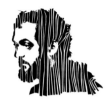

04 Nathan Jobe

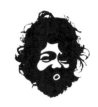

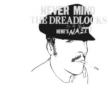

06 HKI - Hellohikimori

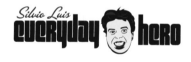

07 Zinc

01 YOK

05 Attak

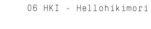

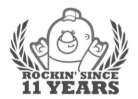

08 Masa

09 Clrqa

10 Yo Freeman

11 Caótica

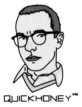

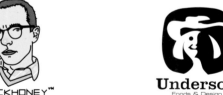

12 QuickHoney

13 underson

14 Emil Hartvig

15 DigitalPlayground Studio

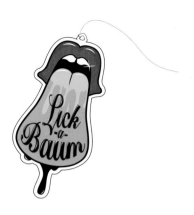

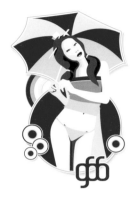

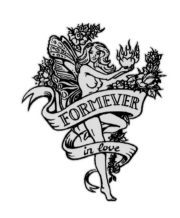

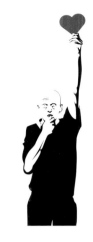

01 Norwegian Ink

02 2Advanced Studios

03 Formgeber

04 Attak

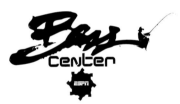

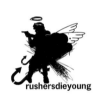

05 iaah

06 Kosta Lazarevski / rdy

07 Cupco!

08 BEK03

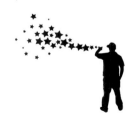

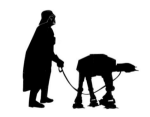

09 hijack graphics

10 Magma

11 Sellout Industries

12 Plastic Kid

01 Sensus Design Factory

02 Sensus Design Factory

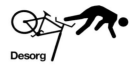

03 Shintaro Yarimizo

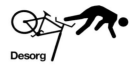

04 Flavio Bagioli

05 kw43

06 44 flavours

07 Shivamat

08 iaah

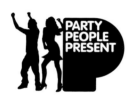

09 Crush Design

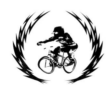

10 Nathan Jobe

11 Matthias Gephart

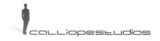

12 Calliope Studios

13 Dennis Eriksson

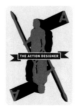

14 actiondesigner

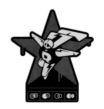

15 Shivamat

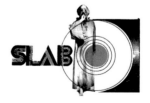

16 Insect

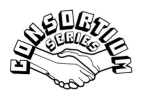

01 Nathan Jobe

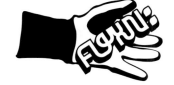

02 Flexn / BANK™

03 Dr. Alderete

04 Masa

05 Mikkel Grafixico Westrup

06 underson

07 Hula Hula

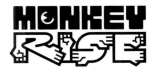

08 Furi Furi Company

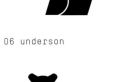

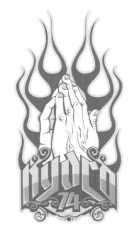

09 Hydro74

10 Lapin

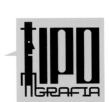

11 Dr. Alderete

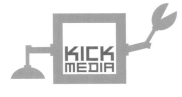

12 Braveland Design

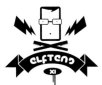

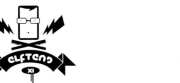

13 I&Eye

14 kw43

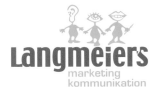

15 Felix Braden

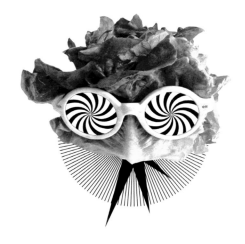

01 Tohyto

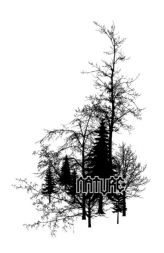

02 Karoly Kiralyfalvi

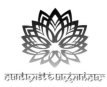

03 usugrow

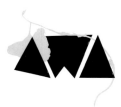

04 Nuuro

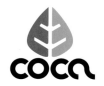

05 Keloide.net

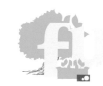

06 Christian Rothenhagen

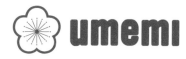

07 Fupete Studio

08 onrushdesign

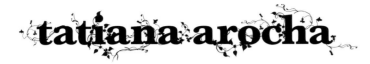

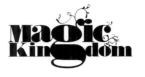

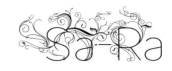

01 Tatiana Arocha

02 Deanne Cheuk

03 Deanne Cheuk

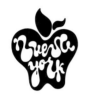

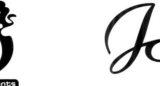

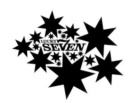

04 Razauno

05 Extraverage Productions

06 Coutworks

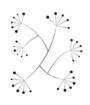

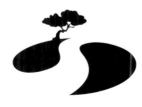

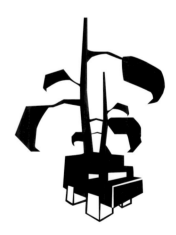

07 Salon Vektoria

08 Felix Braden

09 Norwegian Ink

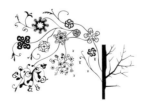

10 Blink Blink

11 Blu Design

12 Resin[sistem] design

13 Keloide.net

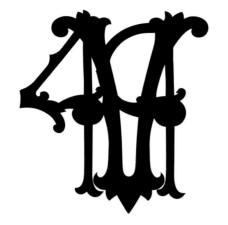

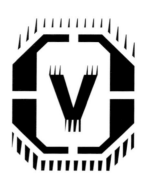

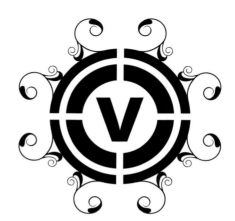

01 Vault49

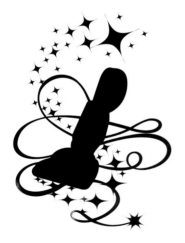

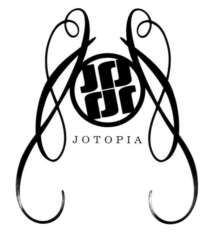

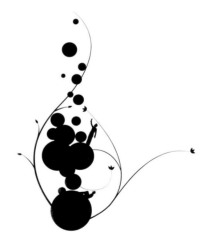

02 redaktion »echtzeit«   03 Formgeber   04 ROM studio

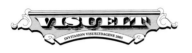

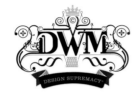

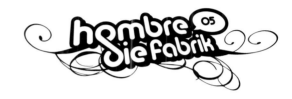

01 Skin Design

02 AmorfoDesignlab™

03 DigitalPlayground Studio

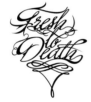

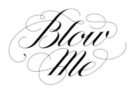

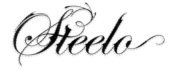

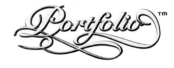

04 Hydro74

05 radargraphics

06 Hydro74

07 Labor f. visuelles Wachstum™

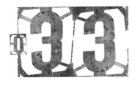

08 FL@33

09 Out Of Order

10 Cape Arcona Typefoundry

11 Niels Shoe Meulman

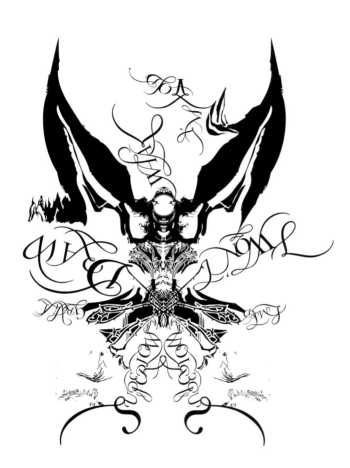

02 Sarah Grimaldi

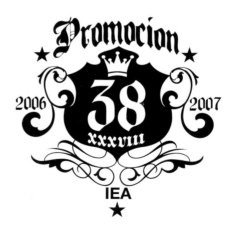

01 Superlow

03 BEK03

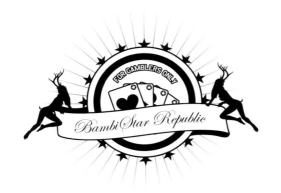

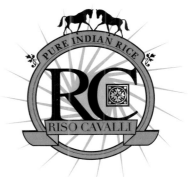

01 Sarah Grimaldi

02 Designkitchen

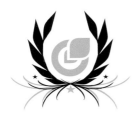

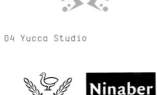

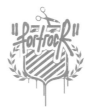

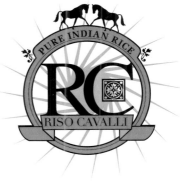

03 Dimomedia Lab

04 Yucca Studio

05 Karoly Kiralyfalvi

06 Tsutomu Umezawa

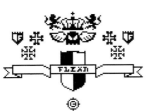

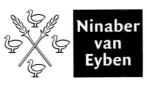

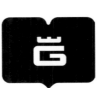

07 Flexn

08 Otherways 5th Floor Studio

09 Labor f. visuelles Wachstum™

10 Microbot David Fuhrer

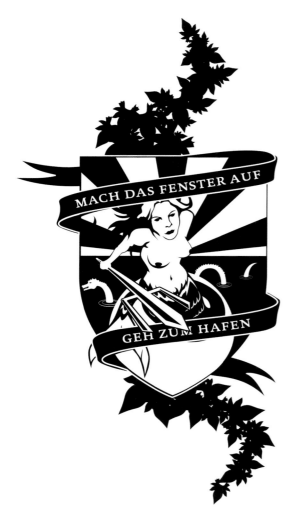

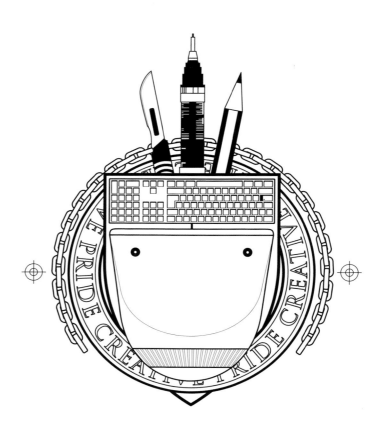

01 redaktion »echtzeit«

02 Creative Pride

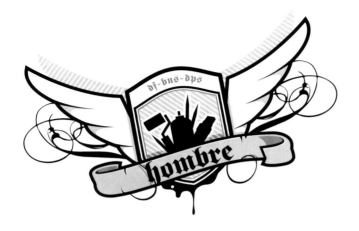

01 DigitalPlayground Studio

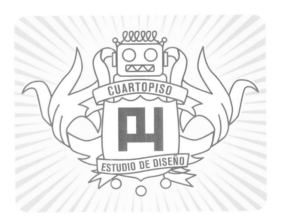

02 DigitalPlayground Studio

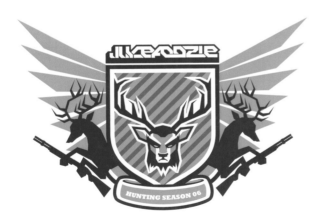

03 DigitalPlayground Studio

04 Cuartopiso

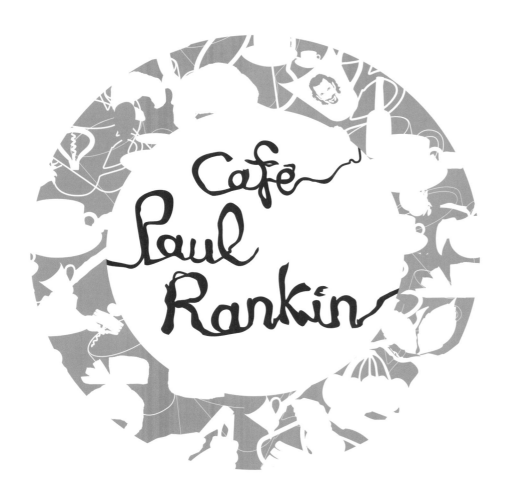

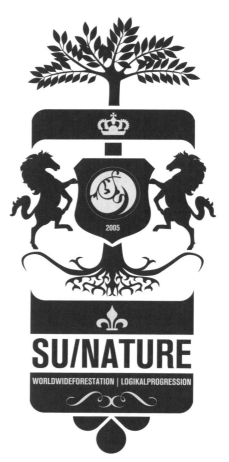

01 Peter Anderson

02 Karoly Kiralyfalvi

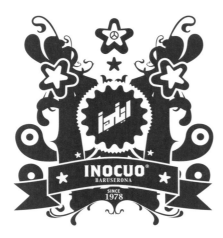

01 Inocuodesign

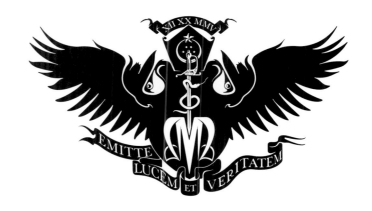

02 Nando Costa

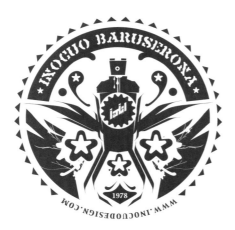

03 Inocuodesign

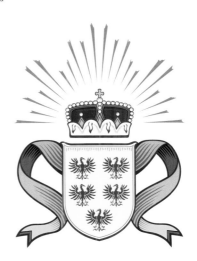

04 Instant

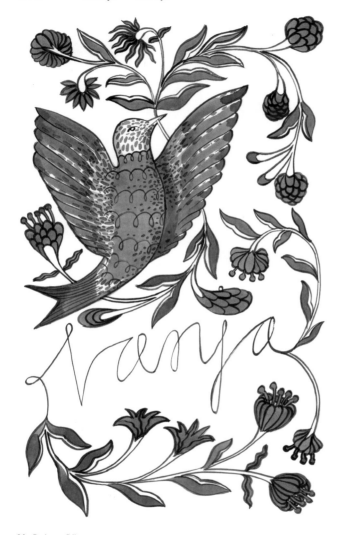

01 Petra Börner

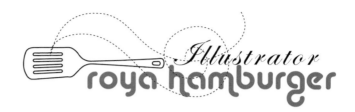

02 Roya Hamburger

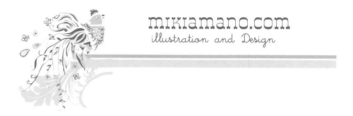

03 Miki Amano

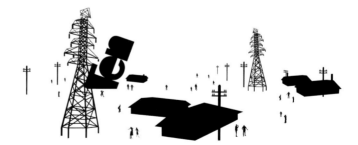

04 Joe A. Scerri

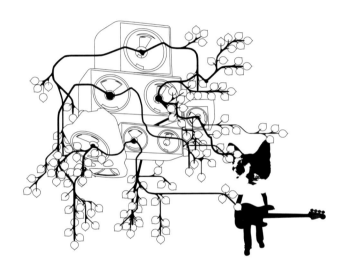

01 Molho

02 Formgeber

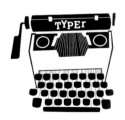

03 Ashi & office Greminger

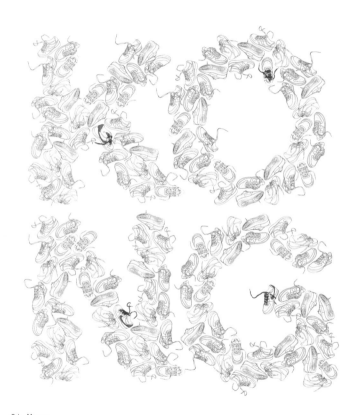

04 Masa

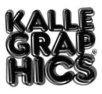

01 Kallegraphics

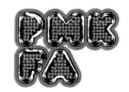

02 PMKFA

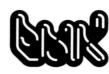

03 PMKFA

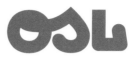

04 Oscar Salinas Losada

05 JDK

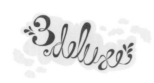

06 3 deluxe

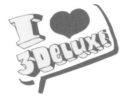

07 3 deluxe

08 Sellout Industries

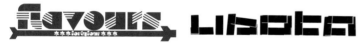

09 44 flavours

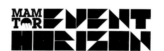

10 Carsten Raffel

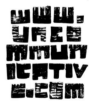

11 Muller

12 Jawa and Midwich

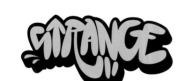

13 Karoly Kiralyfalvi

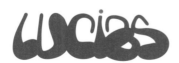

14 Lucias Westrup

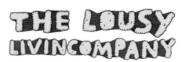

15 Lousy Livincompany

16 Adam Cruickshank

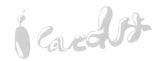

01 Fons Schiedon

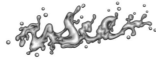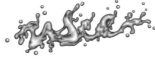

02 The Skull Dezain

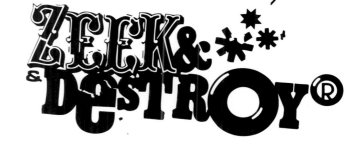

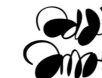

03 Fons Schiedon

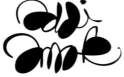

04 Oc/Om/Oy/Ok

05 Zeek&Destroy

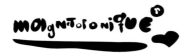

06 Magnetofonica

07 Parra

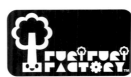

08 Furi Furi Company

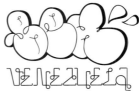

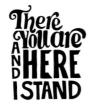

09 Parra

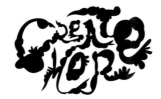

10 I-Manifest

11 BEKO3

12 Mikkel Grafixico Westrup

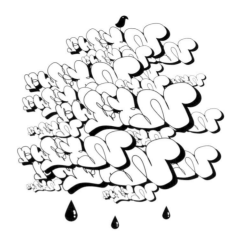

02 Flexn / BANK™

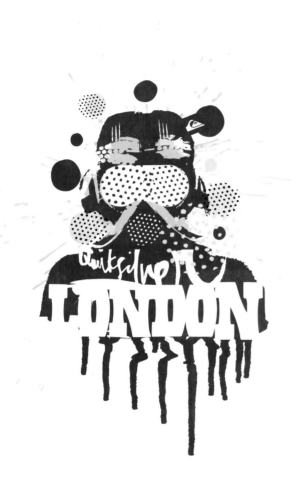

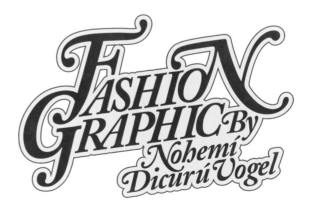

01 Insect Design

03 Nohemi Dicuru-fashiongraphic

01 :g / studio-gpop

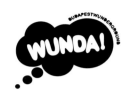

02 Extraverage Productions

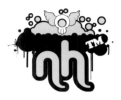

03 Koadzn

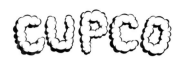

04 Cupco!

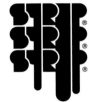

05 Syrup Helsinki

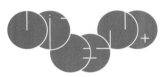

06 Amseldrossel

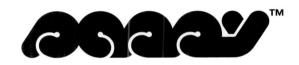

07 viagrafik

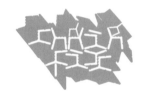

08 Studio Oscar

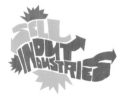

09 Norwegian Ink

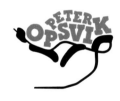

10 Sellout Industries

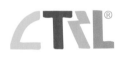

11 Yo Freeman

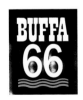

12 Yo Freeman

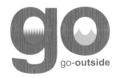

13 YellowToothpick

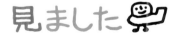

14 Akinori Oishi

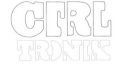

15 Yo Freeman

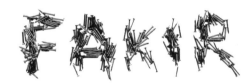

01 Fakir

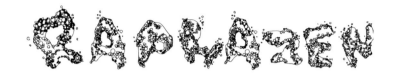

02 Raphazen

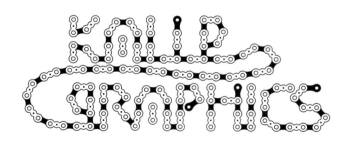

03 Kallegraphics

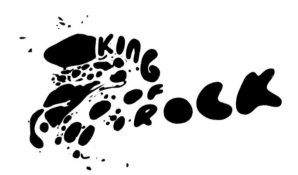

04 Deanne Cheuk

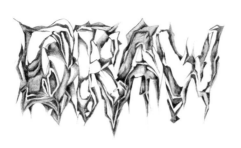

01 Superlow

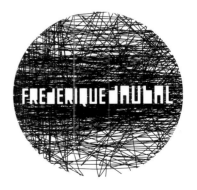

02 Cybu Richli

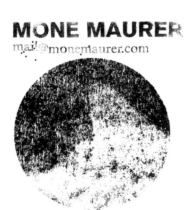

03 Mone Maurer

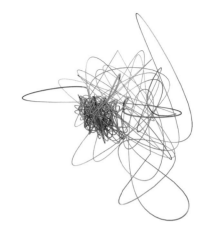

04 Frederique Daubal

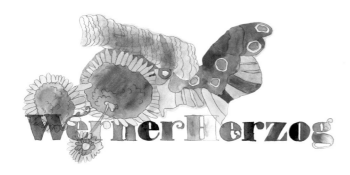

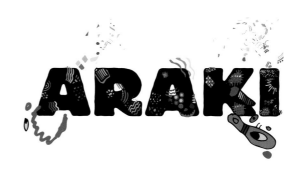

01 Deanne Cheuk

02 Deanne Cheuk

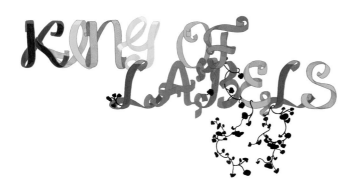

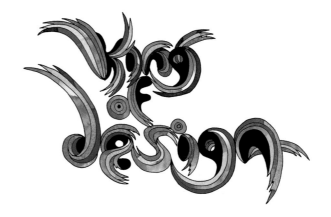

03 Deanne Cheuk

04 Deanne Cheuk

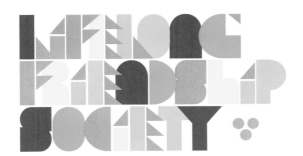

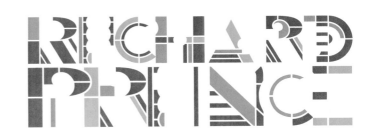

01 lifelong friendship society

02 Deanne Cheuk

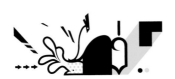

03 Miha Artnak

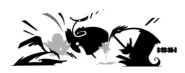

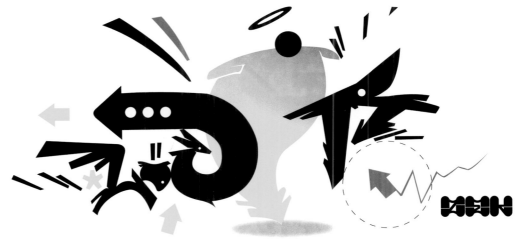

04 Miha Artnak

05 Miha Artnak

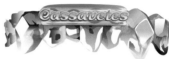

02 Laundry

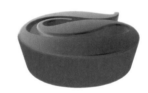

03 Tilt

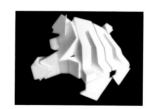

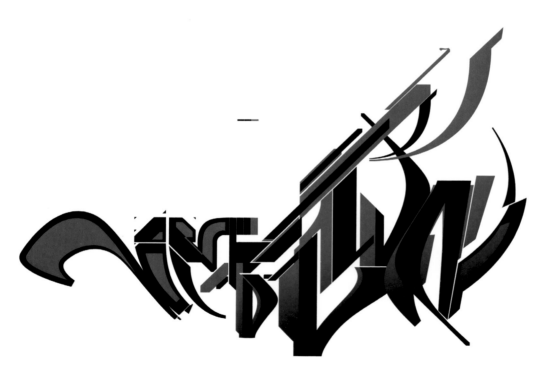

01 Inocuodesign

04 BEKO3

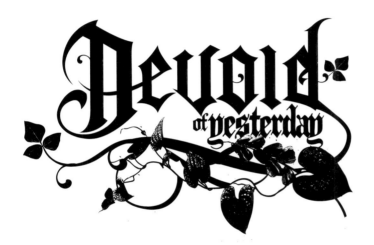

01 Hydro74

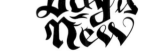

02 Carsten Raffel

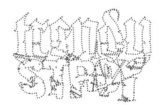

03 dzgnbio

04 I-Manifest

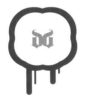

05 dzgnbio

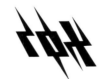

06 Extraverage Productions

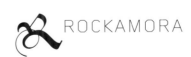

07 3 deluxe

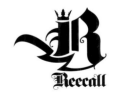

08 Hydro74

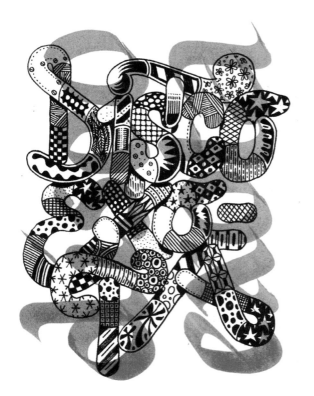

01 Unit c.m.a.

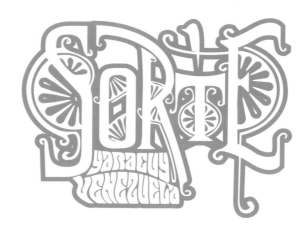

02 Keloide.net

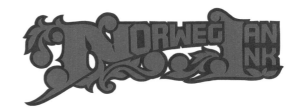

03 WGD

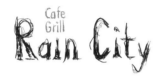

01 Peter Anderson

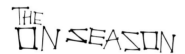

02 The Vacuum Design

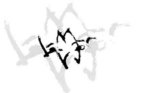

04 Leon Vymenets

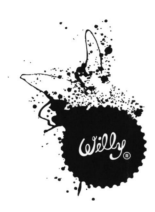

03 William Morrisey

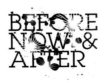

05 I-Manifest

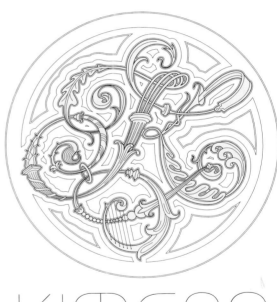

06 Kimera

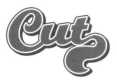 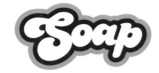 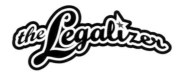 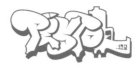

01 Instant

02 Sesame Studio

03 the Legalizer ApS

04 Mikkel Grafixico Westrup

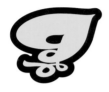 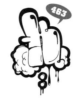

05 the Legalizer ApS

06 Slang

07 Matthias Gephart

08 Keloide.net

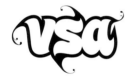 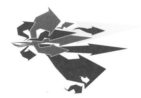 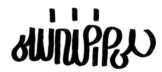

09 Keep Left Studio

10 Resin[sistem] design

11 Resin[sistem] design

12 ehquestionmark

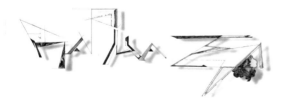 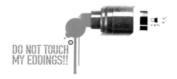 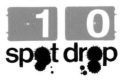

13 Raphazen

14 Lapin

15 surround

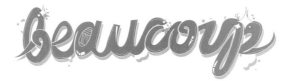

01 Laundry

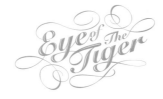

02 Norwegian Ink

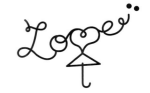

03 Takora

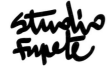

04 Underware

05 Underware

06 Jun Watanabe

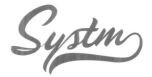

07 Analog.Systm

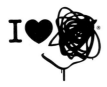

08 Fupete Studio

09 Zeek&Destroy

10 Mattisimo

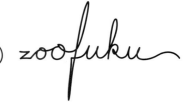

11 lindedesign

12 Plastic Kid

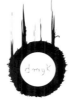

13 Kosta Lazarevski / rdy

14 christian walden

15 Supermundane

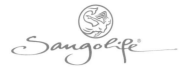

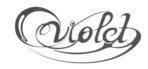

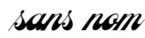

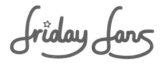

01 Felix Braden

02 Nando Costa

03 Studio Sans Nom

04 onrushdesign / front

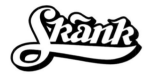

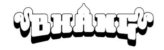

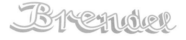

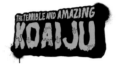

05 inkgraphix

06 Crush Design

07 Büro Brendel

08 Koadzn

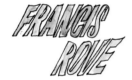

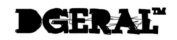

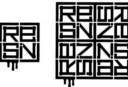

09 Dennis Eriksson

10 Neasden Control Centre

11 Nuuro

12 Resin[sistem] design

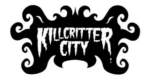

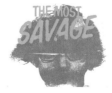

13 Kallegraphics

14 Digart Graphics

15 Zion Graphics

16 Yo Freeman

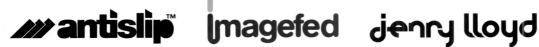

01 viagrafik

02 Ninjacruise

03 Keep Left Studio

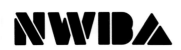

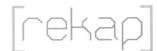

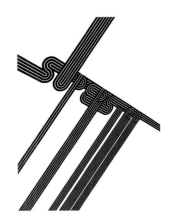

04 Adapter

05 SignalStrong

06 dzgnbio

07 boris dworschak

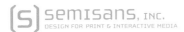

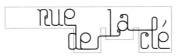

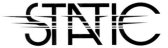

08 Semisans

09 Abraka design

10 29 degres

11 Hydro74

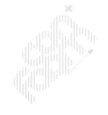

12 Hydro74

13 Attaboy

14 cubemen studio

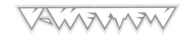

15 Axel Peemöller

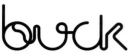

01 Hayato Kamono

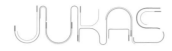

02 Mikkel Grafixico Westrup

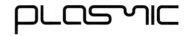

03 Flink

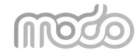

04 projekttriangle

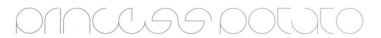

05 Raffaele Primitivo

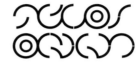

07 0c/0m/0y/0k

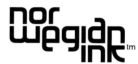

08 modo

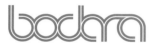

09 Bodara, Büro für Ge-

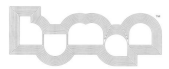

10 viagrafik

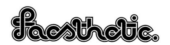

11 Supermundane

12 Norwegian Ink

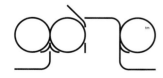

13 SignalStrong

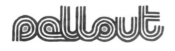

14 Sellout Industries

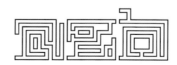

15 Zetuei Fonts

16 june

01 Magnetofonica

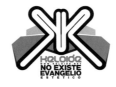

02 Magnetofonica

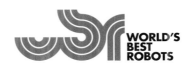

03 Muller

04 paulroberts.tv

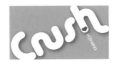

05 Bionyc Industries

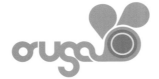

06 Clrqa

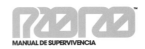

07 Clrqa

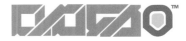

08 Clrqa

09 Mode

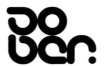

10 Joe A. Scerri

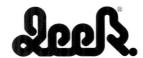

11 Zeek&Destroy

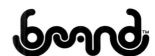

12 AmorfoDesignlab™

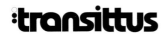

13 Transittus

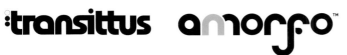

14 AmorfoDesignlab™

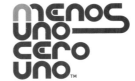

15 AmorfoDesignlab™

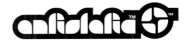

16 viagrafik

kahle,

01 310k

Made.

02 Made

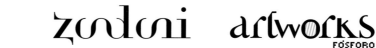

03 Hydro74

CIVILIANAIRE

04 The KDU

camilaarocha

05 Tatiana Arocha

zurdoni

06 Salon Vektoria

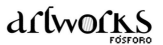

07 FÓSFORO

KONTRAPUNKT

08 Kontrapunkt

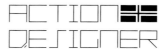

09 actiondesigner

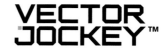

10 Accident Grotesk!

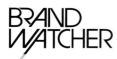

11 Rocholl Selected Designs

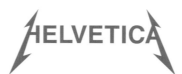

12 Attak

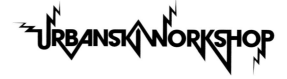

13 Urbanskiworkshop

: schoninghwulffraat

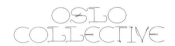

OSLO COLLECTIVE

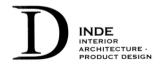

01 Julie Joliat

02 Typosition

03 Superlow

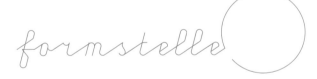

krvkurva

04 Amen

05 Krv Kurva

06 Rocholl Selected Designs

simian™

dvi-hdtv®

DRELLA

D INDE
INTERIOR
ARCHITECTURE ·
PRODUCT DESIGN

07 Simian

08 june

09 Sunday-Vision

10 derek johnson

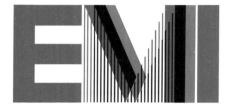

15 Emmi Salonen

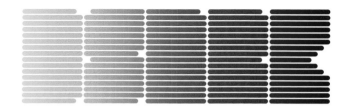

16 Designanorak / DSNRK

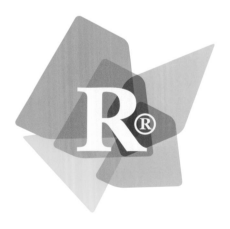

13 Insect

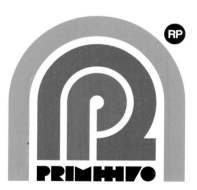

11 Raffaele Primitivo

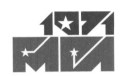

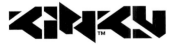

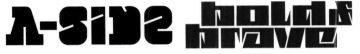

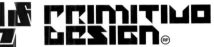

01 Raffaele Primitivo

02 A-Side Studio

03 Attak

04 Raffaele Primitivo

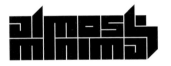

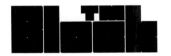

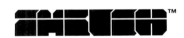

05 Mitch Paone

06 Neubau.

07 Ketchup Arts

08 viagrafik

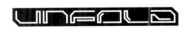

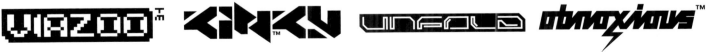

09 viagrafik

10 viagrafik

11 viagrafik

12 viagrafik

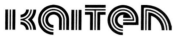

01 Sito

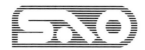

02 Sito

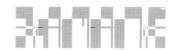

03 SignalStrong

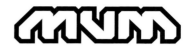

04 MvM / Maarten van Maanen

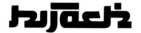

05 hijack graphics

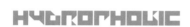

06 Raffaele Primitivo

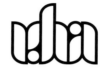

07 Emil Hartvig

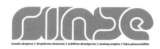

08 Extraverage Productions

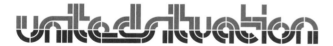

09 Plasticbag

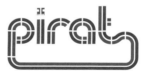

10 mateuniverse

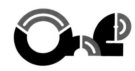

11 Sat One

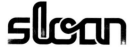

12 Mark Sloan

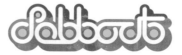

13 Sellout Industries

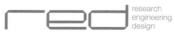

14 projekttriangle

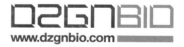

15 dzgnbio

Design   Design

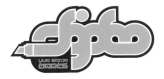

01 Clrqa

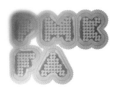

02 PMKFA

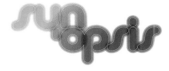

03 Mode

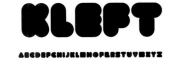

04 Keep Left Studio

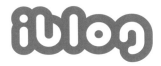

05 fireondesign / herborize

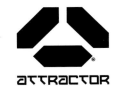

06 2Advanced Studios

07 Out Of Order

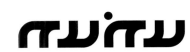

08 NYK

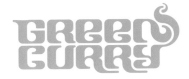

09 Salon Vektoria

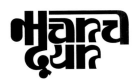

10 HandGun

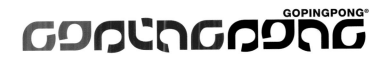

11 the Legalizer ApS

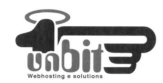

01 Nuuro

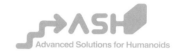

02 Dimomedia Lab

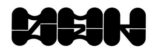

03 Miha Artnak

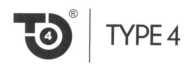

04 Ash

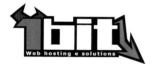

05 Dimomedia Lab

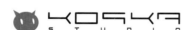
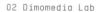

06 NYK

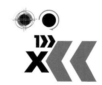

07 La Superagencia ®

08 Tabas

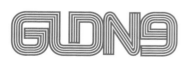

09 Mikkel Grafixico Westrup

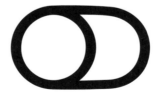

10 NYK

11 moxi

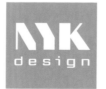

12 Toko

01 Keep Left Studio

02 SignalStrong

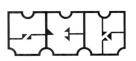

03 Miha Artnak

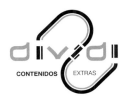

04 Keloide.net

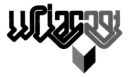

05 Lucias Westrup

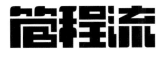

06 Furi Furi Company

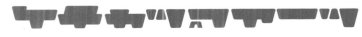

07 Ketchup Arts

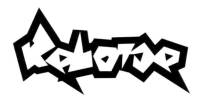

08 Keloide.net

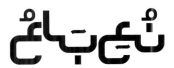

09 Mule Industry

10 Mattisimo

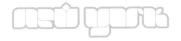

11 Axel Peemöller

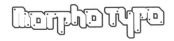

12 Keloide.net

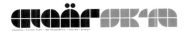

13 Karoly Kiralyfalvi

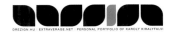

14 Karoly Kiralyfalvi

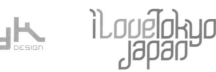

01 NYK

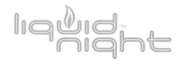

02 Hayato Kamono

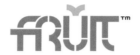

03 viagrafik

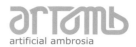

04 DigitalPlayground Studio

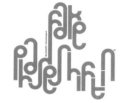

05 Karoly Kiralyfalvi

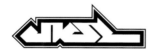

06 Karoly Kiralyfalvi

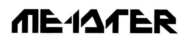

07 Labor f. visuelles Wachstum

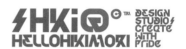

08 HKI - Hellohikimori

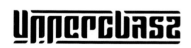

09 I&EYE

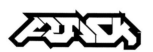

10 I&EYE

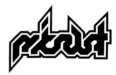

11 3volt Design

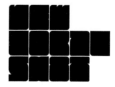

12 Microbot David Fuhrer

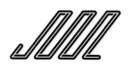

13 Floor Wesseling Ix Opus

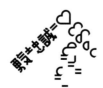

14 jum

15 SignalStrong

16 Jan-Kristof Lipp

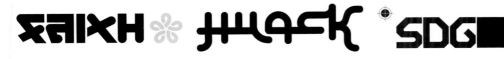

01 Faith

02 hijack graphics

03 La Superagencia ®

04 Flexn / BANK™

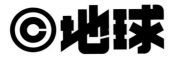

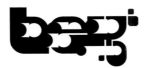

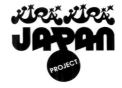

05 Furi Furi Company

06 BEK03

07 Takora

08 hijack graphics

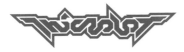

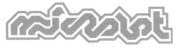

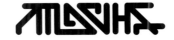

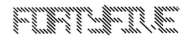

09 Microbot David Fuhrer

10 Microbot David Fuhrer

11 hijack graphics

12 SignalStrong

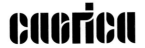

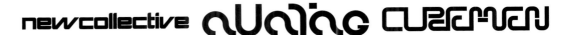

13 Caótica

14 Coutworks

15 cubemen studio

16 cubemen studio

01 asmallpercent

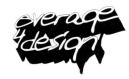

02 Tender

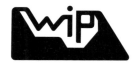

03 HKI - Hellohikimori

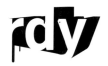

04 Kosta Lazarevski / rdy

05 Intercity

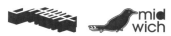

06 Jawa and Midwich

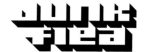

07 Yucca Studio

08 Keloide.net

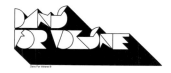

09 Grandpeople

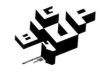

10 Karoly Kiralyfalvi

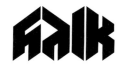

11 Jun Watanabe

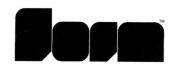

12 Neubau.

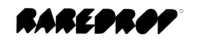

13 Raredrop

14 Maak

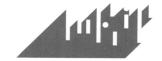

15 Miha Artnak

16 Studio Oscar

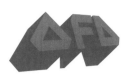

01 HKI - Hellohikimori

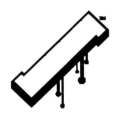

02 viagrafik

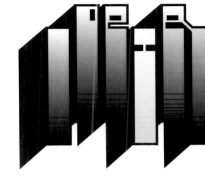

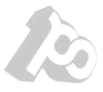

03 Keloide.net

04 Station

05 Miha Artnak

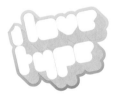

06 Designanorak / DSNRK

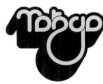

07 Extraverage Productions

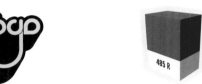

08 Axel Peemöller

09 Resin[sistem] design

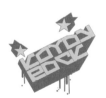

10 cisma

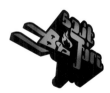

11 Escobas

12 Shivamat

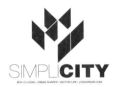

13 Karoly Kiralyfalvi

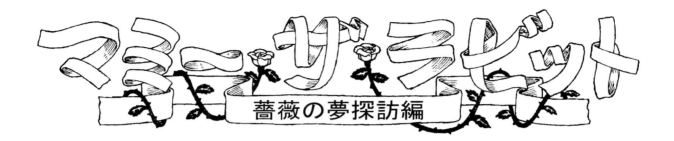

01 Furi Furi Company

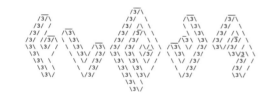

02 FL@33

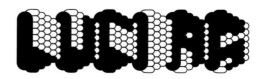

03 Erik Jarlsson

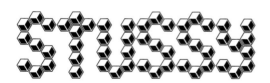

04 Studio Oscar

05 Lucias Westrup

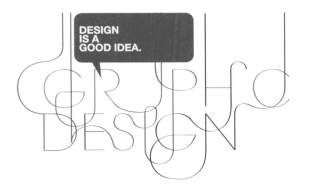

01 Team Manila

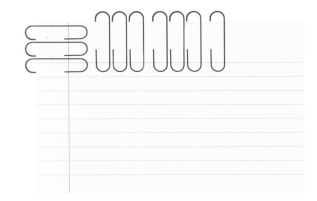

02 Emmi Salonen

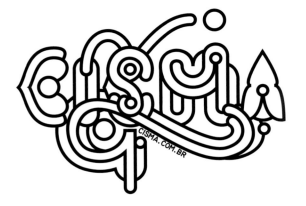

03 cisma

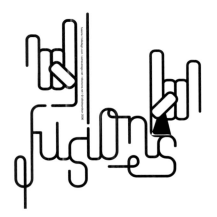

04 Extraverage Productions

01 Mitch Paone

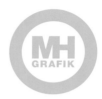

02 Ketchup Arts

03 Kallegraphics

04 MH grafik

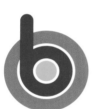

05 Yuu Imokawa

06 Attak

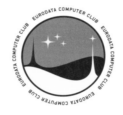

07 Retron / Richard Øiestad

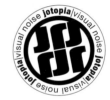

08 Attak

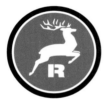

09 Resin[sistem] design

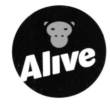

10 Lindedesign

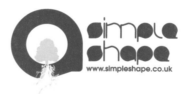

11 Jawa and Midwich

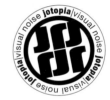

12 Formgeber

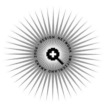

13 David Clavadetscher

14 Dimomedia Lab

15 Ashi & office Greminger

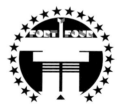

16 44 flavours

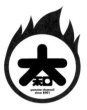

01 Shintaro Yarimizo

02 Shintaro Yarimizo

03 Shintaro Yarimizo

04 Shintaro Yarimizo

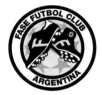

05 Fase

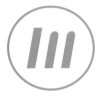

06 Shintaro Yarimizo

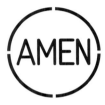

07 Amen

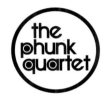

08 :phunk studio

09 FireGirl

10 resistro®

11 Positron

12 David Maloney

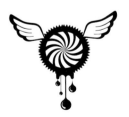

13 Tohyto

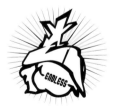

14 Matthias Gephart

15 Laborator

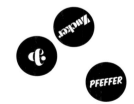

16 zucker und pfeffer

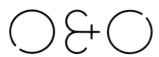

01 e-Types A/S

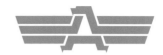

02 44 flavours

03 Mattisimo

04 Attak

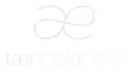

05 Jawa and Midwich

06 Accident Grotesk!

07 The KDU

08 Karoly Kiralyfalvi

09 Georg Schatz

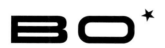

10 Borsellino & Co.

11 Chris Rubino

12 Braveland Design

13 Mwmcreative

14 Chris Rubino

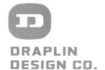

15 Draplin

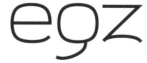

16 Simian

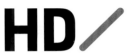

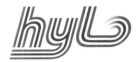

01 Hyl Design

02 Chris Rubino

03 Hyl Design

04 Hyl Design

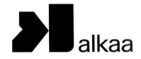

05 jl-prozess

06 Pep Karsten

07 fatbob

08 Ketchup Arts

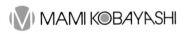

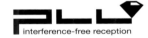

09 Coldwater Graphiix

10 Maniackers Design

11 june

12 june

13 2098

14 Sesame Studio

15 Sesame Studio

16 Transittus

01 Fellow Designers

02 Salon Vektoria

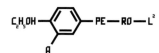

03 Salon Vektoria

04 Salon Vektoria

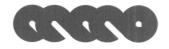

05 44 flavours

06 Attak

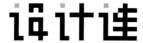

07 archetype : interactive

08 SignalStrong

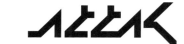

09 Mattisimo

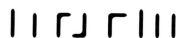

10 Attak

11 selanra grafikdesign

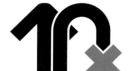

12 Typosition

13 Chris Rubino

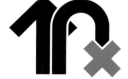

14 La Superagencia ®

15 toxi

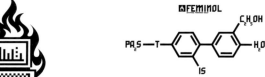

16 Mattisimo

01 Nando Costa

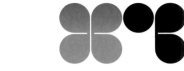

02 :g / studio-gpop

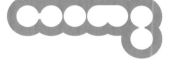

03 Axel Peemöller

04 NYK

05 2Advanced Studios

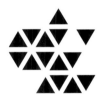

06 Tnop™ & ®bePOS|+|VE

07 Furi Furi Company

08 2Advanced Studios

09 Superfamous

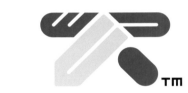

10 Shintaro Yarimizo

11 decoylab

12 Zetuei Fonts

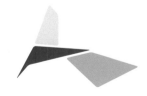

13 Tohyto

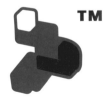

14 Tohyto

15 Engine

16 Maak

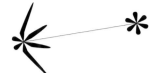

02 dextro.org

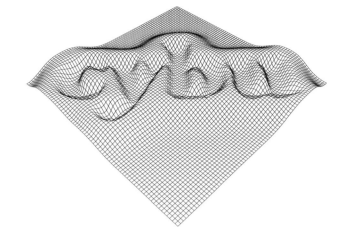

06 Cybu Richli

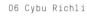

03 Shintaro Yarimizo

04 Shintaro Yarimizo

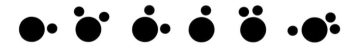

07 Lucias Westrup

05 Polygraph

08 cisma

01 Raphazen

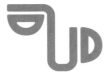

01 eP_ design in progress

02 Ketchup Arts

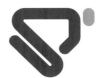

03 dzgnbio

04 Blu Design

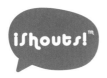

05 Jun Xu

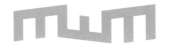

06 Mwmcreative

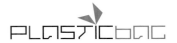

07 Muller

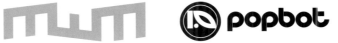

08 Plasticbag

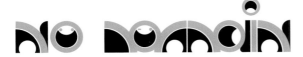

09 No-Domain

10 decoylab

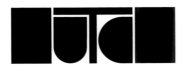

11 Chris Hutchinson

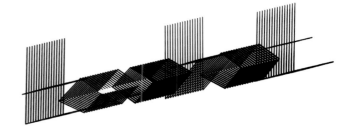

12 Danny Franzreb

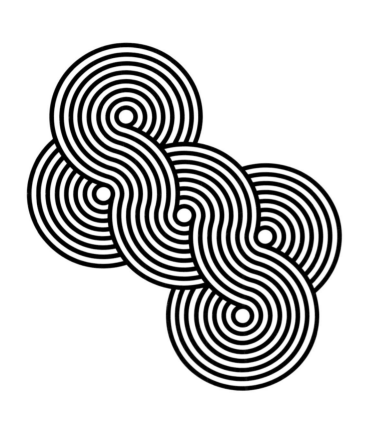

01 Tohyto

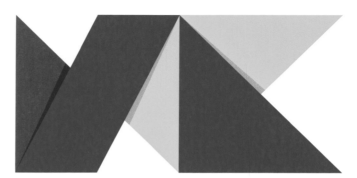

02 Nando Costa

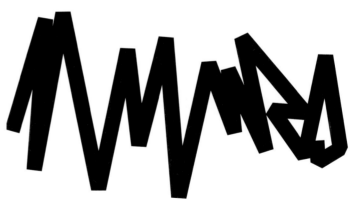

03 Nuuro

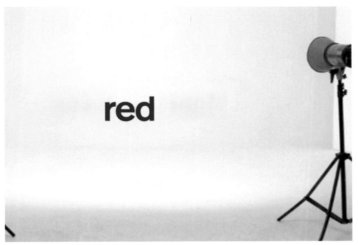

01 red design

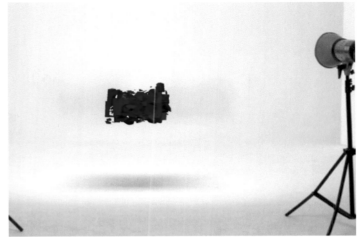

02 red design

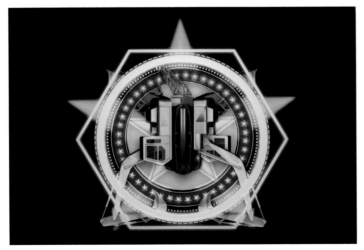

04 BEK03

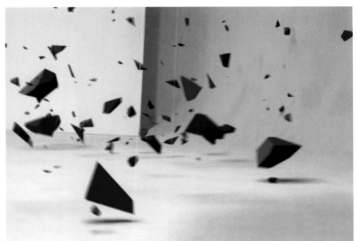

03 red design

FASHION

DAVID AND GOLIATH

When it comes to their trademarks, successful high fashion labels exercise restraint. Their strategies incorporate seductive messages conveyed by lascivious models. But the logo? Please don't touch! Things are different with the young wild ones. Unafraid to take chances, they allow to explode in a veritable orgy of images. But not without strategic calculations: when the marketing budget does not stretch to a double spread in VOGUE or ELLE, the logo has to do more work. The keyword is attention-getting value.

SIMPLICITY VERSUS COMPLEXITY

Fast food, but rich trimmings.

German philosopher Peter Sloterdijk commented in the magazine FOCUS[1]: "To begin with, more communication primarily means more conflict." This thesis could help to explain another phenomenon that is revealed by the analysis of the new symbols: a weakening of the meta level and decline in abstraction. There is less interpretation. Everything is simply the way it is, just as it presents itself - and just as it is expected to be. But if things are really that simple, then the intellectual challenge of deciphering images is defused, and discussions of content become trivial - and conflict is thereby avoided. (Cf. Sloterdijk.) At the same time, however, the complexity of the logo increases at an almost disproportionate degree: its total content, its concentrated charge of information, becomes visible on a surface that conceals far less.

1.   FOCUS 10, 2006

REDFERN, AUSTRALIA
LUCA IONESCU

Street Art inspires the symbols.

Designer Luca Ionescu sees exciting prospects in the exploration of different scenes. "Crossover" is among his favourite words. "There are some great illustrators and typographers coming up from a purely street art background, having crossed over from spraying to hand illustration and logo work. Although they were already illustrating beforehand, it is now more accessible to artists who share their work through blogs, etc. So I think there is a great creative environment at the moment which inspires me to create."

Since his youth, Luca has drawn his inspiration from the most diverse sources. He was fortunate enough to be raised by a grandmother who was a great film buff: she would pick Luca up from school and take him directly to the movies. "That period in my life exposed me to lots of movie titles and different genres, and I think that has taught me a lot about colour use, and what style of type should go with what mood or piece."

Then came the period of academy training. Luca discovered tradition. He immersed himself in the works of internationally-known designers like Müller-Brockmann, Paul Rand, Yusaku Kamekura, Herb Lubalin, Seymour Chwast and Milton Glaser. He browsed old issues of Graphis, Modern Punlicity, One Zero. He studied old font catalogues. Luca drew inspiration from this fund, just as he did from the works of contemporary designers. Crossover.

In his own projects, Luca likes to experiment. For him, this means expeditions into new realms. Upon his return, his designs resonate with all the things he has experienced along the way. Occasionally, clients are sceptical of innovative solutions. Why change things when the familiar is already working so well? The blade cuts two ways: you have to avoid letting your work become repetitive, says Luca, and you have to fulfil the customer's brief while persuading him of the desirability of setting new accents.

And it really works: "For example, I was recently invited to re-brand Nike Air Flight, Force and Uptempo. The commission was to look at the existing logos produced earlier and take them further. Create the new generation of logos to carry the 'Nike Silos" (Nike's designation for various types of sub-brands) into the near future. So I started by studying the current designs, then developed a more streamlined and minimalist design to help propel the Silos into the future and appeal to a new generation of athletes and buyers, and to avoid alienating the older generation who are familiar with the brand. The logos will soon be released on shoes and related items."

MODE

DAVID UND GOLIATH

Die arrivierten Edelmodemarken üben sich in Zurückhaltung, wenn es um ihre Markenzeichen geht. Verführerische Kommunikation mit lasziven Models gehört zur Strategie. Aber das Logo? Please don't touch! Anders die jungen Wilden. Die lassen es knallen. Da explodieren die Zeichen in veritablen Bilderorgien. Nicht ohne strategisches Kalkül: Wenn das Budget (noch) keine Doppelseite im VOGUE oder in der ELLE erlaubt, muss das Logo mehr leisten. Stichwort Aufmerksamkeitswert.

EINFACHHEIT VERSUS KOMPLEXITÄT

Fastfood, aber reich garniert.

Peter Sloterdijk, der deutsche Philosoph, meinte kürzlich im Magazin FOCUS[1] „Mehr Kommunikation bedeutet zunächst einmal vor allem mehr Konflikte." Diese These könnte zur Erklärung eines weiteren Phänomens beitragen, das bei einer Analyse der neuen Zeichen deutlich wird: Schwächere Metaebene und sinkender Abstraktionsgrad. Interpretationen finden seltener statt. Alles ist, wie es ist: genau so wie es sich präsentiert - und es wird auch so antizipiert. Wenn aber alles so einfach ist, wird die mentale Herausforderung beim Dechiffrieren der Bilder entschärft, der Diskurs über Inhalte verharmlost - und damit der Konflikt vermieden. Siehe Sloterdijk. Parallel dazu nimmt jedoch die Komplexität der Logos fast überproportional zu: Der volle Gehalt, die geballte Ladung an Information zeigt sich an der Oberfläche, hinter der sich aber weniger verbirgt als auch schon.

1.   FOCUS 10, 2006

REDFERN, AUSTRALIEN
LUCA IONESCO

Street Art inspiriert die Zeichen.

Der Gestalter Luca Ionesco sieht in der Durchdringung verschiedener Szenen spannende Aspekte. Crossover gehört zu seinen Lieblingswörtern. „Es gibt einige große Illustratoren und Typografen mit reinem Street-Art-Background. Sie haben den Sprung vom Sprayer zur Illustration und zum Logodesign geschafft. Obwohl sie bereits vorher Illustrationen kreiert haben, ist der Zugang etwa durch Blogs für Gestalter und Künstler leichter geworden ... Im Moment existiert ein großes kreatives Environment, das mich zum Gestalten inspiriert."

Luca bezog seine Inspirationen seit jeher aus unterschiedlichen Quellen. Das fing in der Jugendzeit an. Er hatte das Glück, dass seine ihn aufziehende Großmutter eine große Filmliebhaberin war: Sie holte Luca von der Schule ab - und dann gingen sie ins Kino. „In dieser Zeit habe ich Bekanntschaft mit vielen Filmtiteln unterschiedlichster Genres gemacht. Ich denke, das hat mich einiges darüber gelehrt, wie man mit Farben umgeht und welcher Schriftstil mit welcher Stimmung und welcher Geschichte geht."

Dann kam die Ausbildungs- und Collegezeit. Luca entdeckte die Tradition. Er vertiefte sich in die Arbeiten internationaler Designer wie Müller-Brockmann, Paul Rand, Yusaku Kamekura, Herb Lubalin, Seymour Chwast, Milton Glasser. Er durchblätterte alte Nummern von Graphis, Modern Punlicity, One Zero. Er studierte alte Schriftenkataloge. Luca schöpft aus diesem Fundus ebenso seine Inspirationen wie aus den Arbeiten zeitgenössischer Designer. Crossover eben.

Bei eigenen Projekten experimentiert Luca gerne. Für ihn sind das Entdeckungsreisen in neue Räume. Wenn er zurückkommt, schwingt in seiner Gestaltung etwas mit von dem, was er in diesen Räumen gesehen hat. Kunden sind gelegentlich skeptisch gegenüber innovativen Lösungen. Sie fragen sich, warum groß etwas verändern, wenn wir mit dem Bestehenden gut gefahren sind. Das ist ein zweischneidiges Schwert: Du musst aufpassen, dass deine Arbeit nicht repetitiv wird, meint Luca, du musst das Briefing des Kunden erfüllen - ihn aber überzeugen, dass es richtig ist neue Akzente zu setzen.

Das funktioniert: „Kürzlich war ich eingeladen, Nike Air, Flight, Force und Uptempo zu re-branden. Das Briefing lautete, die existierenden Logos zu überprüfen und weiterzuentwickeln, um die ‚Nike Silos' (Nike-Bezeichnung für verschiedene Typen von Subbrands) zukunftskompatibel zu machen. Ich begann damit, das bestehende Design zu analysieren. Dann entwickelte ich ein mehr ‚stromlinienförmiges', minimalistisches Design, das helfen soll die Silos in die Zukunft zu katapultieren und eine neue Generation von Athleten und Konsumenten anzusprechen, ohne die alten Kunden der Marke zu entfremden. Die Logos kommen bald auf den Markt - appliziert auf Schuhe und andere Artikel."

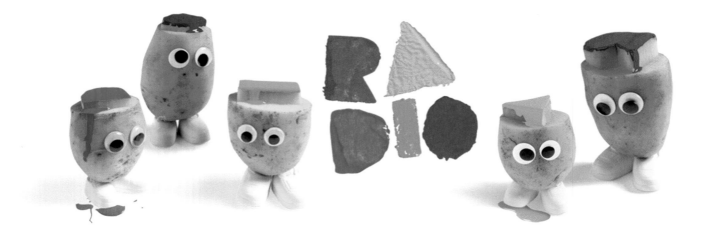

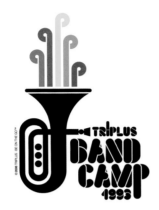

01 viagrafik

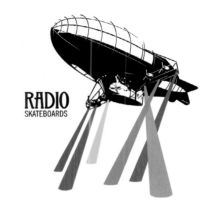

02 blackjune

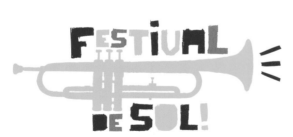

03 A-Side Studio

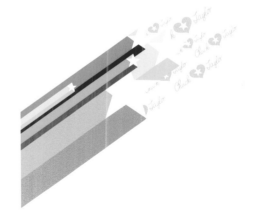

04 blackjune

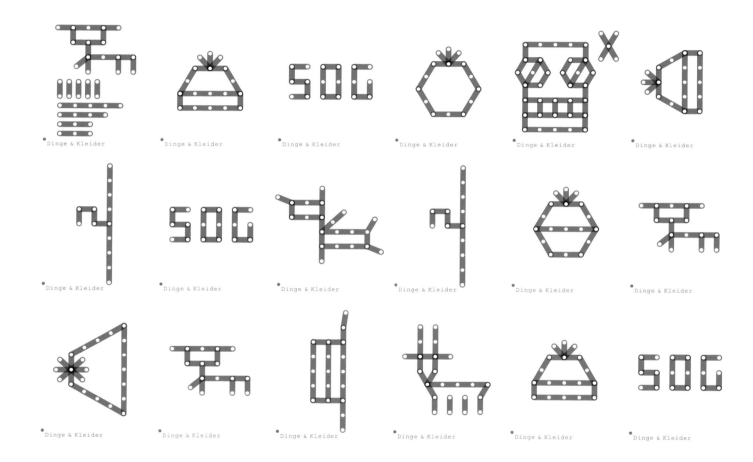

Dinge & Kleider

Dinge & Kleider

Dinge & Kleider

Dinge & Kleider

Dinge & Kleider

Dinge & Kleider

Dinge & Kleider

Dinge & Kleider

Dinge & Kleider

Dinge & Kleider

Dinge & Kleider

Dinge & Kleider

Dinge & Kleider

Dinge & Kleider

Dinge & Kleider

Dinge & Kleider

Dinge & Kleider

Dinge & Kleider

01 Theres Steiner

BBUILD

BBUILD

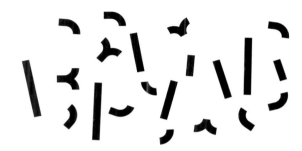

01 News

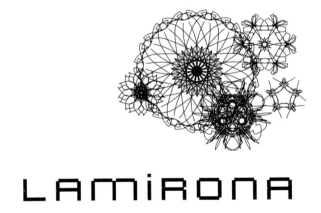

LAMIRONA

02 La Mirona

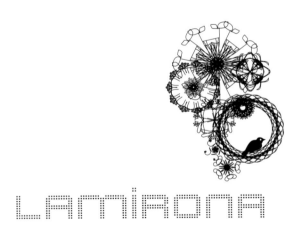

LAMIRONA

03 La Mirona

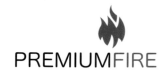

01 blackjune

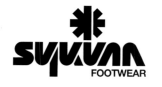

02 Kjetil Vatne

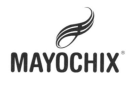

03 Karoly Kiralyfalvi

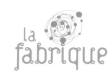

04 Abraka Design

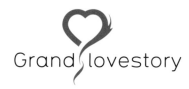

05 viagrafik

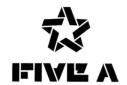

06 viagrafik

07 flat

08 The Skull Dezain

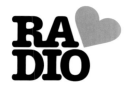

09 blackjune

10 GWG

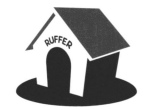

11 Visual Mind Rockets

12 Borsellino & Co.

01 Yuu Imokawa

02 Amore Hirosuke

03 asmallpercent

04 Vrontikis Design Office

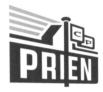

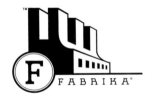

05 Axel Domke

06 Futro

07 Zion Graphics

08 KesselsKramer

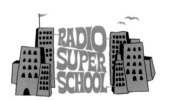

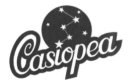

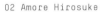

09 blackjune

10 Iván Solbes

11 artless Inc

12 Inksurge

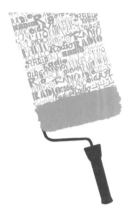

01 blackjune

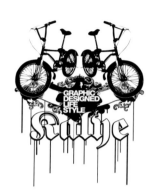

02 Team Manila

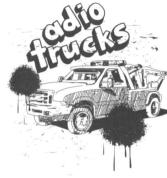

03 jeremyville

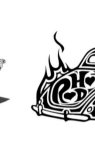

04 Studio Oscar

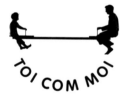

05 FL@33

06 Tsai-Fi

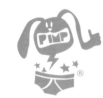

07 Raffaele Primitivo

08 Studio Oscar

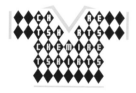

09 Fase

10 Neeser & Müller

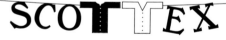

11 Miki Amano

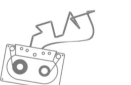

01 chemicalbox

02 tstout inc.

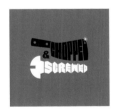

03 Christian Rothenhagen

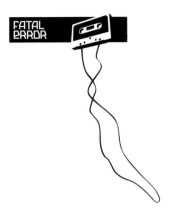

04 Raffaele Primitivo

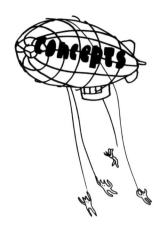

05 The Skull Dezain

06 backyard 10

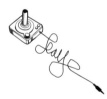

07 Sellout Industries

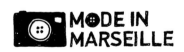

08 Tabas

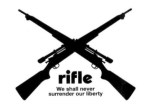

09 underson

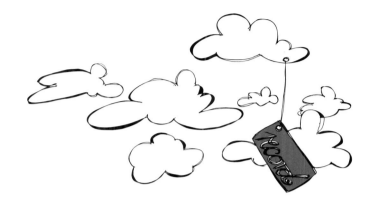

10 Grotesk

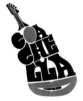

11 Tohyto

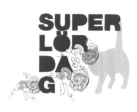

01 bleed

02 Die Seiner

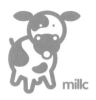

03 Yorgo Tloupas

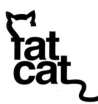

04 Intercity

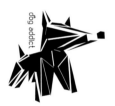

05 Canefantasma Studio

06 dopepope

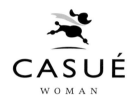

07 Simon & Goetz Design

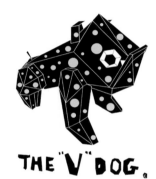

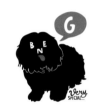

08 june

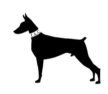

09 Parra

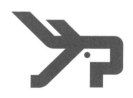

10 projekttriangle

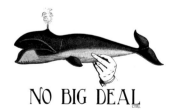

11 Henrik Vibskov

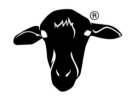

12 Raffaele Primitivo

13 DTM_INC

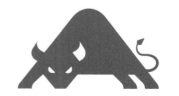

14 viagrafik

15 Yo Freeman

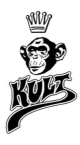

01 Jun Watanabe

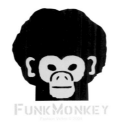

02 GWG

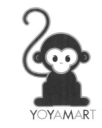

03 Hammarnäs

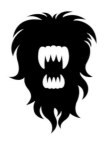

04 Magma

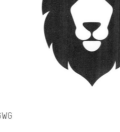

05 Jason Kochis

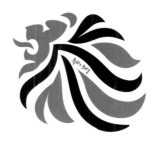

06 Calliope Studios

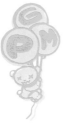

07 Furi Furi Company

08 DED Associates

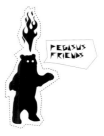

09 austrianilllustration.com

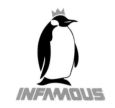

01 Nish

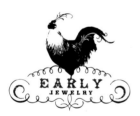

02 K-Berg Projects

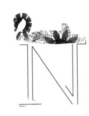

03 cabina

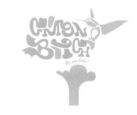

04 No-Domain

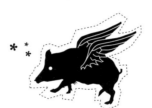

05 decoylab

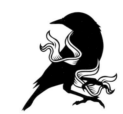

06 austrianilllustration.

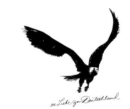

07 HandGun

08 Lloyd & Associates

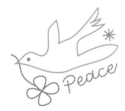

09 Yuu Imokawa

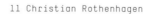

10 Upnorth

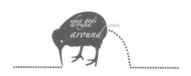

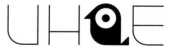

11 Christian Rothenhagen

12 Carsten Raffel

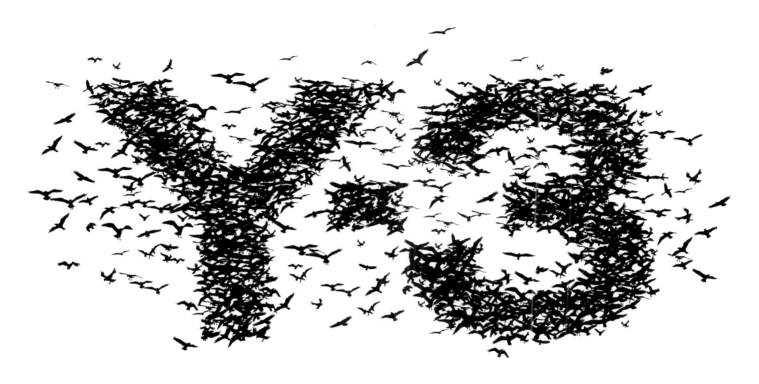

01 Graeme McMillan

02 urbn;

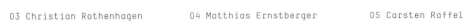

03 Christian Rothenhagen

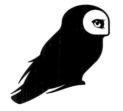

04 Matthias Ernstberger

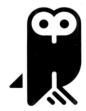

05 Carsten Raffel

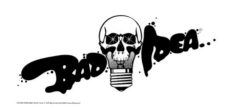

01 Keep Left Studio

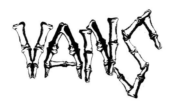

02 Hydro74

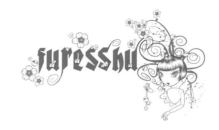

03 Jules

04 Masa

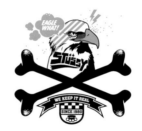

05 123klan

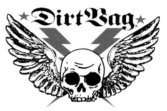

06 Jason Kochis

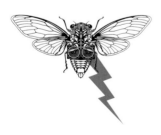

07 Polygraph

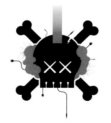

08 AmorfoDesignlab™

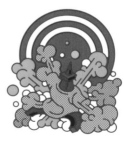

09 Tsuyoshi Hirooka

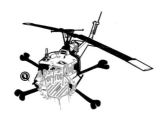

01 Karoly Kiralyfalvi

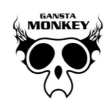

02 zookeeper

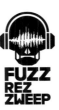

03 Positron

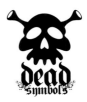

04 zookeeper

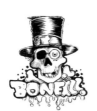

05 Keep Left Studio

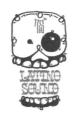

06 Masa

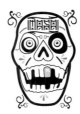

07 Masa

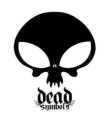

08 zookeeper

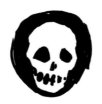

09 Formgeber

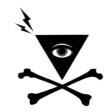

10 Ninjacruise

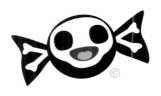

11 Tokidoki LLC

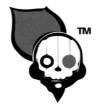

12 The Skull Dezain

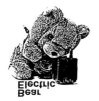

01 Tsuyoshi Hirooka

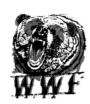

02 Tsuyoshi Hirooka

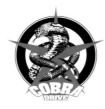

03 The Skull Dezain

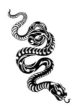

04 Formgeber

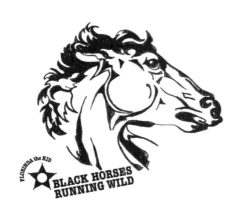

05 substrat

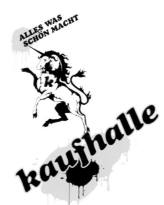

06 raum mannheim

07 Plastic Kid

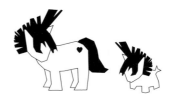

08 austrianilllustration.com

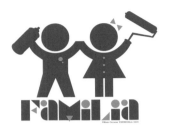

01 Masa

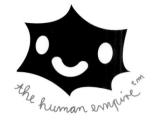

02 human empire

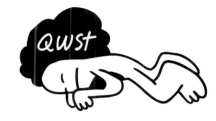

03 tstout inc.

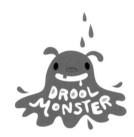

04 Meomi

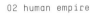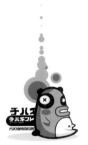

05 zookeeper

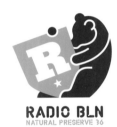

06 blackjune.

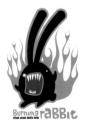

07 zookeeper

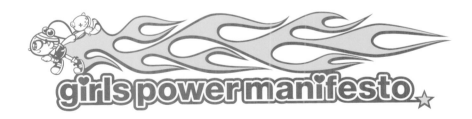

08 Furi Furi Company

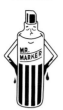

01 Grotesk

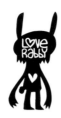

02 Jon Burgerman

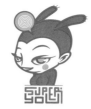

03 jeremyville

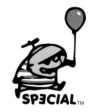

04 jum

05 jewboy Corporation™

06 Maniackers Design

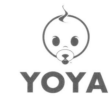

07 Calliope Studios

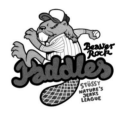

08 derek johnson

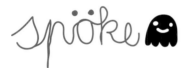

09 human empire

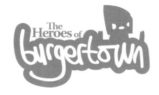

10 Jon Burgerman

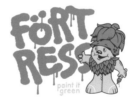

11 Flying Förtress

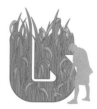

12 Flying Förtress

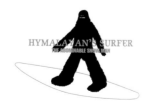

13 Gianni Rossi

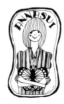

14 Naho Ogawa

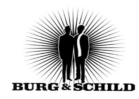

15 Fiftyeight3d

16 automatic art and design

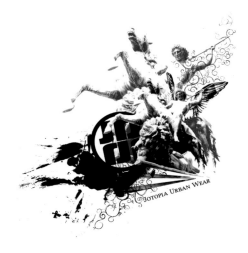

01 Formgeber

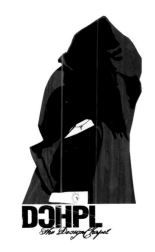

02 DesignChapel

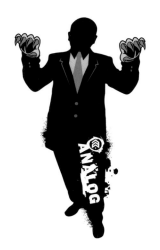

03 automatic art and design

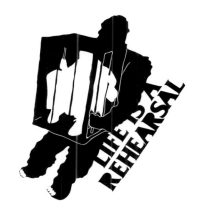

04 Kingsize

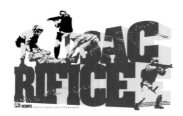

01 The Skull Dezain

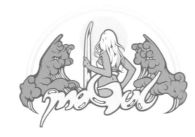

02 Sat One

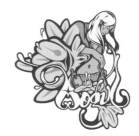

03 Sat One

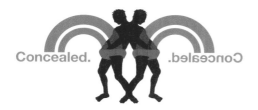

04 William Morrisey

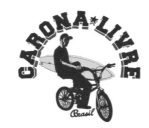

05 A-Side Studio

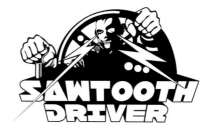

06 Positron

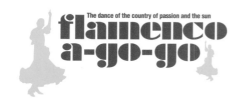

07 underson [Tsutomu Horiguchi]

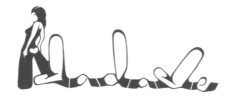

08 Sat One

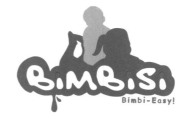

09 Dimomedia Lab

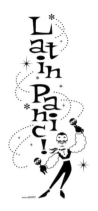

01 Amore Hirosuke

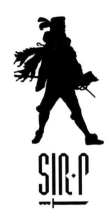

02 Syrup Helsinki

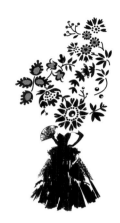

03 the red is love

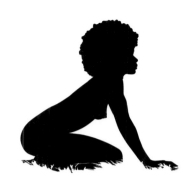

04 Out Of Order

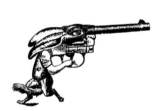

05 Lynn Hatzius

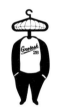

06 Grotesk

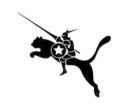

07 Polygraph

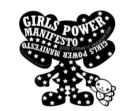

08 Furi Furi Company

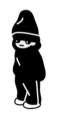

09 Fellow Designers

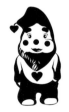

10 the red is love

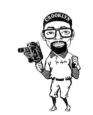

11 Grotesk

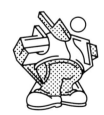

12 Tsuyoshi Hirooka

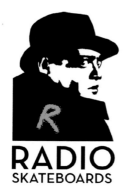

01 blackjune

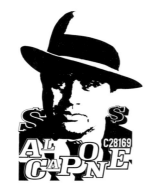

02 Jason Kochis

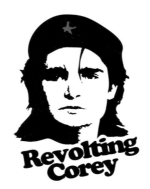

03 Jason Kochis

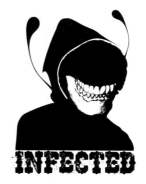

04 Insect Design

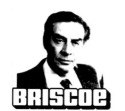

05 Jason Kochis

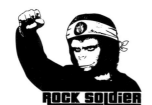

06 Jason Kochis

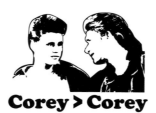

07 Jason Kochis

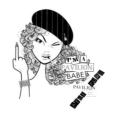

08 Ashi & office Greminger

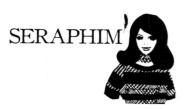

09 Miki Amano

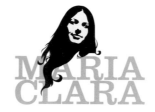

10 Team Manila

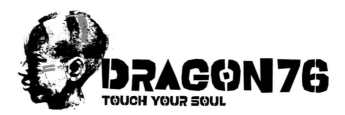

11 dragon

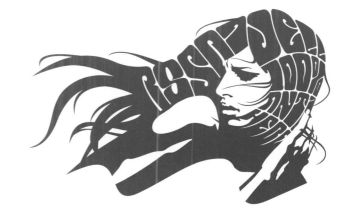

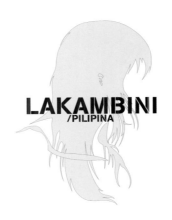

01 Out Of Order

02 The Skull Dezain

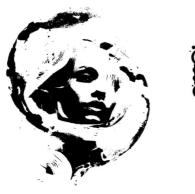

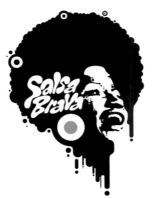

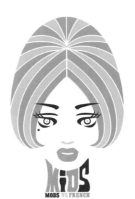

03 Zion Graphics

04 Masa

05 Team Manila

06 Amore Hirosuke

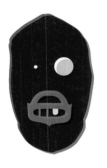

01 Masa

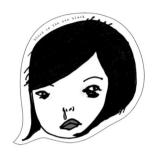

02 Christian Rothenhagen

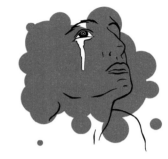

03 Keren Richter

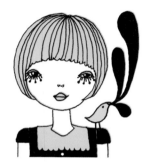

04 Keren Richter

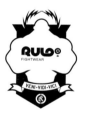

05 NeoDG

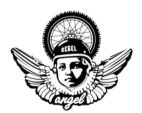

06 seacreative

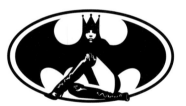

07 Lunatiq

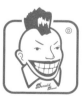

08 The Skull Dezain

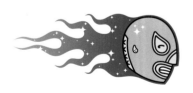

09 Hula Hula

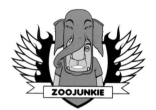

10 Magma

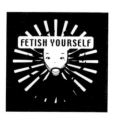

11 Akiza

12 KesselsKramer

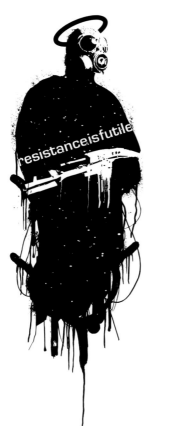

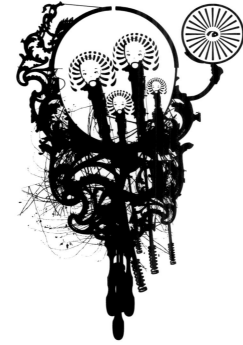

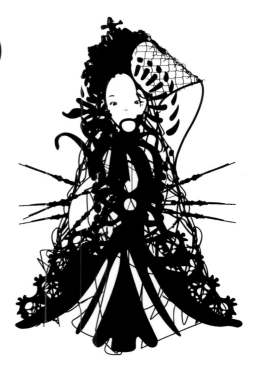

01 dzgnbio

02 Akiza

03 Akiza

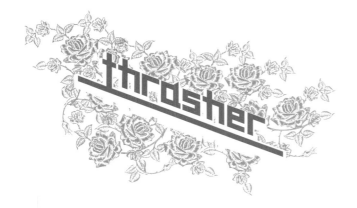

01 bleed

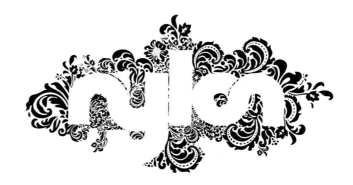

02 Keep Left Studio

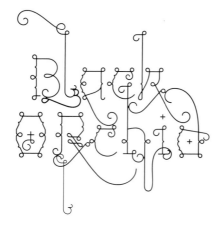

03 Deanne Cheuk

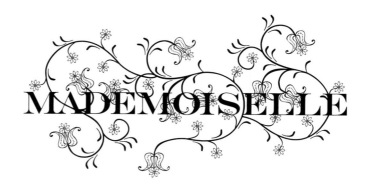

04 Faith

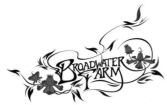

01 red design

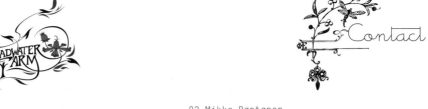

02 Mikko Rantanen

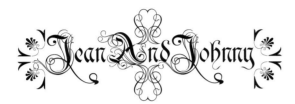

03 Deanne Cheuk

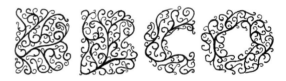

04 Stockbridge International

05 Studio Output

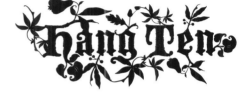

06 Studio 3

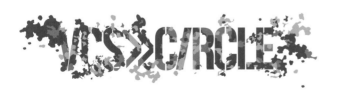

17 The Skull Dezain

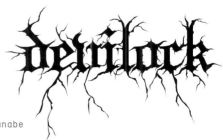

08 Jun Watanabe

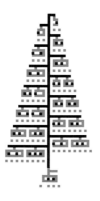

01 ten_do_ten

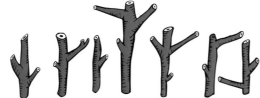

02 Karoly Kiralyfalvi

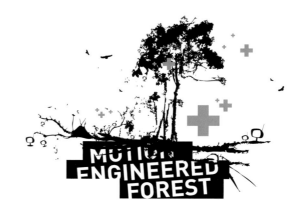

03 chemicalbox

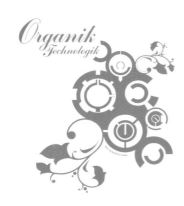

04 Tohyto

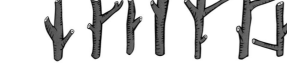

05 The Skull Dezain

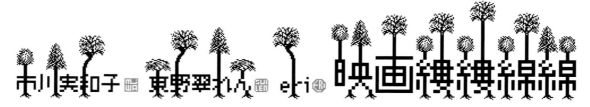

06 ten_do_ten

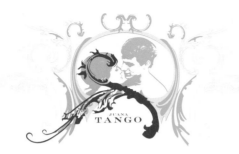

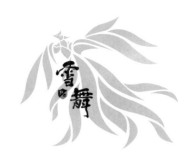

01 cabina

02 Zion Graphics

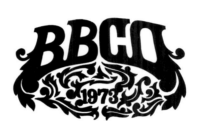

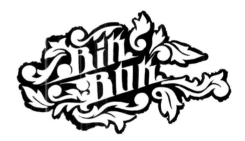

03 struggle inc.

04 Studio 3

05 Studio 3

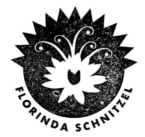

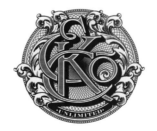

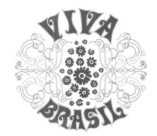

06 substrat

07 Razauno

08 A-Side Studio

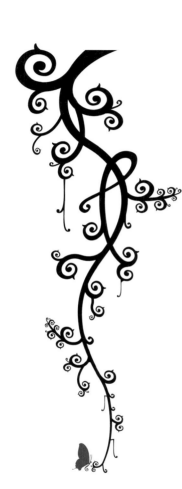

01 derfaber

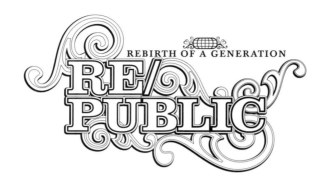

02 Team Manila

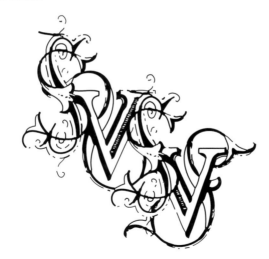

04 The KDU

03 Faith

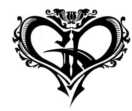

05 Furi Furi Company

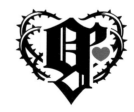

06 Furi Furi Company

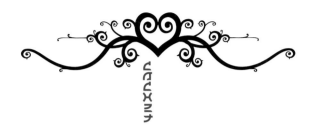

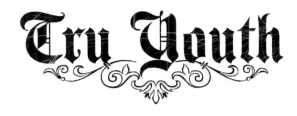

01 derfaber

02 Team Manila

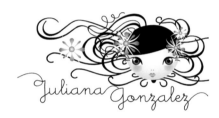

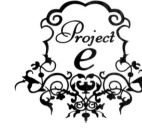

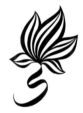

03 Catalina Estrada Uribe

04 Jason Kochis

05 usugrow

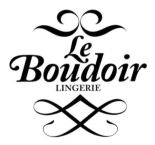

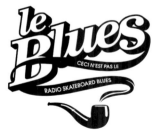

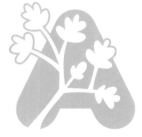

06 Nohemi Dicuru-fashiongraphic

07 blackjune

08 Studio Output

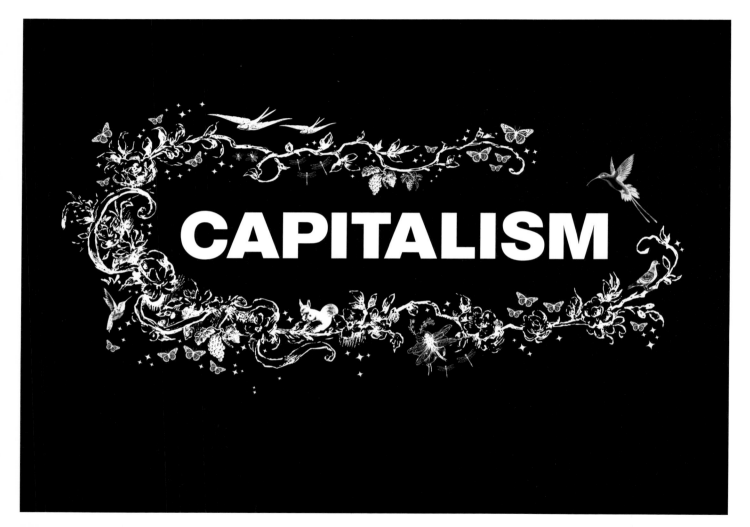

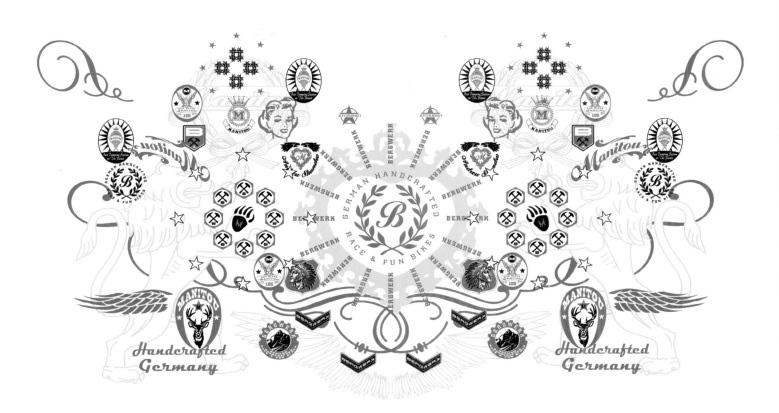

01 Magma

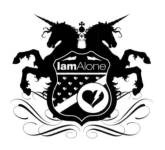

01 HandGun

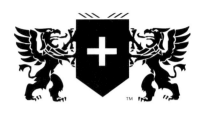

02 K-Berg Projects

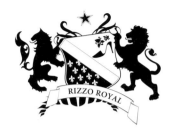

03 Supershapes

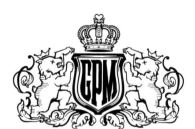

04 Furi Furi Company

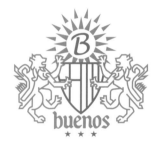

05 Yuu Imokawa

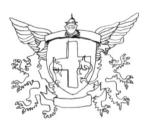

06 Maak

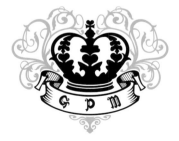

07 Furi Furi Company

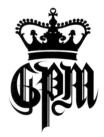

08 Furi Furi Company

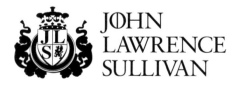

09 Sunday-Vision

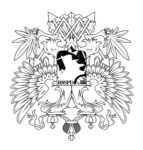

01 The Skull Dezain

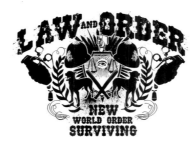

02 Stockbridge International

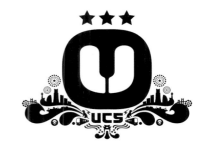

03 TGB design

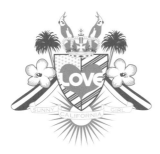

04 Yuu Imokawa

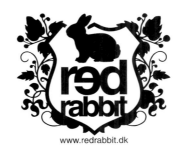

05 Palle Bruun Rasmussen

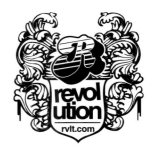

06 Palle Bruun Rasmussen

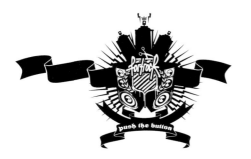

07 Karoly Kiralyfalvi

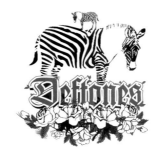

08 AmorfoDesignlab™

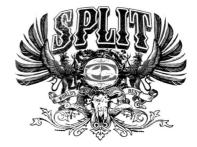

09 Hydro74

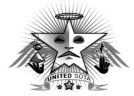

01 jum

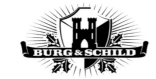

02 Fiftyeight3d

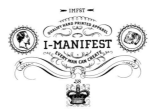

03 I-Manifest

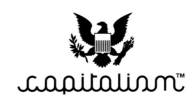

04 Lloyd & Associates

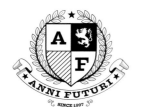

05 Binatural

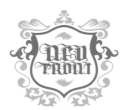

06 Nohemi Dicuru

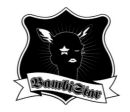

07 Sarah Grimaldi

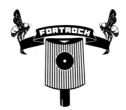

08 Extraverage Productions

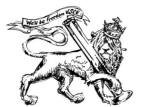

09 The Skull Dezain

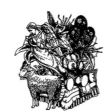

10 Tsuyoshi Hirooka

11 ehquestionmark

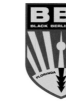

12 substrat

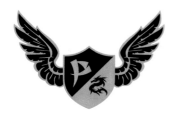

13 Zion Graphics

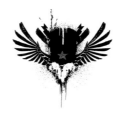

14 dzgnbio

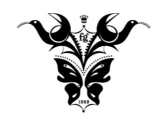

15 A-Side Studio

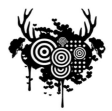

16 Resin[sistem] design

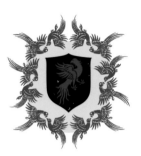

01 Flexn / BANK™

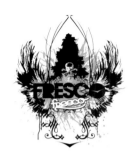

02 AmorfoDesignlab™

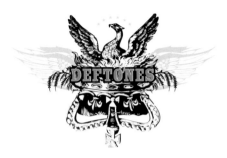

03 AmorfoDesignlab™

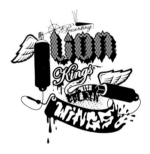

04 Lucias Westrup

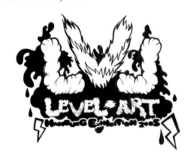

05 Koadzn

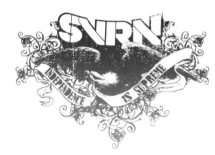

06 Hydro74

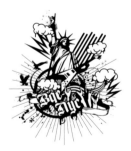

07 Power Graphixx

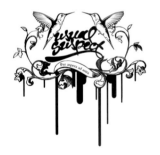

08 backyard 10

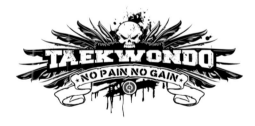

09 NeoDG

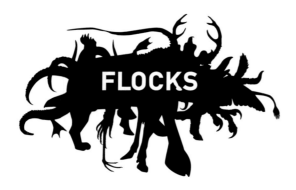

01 Julie Joliat

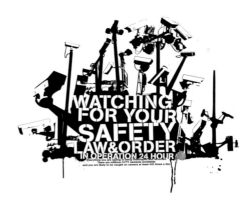

02 Stockbridge International

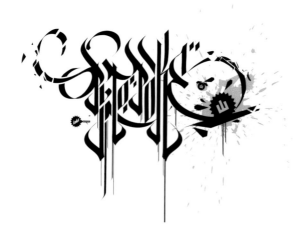

03 Inocuodesign

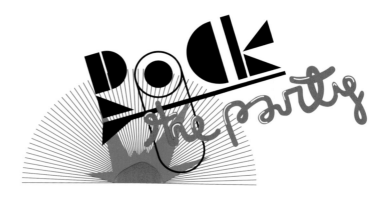

04 Tohyto

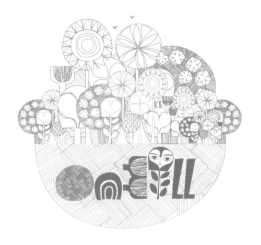

01 Keep Left Studio

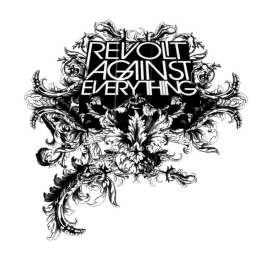

02 Hydro74

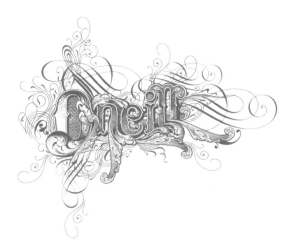

03 Keep Left Studio

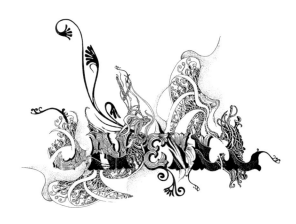

04 Keep Left Studio

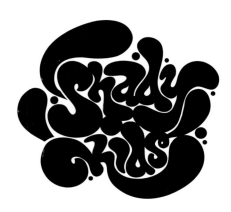

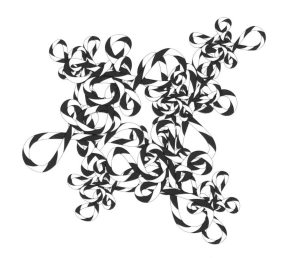

01 Keep Left Studio

02 Henrik Vibskov

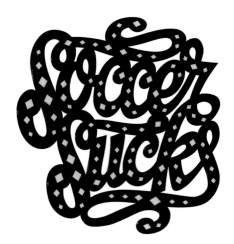

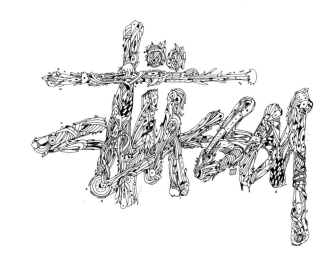

03 Niels Shoe Meulman

04 Michael Genovese

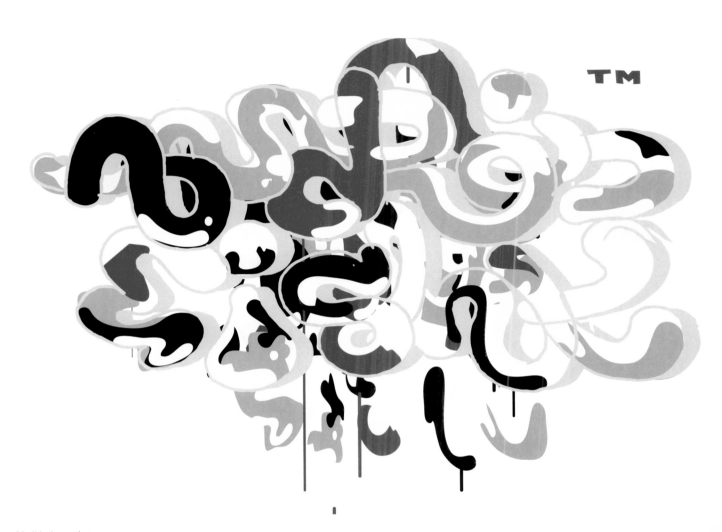

01 Ninjacruise

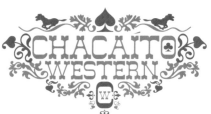

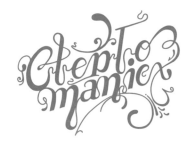

01 Masa

02 Lousy Livincompany

03 Niels Shoe Meulman

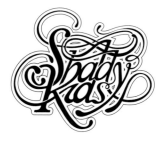

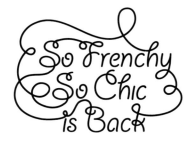

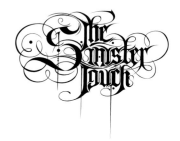

04 Keep Left Studio

05 Keep Left Studio

06 Keep Left Studio

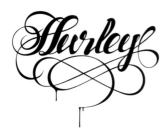

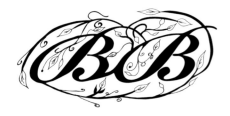

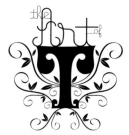

07 The Skull Dezain

08 WGD

09 Faith

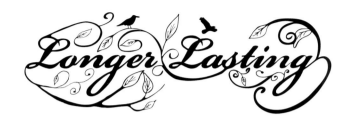

01 WGD

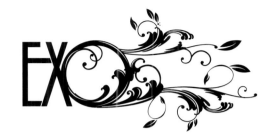

02 Hydro74

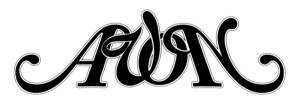

03 Nohemi Dicuru

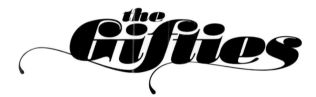

04 Mitch Paone

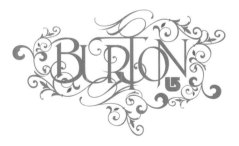

05 Keep Left Studio

06 Hydro74

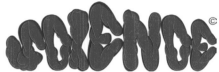

01 Koadzn

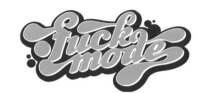

02 Out Of Order

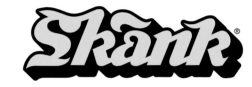

03 inkgraphix

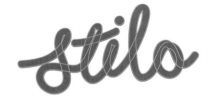

04 A-Side Studio

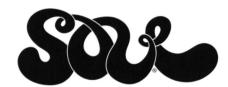

05 Keep Left Studio

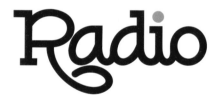

06 blackjune

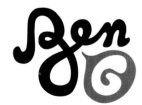

07 Parra

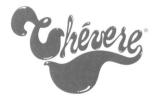

08 Razauno

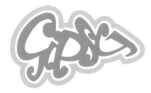

09 Salon Vektoria

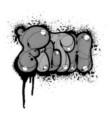

01 Keep Left Studio

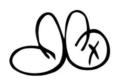

02 Koadzn

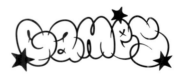

03 backyard 10

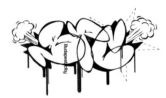

04 Axel Peemöller

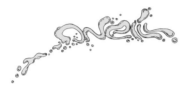

05 JB CLASSICS

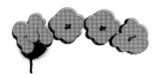

06 123klan

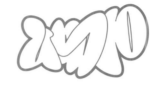

07 The Skull Dezain

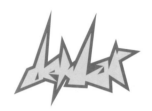

08 Karoly Kiralyfalvi

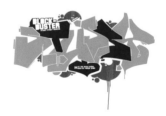

09 Masa

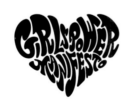

10 Furi Furi Company

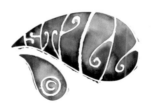

11 Typeholics.

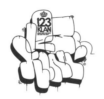

12 123klan

01 Koadzn

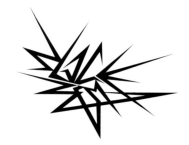

02 bandage

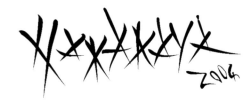

03 Raphazen

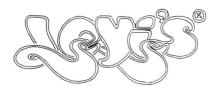

04 Studio Oscar

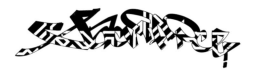

05 The Skull Dezain

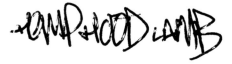

06 310k

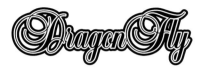

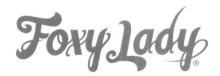

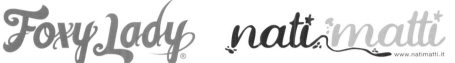

01 Magma

02 Adhemas

03 Dimomedia Lab

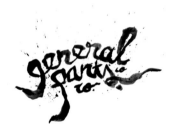

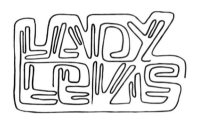

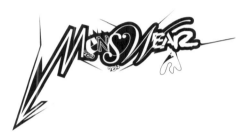

04 Keep Left Studio

05 Studio Oscar

06 ZIP Design

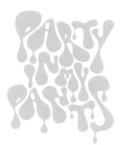

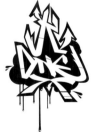

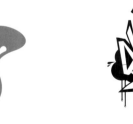

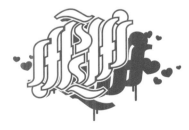

07 Raffaele Primitivo

08 Raffaele Primitivo

09 Matthias Gephart

10 Formgeber

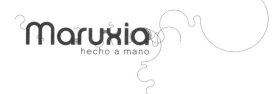

01 Carlos Bêla

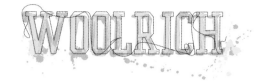

02 Stockbridge International

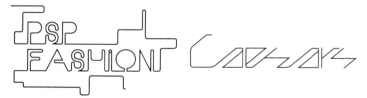

03 FL@33

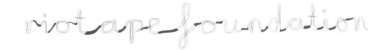

04 christian walden

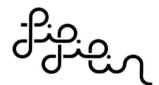

05 sophie toporkoff

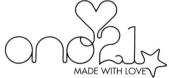

06 Retron

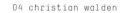

07 Binatural

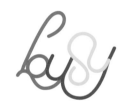

08 Lousy Livincompany

09 Labor f. visuelles Wachstum™

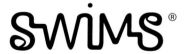

10 Zetuei Fonts

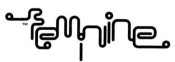

11 newoslo

12 viagrafik

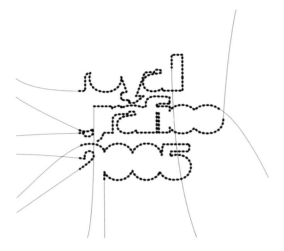

01 0c/0m/0y/0k

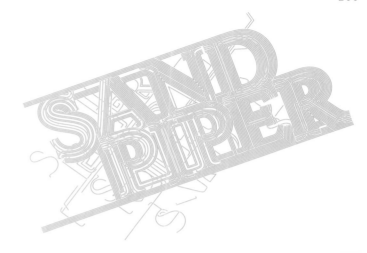

02 Caótica

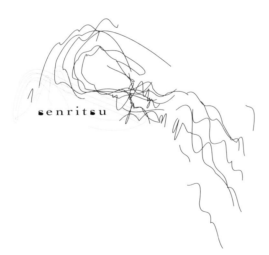

03 evaq studio

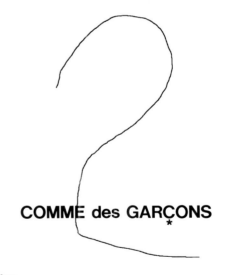

04 Marc Atlan

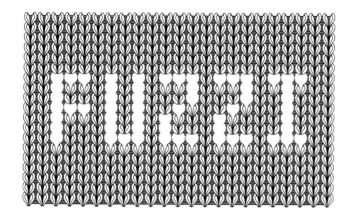

01 milchhof : atelier

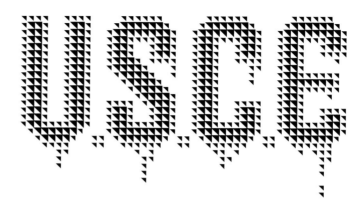

02 The Skull Dezain

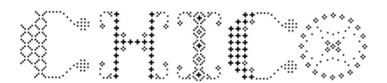

03 ten_do_ten

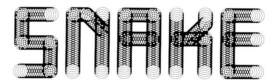

04 Tsuyoshi Hirooka

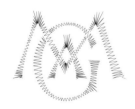

05 Niels Shoe Meulman

06 Studio Output

07 I-Manifest

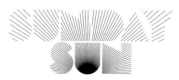

08 Vår

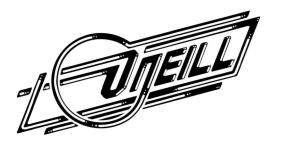

01 Keep Left Studio

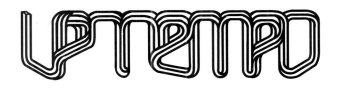

02 Keep Left Studio

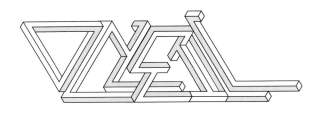

03 Keep Left Studio

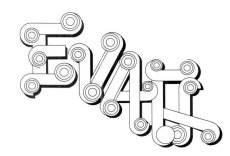

04 evaq studio

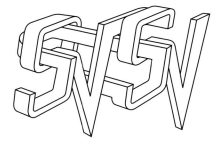

05 The KDU

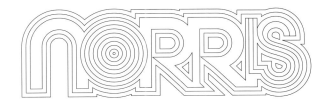

06 Emil Kozak

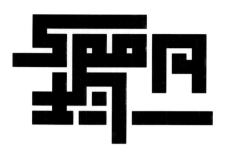

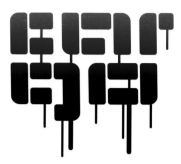

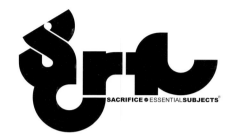

01 Zetuei Fonts

02 Carsten Raffel

03 The Skull Dezain

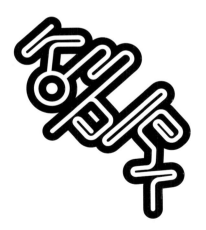

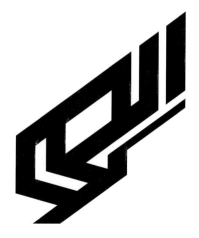

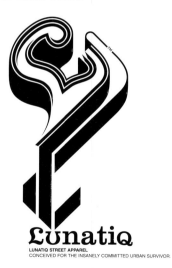

04 0c/0m/0y/0k

05 Jun Watanabe

06 Lunatiq

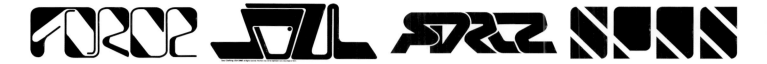

01 Keep Left Studio

02 Keep Left Studio

03 Keep Left Studio

04 Jun Watanabe

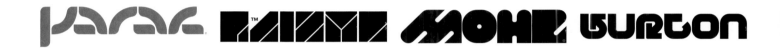

05 Coldwater Graphiix

06 viagrafik

07 Neubau.

08 Hydro74

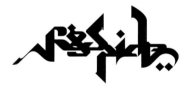

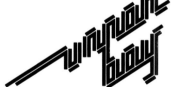

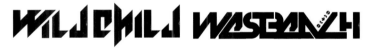

09 The Skull Dezain

10 Tsuyoshi Hirooka

11 Jun Watanabe

12 Hydro74

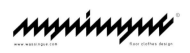

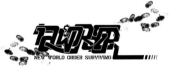

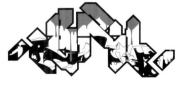

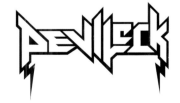

13 Atelier télescopique

14 Stockbridge International

15 The Skull Dezain

16 Jun Watanabe

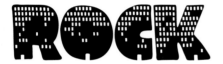

01 Parra

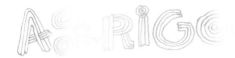

02 cabina

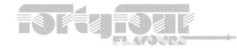

03 44 flavours

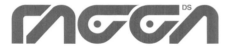

04 Raffaele Primitivo

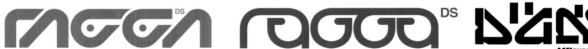

05 Raffaele Primitivo

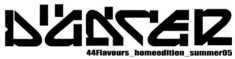

06 44 flavours

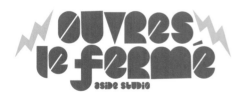

07 A-Side Studio

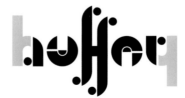

08 fatbob

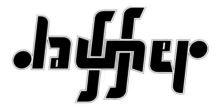

09 fatbob

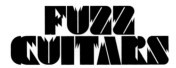

01 No-Domain

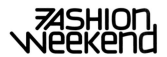

02 Paco Aguayo

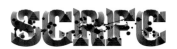

03 The Skull Dezain

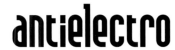

04 Tsuyoshi Hirooka

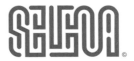

05 Kallegraphics

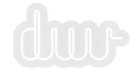

06 Axel Peemöller

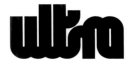

07 Karen Jane

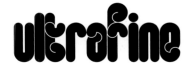

08 Karen Jane

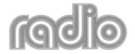

09 blackjune

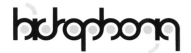

10 Clrqa

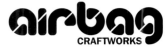

11 viagrafik

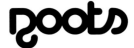

12 Emil Kozak

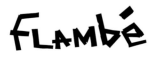

13 :phunk studio

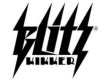

14 Attak

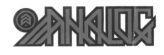

15 automatic

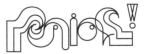

16 cisma

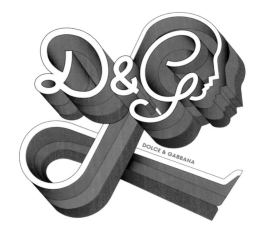

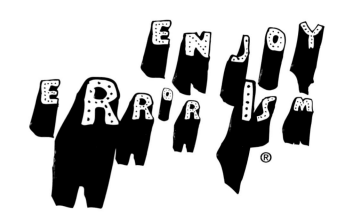

01 Hammarnäs

02 viagrafik

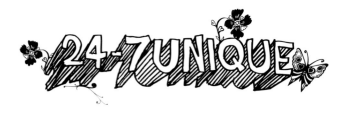

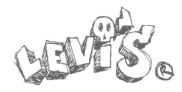

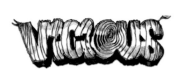

03 44 flavours

04 backyard 10

05 The Skull Dezain

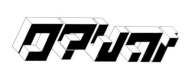

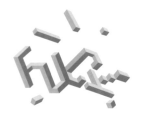

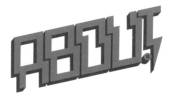

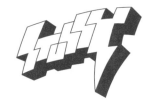

06 Axel Peemöller

07 DTM_INC

08 Raffaele Primitivo

09 Flying Förtress

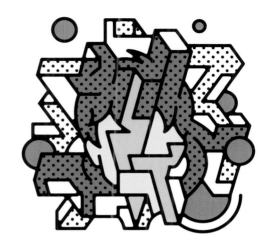

02 Tsuyoshi Hirooka

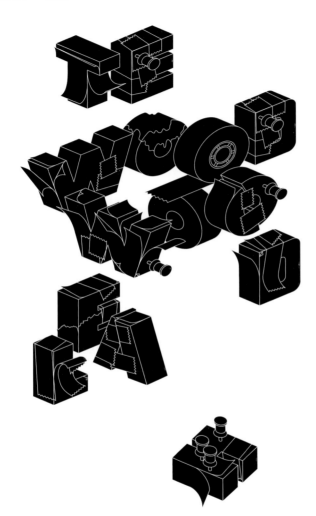

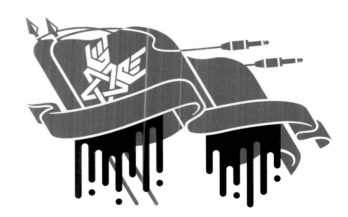

01 PMKFA

03 Power Graphixx

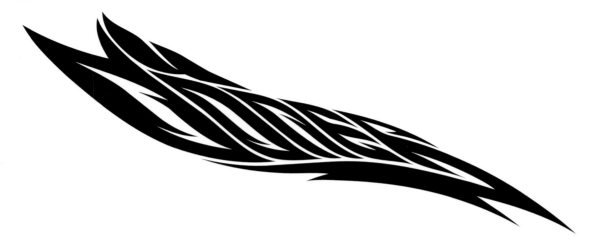

01 bandage

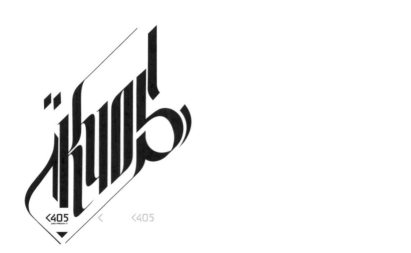

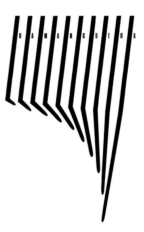

02 Inocuodesign   03 Büro Otto Sauhaus

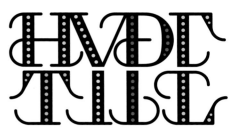

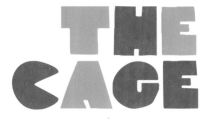

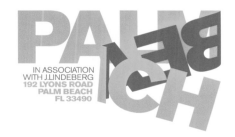

01 Niels Shoe Meulman

02 blackjune

03 Zion Graphics

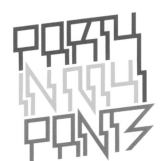

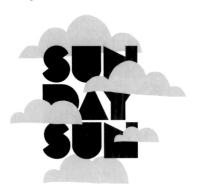

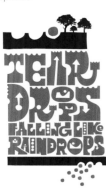

04 Raffaele Primitivo

05 Vår

06 struggle inc.

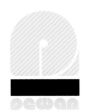

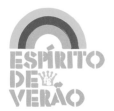

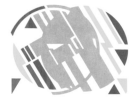

07 Axel Peemöller

08 A-Side Studio

09 :g / studio-gpop

10 Deanne Cheuk

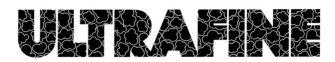

01 Karen Jane

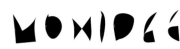

02 Hydro74

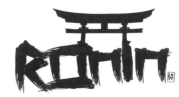

03 Laborator

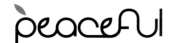

04 usugrow

joey Dee

05 Marc Atlan

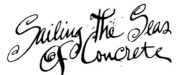

06 blackjune

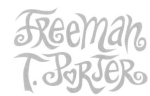

07 Formikula

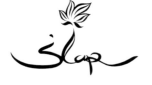

08 Raffaele Primitivo

09 Pandarosa

b.young

10 Designbolaget

club·missya

11 Thomas Nolfi

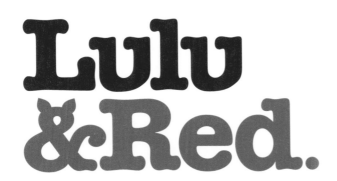

01 stylodesign

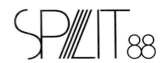

03 Hydro74

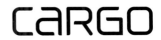

KOPENHAGEN FUR

02 re-public

04 Carsten Raffel

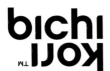

05 AmorfoDesignlab™

siebenschoen

06 Codeluxe

kip farmer design

07 Semisans

marlies|dekkers
UN|DRESSED

08 STUDIO DUMBAR

RENÉ LEZARD

09 Simon & Goetz Design

bianca spender

10 sopp collective

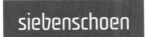

11 MH grafik

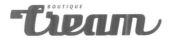

debeaufort

12 Büro Destruct

01 Lloyd & Associates

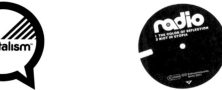

02 blackjune

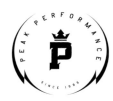

03 Zion Graphics

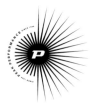

04 Zion Graphics

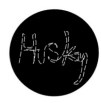

05 Petr Babák, Laborator

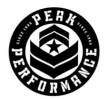

06 Zion Graphics

07 Zion Graphics

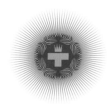

08 Zion Graphics

09 344 Design, LLC

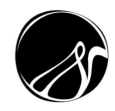

10 Semitransparent Design

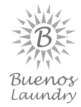

11 Yuu Imokawa

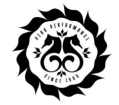

12 Neeser & Müller

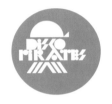

01 Stolen Inc.

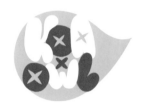

02 Koadzn

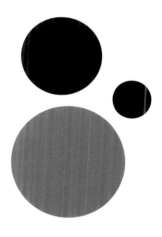

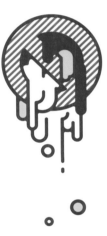

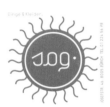

03 Theres Steiner

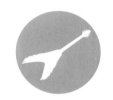

04 Salon Vektoria

05 Flavio Bagioli

06 Tsuyoshi Hirooka

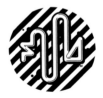

07 viagrafik

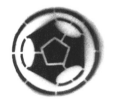

08 Formgeber

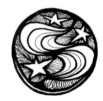

09 Formgeber

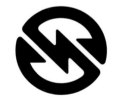

10 The Skull Dezain

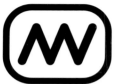

01 Resin[sistem] design

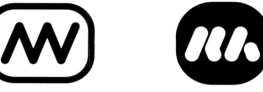

02 Ketchup Arts

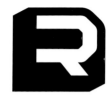

03 3 deluxe

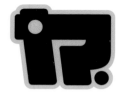

04 Resin[sistem] design

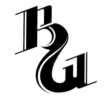

05 Tsuyoshi Hirooka

06 Koadzn

07 Polygraph

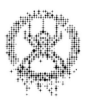

08 The Skull Dezain

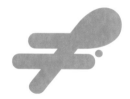

09 Extraverage Productions

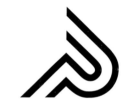

10 Zion Graphics

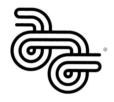

11 Yorgo Tloupas

12 strange//attraktor:

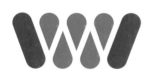

13 Studio Output

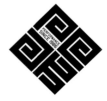

14 Zion Graphics

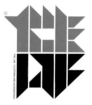

15 Karoly Kiralyfalvi

16 Atomic Attack

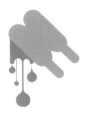

01 Tohyto

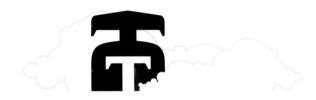

02 Mattisimo

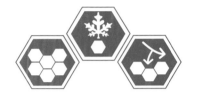

03 310k

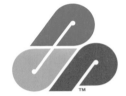

04 backyard 10

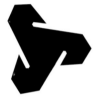

05 Microbot David Fuhrer

06 310k

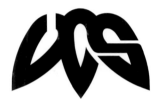

07 The Skull Dezain

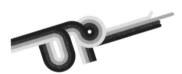

08 Form

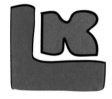

09 Fase

10 Tsuyoshi Hirooka

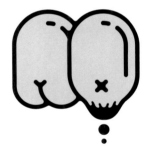

DesignerClobber
Mens.Womens.Online.Oufitters

11 :g / studio-gpop

WOLFSMILCH

12 Balsi Grafik

C-ARROW. THE MONTHLY
MAGAZINE OF FASHION
AND COMPUTER.

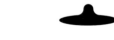

13 sunrise studios

14 Tsuyoshi Hirooka

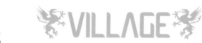
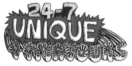

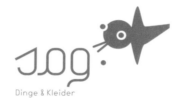

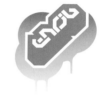

01 44 flavours

02 Christian Albriktsen

03 Theres Steiner

04 DigitalPlayground Studio

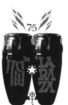

07 Masa

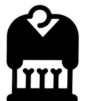

05 struggle inc.

06 Tsuyoshi Hirooka

07 Masa

08 Tsuyoshi Hirooka

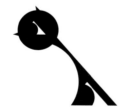

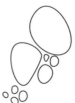
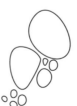

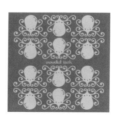

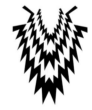

09 Kosta Lazarevski / rdy

10 Keren Richter

11 YellowToothpick

12 Henrik Vibskov

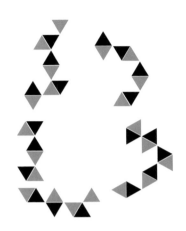

01 Henrik Vibskov

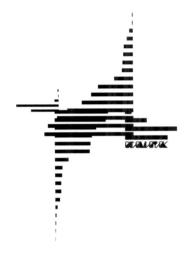

02 0c/0m/0y/0k

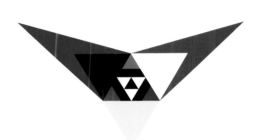

03 Henrik Vibskov

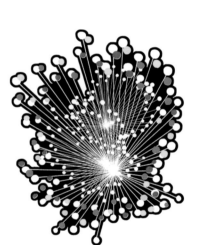

04 Henrik Vibskov

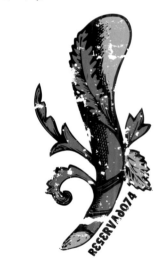

05 the red is love

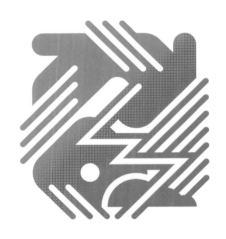

06 Power Graphixx

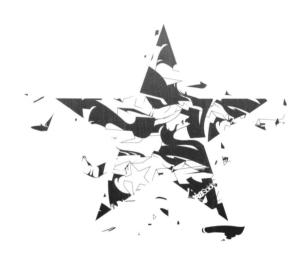

01 The Skull Dezain

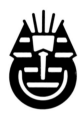

02 The Skull Dezain

03 Fluid Creativity

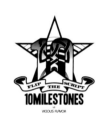

04 Tsuyoshi Hirooka

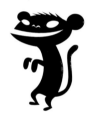

05 Gastón Caba

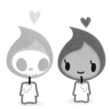

06 Tokidoki LLC

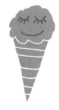

07 Ottograph

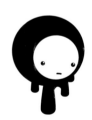

08 Ohio Girl Design

09 Attak

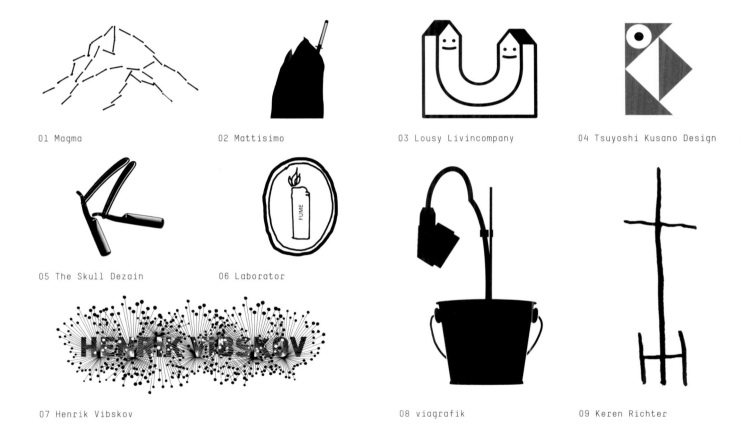

01 Magma

02 Mattisimo

03 Lousy Livincompany

04 Tsuyoshi Kusano Design

05 The Skull Dezain

06 Laborator

07 Henrik Vibskov

08 viagrafik

09 Keren Richter

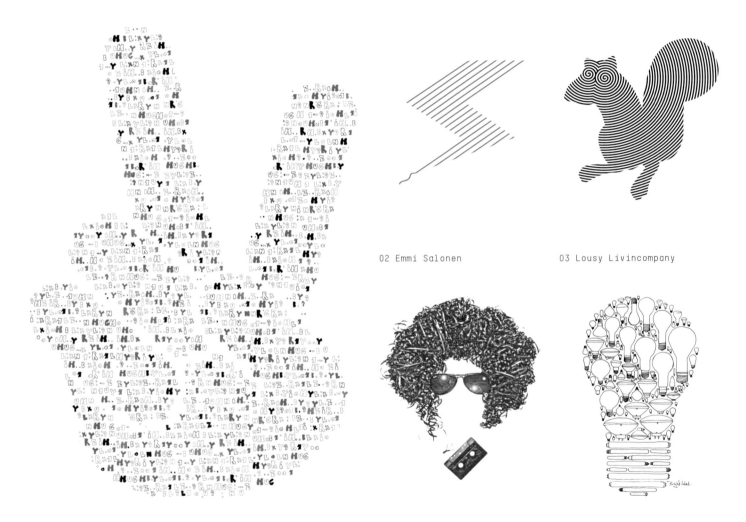

02 Emmi Salonen

03 Lousy Livincompany

01 Henrik Vibskov

04 Tsuyoshi Hirooka

05 Keep Left Studio

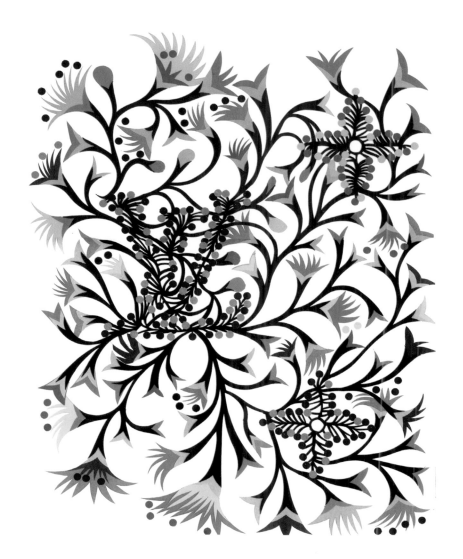

01 Petra Börner

MOTION

VIRTUAL AND MATERIAL

An important topic: illustrations that positively leap out at the beholder. And this is exactly what their designers intended. Logos designed for television and for live streaming on the web often display an aversion to immobility: they would like to run away, yet must behave in a cross-medial fashion in order to function in the static realm of print. Still, they are genuinely in their element only in the virtual realm.

THE SKULL

Fashionable rituals of repression?
He gazes forward meditatively, Paul Cezanne's "Le jeune homme à la tête de mort." Perhaps he is a poet contemplating the finality of human existence, observed by a skull: the advent of Modernism, followed by a deep black hole in time. And now? They look fashionable, canvas Chuck's by Converse, in black, adorned with cute white skulls. Their name is "Hi Skull." In our times, when death and violence are omnipresent in the media, the skull as a symbol needs to be toppled from its massive and portentous pedestal and appropriated as a fashion accessory. That today's designers of signs are also experimenting with this symbol is consistent with contemporary zeitgeist blowing in from Hollywood, where romantic Caribbean pirates are among the latest heroes.

LAUNDRY

Logos are the hierarchy of our society.

Philippe John Richardson is "pj", a designer who runs "Laundry", a studio for motion graphics and design in Beverly Hills together with his partner Anthony Lin. The main focus of their work is on animated graphic sequences and effects for commercials, television stations and music videos. Laundry is also responsible for numerous printed works. The studio was shortlisted by the art director's club Gun 5. Laundry have also been featured in numerous publications like I.D. Magazine, Grafuck, Coast to Coast by Die Gestalten, Wired Magazine and San Francisco MOMA.

Concerning current trends and tendencies in the world of design, pj has his own decisive views: "I think design in the popular sense is shifting towards an illustrative and mood-driven approach to problem-solving. Design as art is quite strong these days, and especially with increased access to faster computers, anyone can become a designer. The volume of less crafted and less educated work is quite high, but the need for strong iconography and simple messages - even if stylised - remains."

In some way, this view – which is shared by pj's partner – determines the working philosophy of Laundry itself: "Our goal is to solve each design assignment via the most experimental and unconventional route possible for the most visible and open-minded clients worldwide." A partial list of current and previous clients corroborates this statement: Coca-Cola, Pepsi, BMW, Nike, Adidas, MTV, VH1, Boost Mobile, Amstel, Microsoft, Sin City, Altoids, Transformers, Samsung, Hugo Boss, Madonna, Ecko, G4 networks, Aol, Yahoo!, Honda, Yaris, Toyota, Absolut, Mastercard, At+t, Bacardi and Cola, HP, Espn, Fine Living Network, Nokia, Red Hot Chili Peppers, Nissan, Wired Magazine, UPS, Kyocera, Google, Cox Communication, Fuse, Air Jordan and the White Stripes.

Among the studio's current projects (as of August 2006) are an artistic interpretation of Colour Magazine for the exhibition "Fabrica: Les Yeux Ouverts," scheduled to open in the autumn of 2006 at the Centre Pompidou in Paris; an animated film inspired by 70s erotica and a logo project for Boost Mobile. On the role of the logo in our society, pj remarks: "A logo can make or break a brand. Logos reveal a society's hierarchy, they distinguish a Holiday Inn from an Ian Schraeger hotel, a pair of Nikes from a pair of Pumas, the White House from the English Parliament. For me, the best logos are the ones where you don't even know what they are for, but the images are so interesting you want to be a part of it."

MOTION

VIRTUELL UND MATERIELL

Wichtiges Thema: Illustrationen, die den Rezipienten förmlich an-springen. Was exakt den Intentionen ihrer Gestalter entspricht. Logos für TV und Live-Streaming im Web drücken gelegentlich eine Aversion gegen den Stillstand aus: Sie möchten gerne davonlaufen, müssen sich aber crossmedial verhalten, um auch im statischen Printbereich zu funktionieren. Doch richtig in ihrem Element sind sie eigentlich in der Virtualität.

TOTENKOPF

Modische Verdrängungsrituale?

Sinnend schaut er vor sich hin, „Le jeune homme à la tête de mort" von Paul Cezanne. Vielleicht ist es ein über die Endlichkeit menschlicher Existenz nachdenkender Poet, beobachtet vom Toten-kopf: Der Beginn der Moderne, der ein tiefes schwarzes Zeitloch folgt. Und jetzt? Einen modischen Eindruck machen sie, die Chucks Canvas aus dem Hause Converse, in Schwarz, mit niedlichen kleinen weißen Totenköpfchen. Ihr Name „Hi Totenkopf". In unserer Zeit, in der Tod und Gewalt in den Medien omnipräsent sind, muss der Totenkopf als Symbol von seinem tonnenschweren Bedeutungssockel gestürzt und als Modeaccessoire vereinnahmt werden. Dass die Gestalter von Zei-chen heute gleichfalls mit diesem Symbol experimentieren, liegt im zeitgeistigen Wind begründet - der aber nicht zuletzt auch aus Rich-tung Hollywood bläst, wo in der Karibik agierende, romantische Pira-ten zu den neuen Helden gehören.

LOS ANGELES, VEREINIGTE STAATEN

LAUNDRY

Logos sind die Hierarchie unserer Gesellschaft.

Philippe John Richardson ist „pj", ein Gestalter, der gemeinsam mit seinem Partner Anthony Lin in Beverly Hills ein Studio für Motion Graphics und Design führt: Laundry. Der Hauptfokus ihrer Arbeit liegt auf bewegten grafischen Sequenzen und Effekten für Commercials, TV-Stationen und Musikvideos. Daneben realisiert Laundry auch zahlreiche Printobjekte. Das Studio wurde vom Art Directors Club Gun 5 nominiert. Laundry war auch Thema in zahlreichen Publikationen: I.D. Magazine, Grafuck publication, Coast to Coast von den Gestalten, Wired Magazine und San Francisco MOMA.

Über die aktuellen Trends und Tendenzen in der Welt des Design hat pj seine eigene, dezidierte Meinung: „Ich glaube, Design im populären Sinn bewegt sich in Richtung einer illustrativen, stimmungsgetriebenen Herangehensweise an die Probleme. Design hat eine starke Präsenz, heutzutage. Durch den Zugang zu immer schnelleren Computern kann heute jeder ein Designer sein. Das Volumen an handwerklich schwächeren, nicht auf solider Ausbildung basierenden Arbeiten ist hoch. Trotzdem bleibt der Bedarf an starker Ikonografie und einfachen, aber stilsicheren Botschaften bestehen." Irgendwie definiert diese Meinung, die von pj's Partner geteilt wird, auch die Arbeitsphilosophie von Laundry selbst: „Unser Ziel ist klar: jeden Designauftrag auf möglichst experimentelle und unkonventionelle Weise lösen - für die am stärksten präsenten und aufgeschlossensten Kunden weltweit." Ein Auszug aus der Liste aktueller und früherer Kunden liest sich wie eine Bestätigung dieser Aussage: Coca Cola, Pepsi, BMW, Nike, Adidas, MTV, VH1, Boost Mobile, Amstel, Microsoft, Sin City, Altoids, Transformers, Samsung, Hugo Boss, Madonna, Ecko, G4 networks, Aol, Yahoo!, Honda, Yaris, Toyota, Absolut, Mastercard, At+t, Bacardi and Cola, HP, Espn, Fine Living Network, Nokia, Red Hot Chili Peppers, Nissan, Wired Magazine, UPS, Kyocera, Google, Cox Communication, Fuse, Air Jordan und die White Stripes.

Zu den aktuellen Projekten des Studios (Stand: August 06) gehören eine künstlerische Interpretation von Color Magazine für die im Herbst 06 im Centre Pompidou von Paris stattfindende Ausstellung „Fabrica: Les Yeux Ouverts", ein von der Erotica der 70er inspirierter Animationsfilm sowie ein Logoprojekt für Boost Mobile. Womit wir beim Logo wären, der, wie pj es nennt, Hierarchie unserer Gesellschaft: „Ein Logo kann eine Marke leben oder sterben lassen. Logos sind die Hierarchie unserer Gesellschaft. Sie machen den Unterschied aus zwischen einem Holiday Inn und einem Ian Schraeger-Hotel, zwischen einem Paar Nikes und einem Paar Pumas, zwischen dem Weißen Haus und dem englischen Parlament. Die besten Logos für mich sind jene, bei denen du nicht einmal weißt, wofür sie stehen. Aber sie sind so interessant, so ‚einnehmend', dass du am liebsten dazugehören, ein Teil von ihnen sein möchtest."

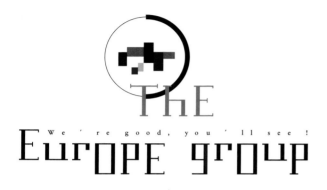

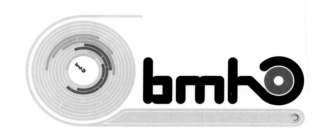

01 Rocholl Selected Designs

02 Salon Vektoria

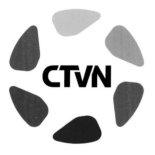

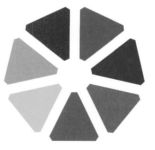

03 TGB design

04 Tsuyoshi Kusano Design

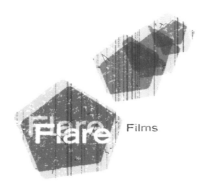

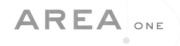

01 weissraum.de(sign)   02 Rocholl Selected Designs

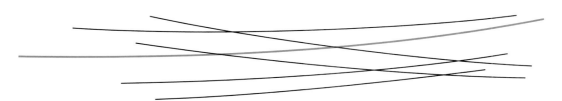

03 weissraum.de(sign)

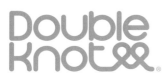

01 stylodesign

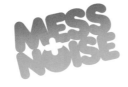

02 Adam Cruickshank

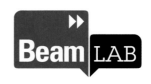

03 Power Graphixx

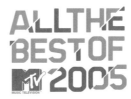

04 310k

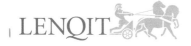

05 Mutabor Design

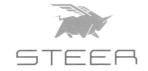

06 Mutabor Design

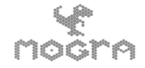

07 Calliope Studios

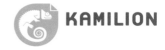

08 Mutabor Design

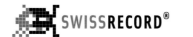

09 29 degres

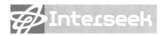

10 Futro

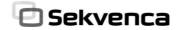

11 Futro

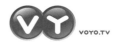

12 Mutabor Design

13 Raredrop

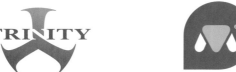

14 Bionic Systems

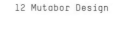

15 Borsellino & Co.

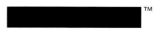

16 Borsellino & Co.

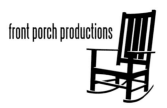

01 David Maloney

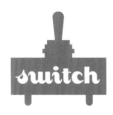

02 jum

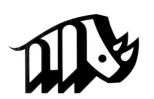

03 Ken Tanabe

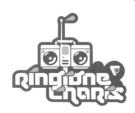

04 Bionic Systems

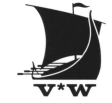

05 Masa

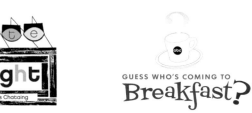

06 Anónimo Studio

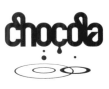

07 Power Graphixx

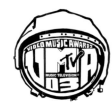

08 JDK

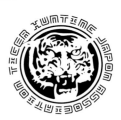

09 Ketchup Arts

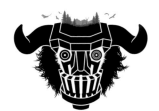

10 Polygraph

11 Emil Hartvig

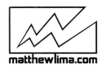

12 JDK

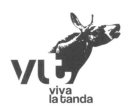

13 cabina

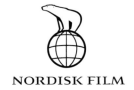

14 Kontrapunkt

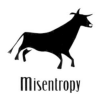

15 luca Marchettoni

16 Sanjai Bhana

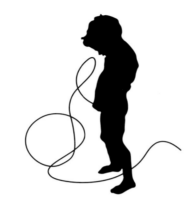

FOTOKOMPAGNIET

FOTOKOMPAGNIET.DK

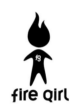

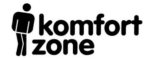

03 FilmGraphik

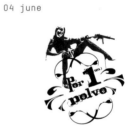

01 Emil Hartvig

02 Futro

04 june

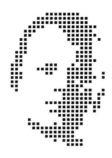

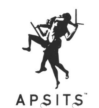

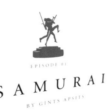

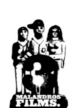

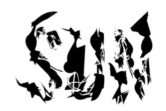

05 Gints Apsits

06 Gints Apsits

07 Masa

08 Magnetofonica

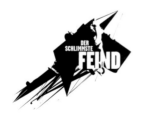

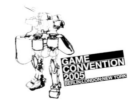

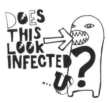

09 FilmGraphik

10 Tsuyoshi Kusano Design

11 sunrise studios

12 A-Side Studio

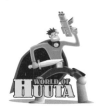

01 La Fusée

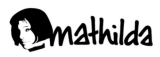

02 jl-prozess

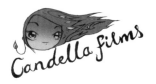

03 Matt Sewell

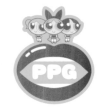

04 JDK

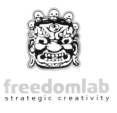

05 ultrafris

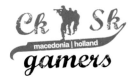

06 Kosta Lazarevski / rdy

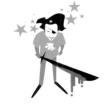

07 29 degres

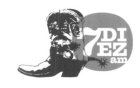

08 Hula Hula

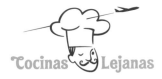

09 Hula Hula

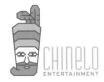

10 Hula Hula

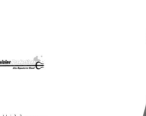

11 David A. Ortiz Villegas

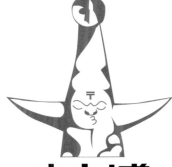

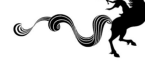

12 Polygraph

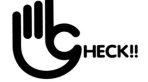

13 Ketchup Arts

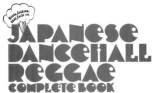

14 Ketchup Arts

15 Ketchup Arts

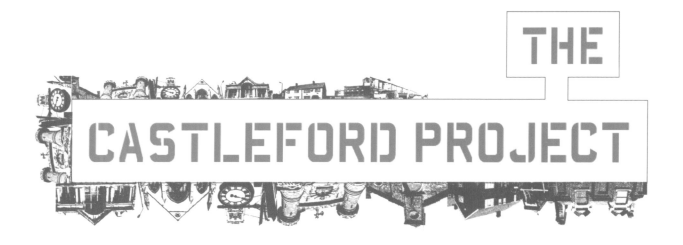

THE CASTLEFORD PROJECT

01 Peter Anderson

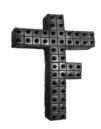 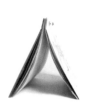 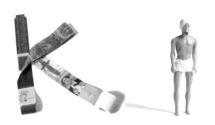 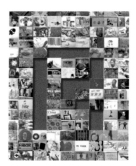

02 Fakir

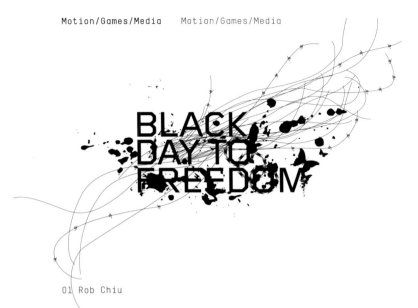

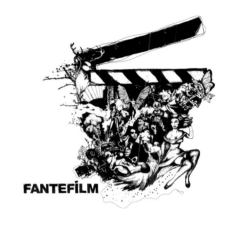

FANTEFILM

01 Rob Chiu   02 bleed

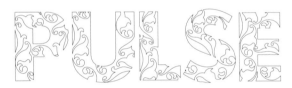

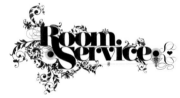

03 Konstantinos Gargaletsos   04 Upnorth   05 Colourmovie

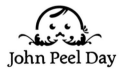

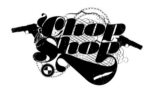

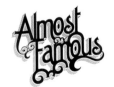

06 Studio Output   07 Upnorth   08 Upnorth   09 Chris Rubino

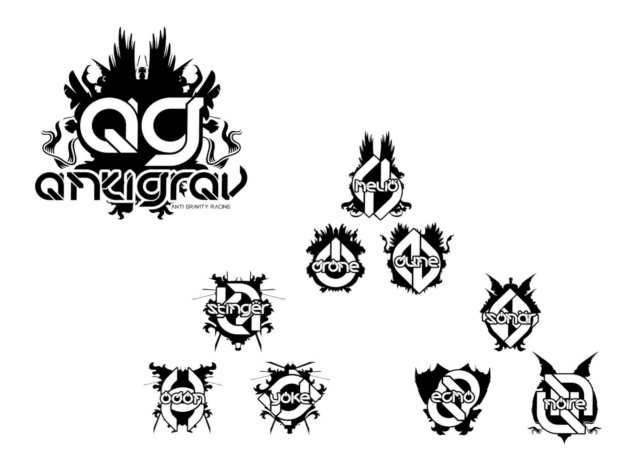

01 HandGun

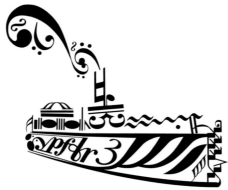

01 No-Domain

02 No-Domain

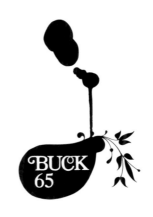

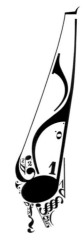

03 Masato Yamaguchi

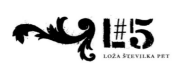

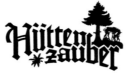

04 Lukatarina

05 FilmGraphik

06 Hugh Morse

07 No-Domain

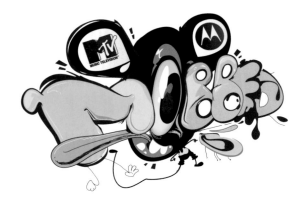

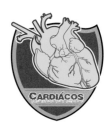

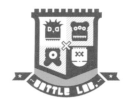

01 Fons Schiedon

02 Sarah Grimaldi

03 Glauco Diogenes

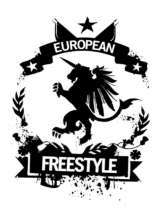

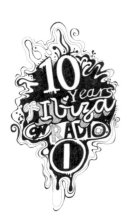

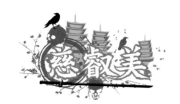

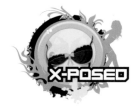

06 Engine

08 Colletivo Design

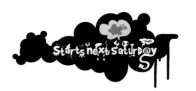

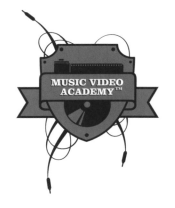

04 FilmGraphik

05 Studio Output

07 Bionyc Industries

09 Engine

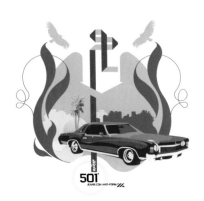

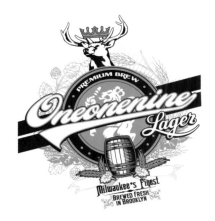

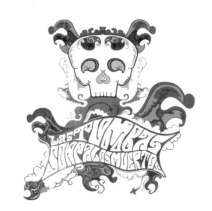

01 No-Domain

02 Upnorth

03 Tohyto

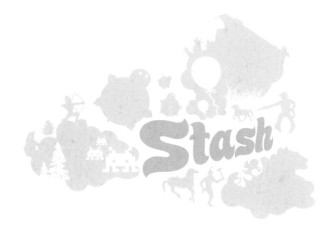

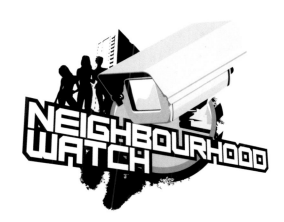

04 interspectacular

05 Engine

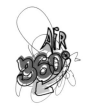

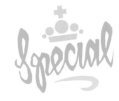

01 Tsuyoshi Hirooka

02 Fase

03 Fons Schiedon

04 Bionic Systems

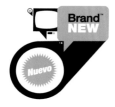

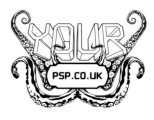

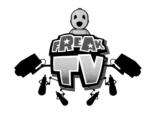

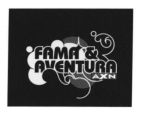

05 Masa

06 NeoDG

07 Insect

08 cisma

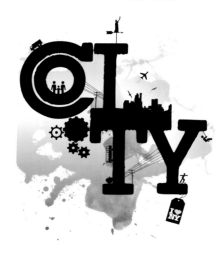

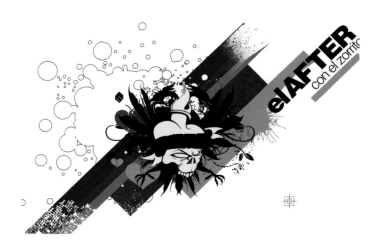

09 Upnorth

10 zinestesia

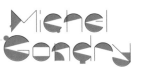

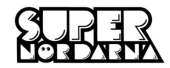

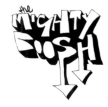

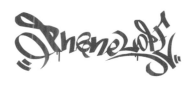

01 Tsuyoshi Hirooka

02 Kingsize

03 JAKe

04 Dimomedia Lab

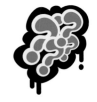

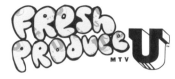

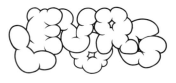

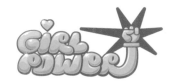

05 Bionyc Industries

06 A-Side Studio

07 Jun Watanabe

08 cisma

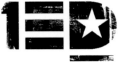

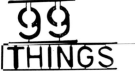

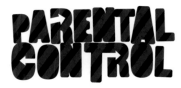

09 Faith

10 A-Side Studio

11 JAKe

12 A-Side Studio

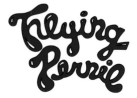

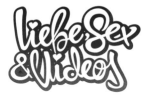

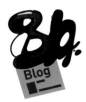

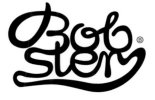

13 No-Domain

14 Etienne Heinrich

15 Fons Schiedon

16 Kingsize

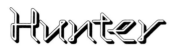

01 Polygraph

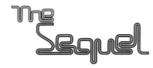

02 Sito

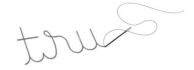

03 A-Side Studio

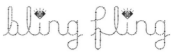

04 A-Side Studio

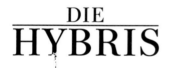

05 Rinzen

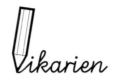

06 Alphabetical Order®

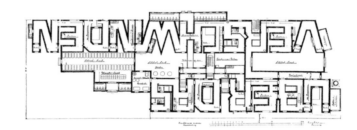

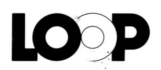

07 FilmGraphik

08 martin kvamme

09 FilmGraphik

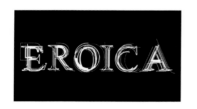

10 Peter Anderson

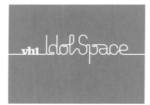

11 loyalkaspar

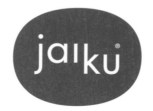

12 Syrup Helsinki

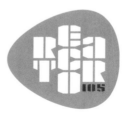

13 Hula Hula

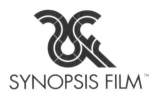

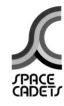

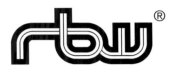

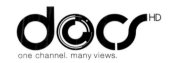

01 Engine

02 Emmi Salonen

03 viagrafik

04 loyalkaspar

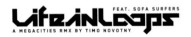

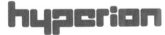

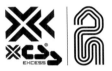

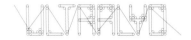

05 Studio Output

06 viagrafik

07 viagrafik

08 Emil Hartvig

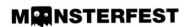

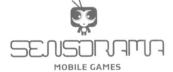

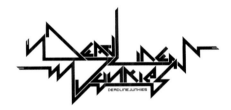

09 Timo Novotny

10 Kallegraphics

11 viagrafik

MONSTERFEST

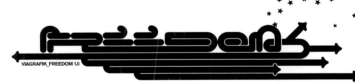

12 Supershapes

13 Adhemas

14 viagrafik

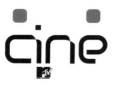

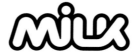

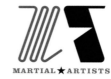

01 Carlos Bêla

02 Plastic Kid

03 Plastic Kid

04 Carsten Raffel

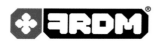

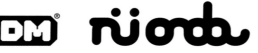

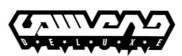

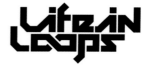

05 viagrafik

06 zinestesia

07 Microbot David Fuhrer

08 Power Graphixx

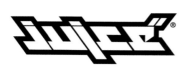

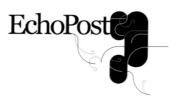

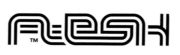

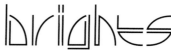

09 viagrafik

10 Dimaquina

11 viagrafik

12 Studio Maverick

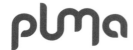

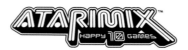

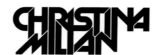

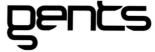

13 Anónimo Studio

14 Polygraph

15 Upnorth

16 Norwegian Ink

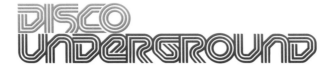

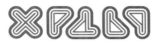

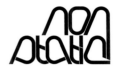

01 Raredrop

02 Laundry

03 Mitch Paone

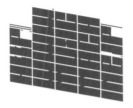

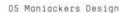

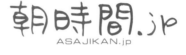

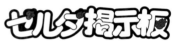

04 Ketchup Arts

05 Maniackers Design

06 Maniackers Design

07 Ketchup Arts

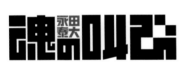

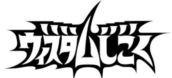

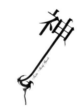

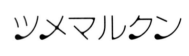

08 Ketchup Arts

09 Raredrop

10 Ketchup Arts

11 Maniackers Design

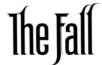

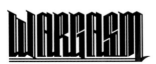

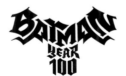

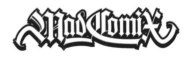

12 344 Design, LLC

13 Tsuyoshi Hirooka

14 Rinzen

15 Mikkel Grafixico Westrup

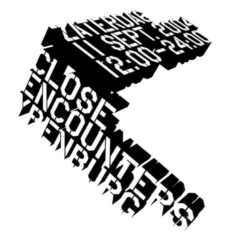

01 Catalogtree

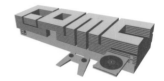

02 viagrafik

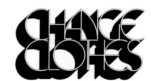

03 Creative Pride

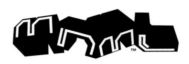

04 viagrafik

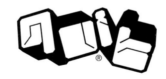

05 Upnorth

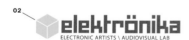

06 zinestesia

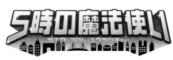

07 Hideaki Komiyama

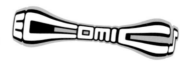

08 Gints Apsits

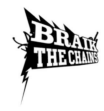

09 Matthias Gephart

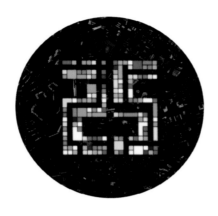

01 Tsuyoshi Kusano Design

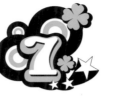

02 anna-OM-line.com

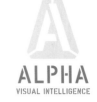

03 archetype : interactive

04 struggle inc.

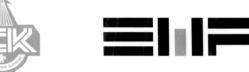

05 Büro Destruct

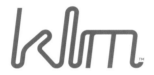

06 blackjune

07 Tnop™ & ®bePOS|+|VE

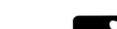

08 Tsuyoshi Kusano Design

09 Faith

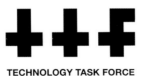

10 asmallpercent

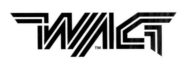

11 viagrafik

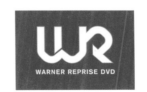

12 Colourmovie

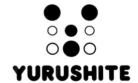

13 Maniackers Design

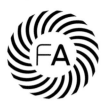

01 Sarah Grimaldi

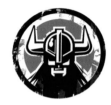

02 Kosta Lazarevski / rdy

03 Carsten Raffel

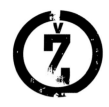

04 Chris Rubino

05 William Morrisey

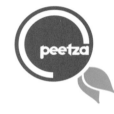

06 viagrafik

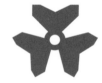

07 the red is love

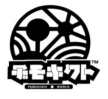

08 Fase

09 automatic

10 Jürgen und ich

11 dainippon

12 2098

13 Studio Maverick

14 Chris Rubino

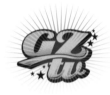

15 Chico Jofilsan

16 Katrin Acklin

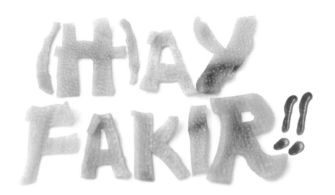

01 Fakir

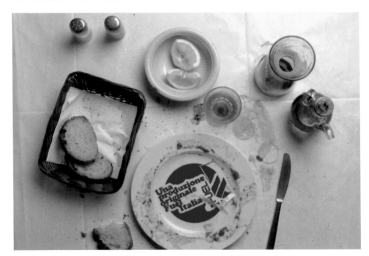

02 zinestesia

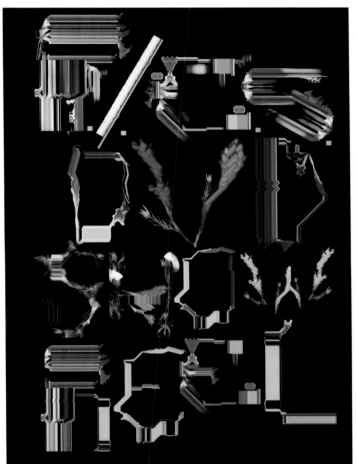

03 Adapter

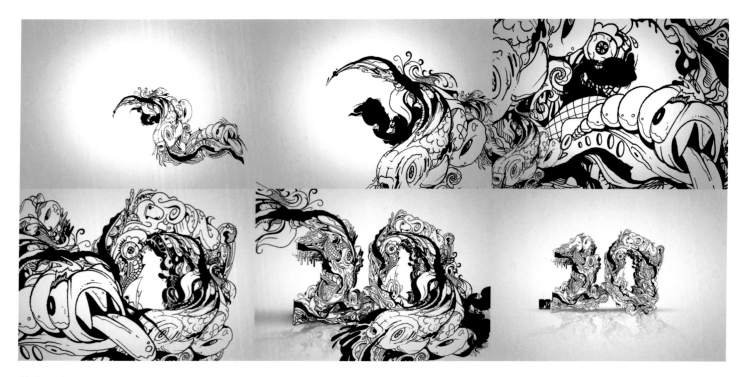

01 Laundry

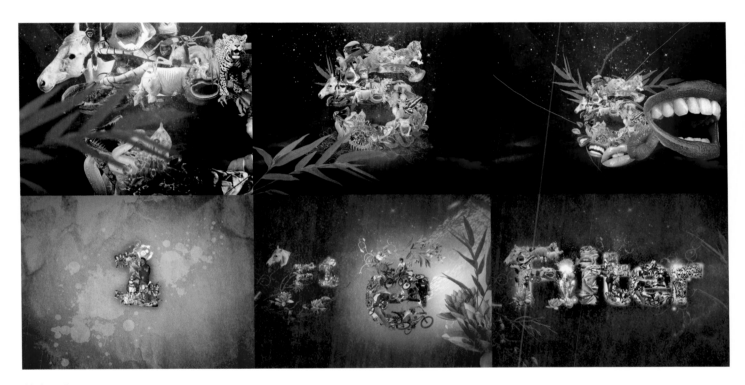

01 Laundry

MUSIC

HOW MANY PEOPLE READY TO ROCK THE HOUSE?

Ask the Gorillaz. The answer from the design scene is unequivocal: "Many!" For the signs of the times once again point toward Rock 'n' Roll, toward the music business. Physical sound storage media are obsolete. Techno is tired. Electronica has retreated into meditative intellectual niches. The consequence for design? The logos are as radically brutal as the sounds are loud. What was typical for Heavy Metal back then is mainstream today.

APPROPRIATION

Designers usurp the symbol.

In the absence of resistance, it happens peacefully: many symbols with conventional content inevitably elude their normal patterns of significance, placed in new contexts by the designers. As components of logos, they suddenly tell completely new stories, ones an indifferent zeitgeist listens to gladly, since popular patterns of behaviour can be derived from them. Preferences for products and services, for example. Under the motto "the pictorial turn," aesthetic theory has investigated whether the image still represents reality realistically, or whether it can do so no longer. In the sphere of private enterprise, designers unavoidably conditioned by pragmatism have long since answered this question.

MONTERREY, MEXICO

AMORFODESIGNLAB

I am a walking disaster.

No, this is not a self-assessment by Mexican designer Ricardo (Rick) Danilo Bracho. It is a motif that appears on one of his countless T-shirt creations, together with flyers and merchandising articles, and worn by internationally known DJs at the hippest parties in every corner of the planet. Entirely consistent with the motto: irony first.

Rick himself is the opposite of depressive, as attested by his life and work philosophy: "My philosophy is balance, to be in equilibrium with myself. Why? It creates harmony, and that is a good feeling. You have to be able to accept the good and the bad and come to terms with both. The simplest things in life are the best. They are the basic concepts. You take it from there, and everything goes right. You have to work hard, of course, but you have to stay relaxed, and allow the ideas to flow in the right direction. You have to be patient, to learn, and to accept risks. Arrogance? It's pointless! Stay humble, but value your own work, help people who need help, they'll do the same for you when you need it."

Rick lives in Monterrey, Mexico's third largest city. He began his career as a designer by working for a number of recognized agencies and design offices in the city: Danilo Black, Zona-Zero, 1:0:1. Apropos 1:0:1. Back then, Rick had already achieved his breakthrough: working in his studio together with his colleagues, he issued Domestica, a cool magazine that set new standards in Mexican graphic design. Especially important for Rick at the time, of course, was "PastillaDigital," an ideal platform for getting international exposure for his own work. His legendary T-shirts, for example.

At some point, Rick – who takes inspiration from music of every conceivable style and type along with street art, contemporary art, philosophy, fast food, film and nature – realised it was time to stand on his own two feet. The result of this decision is called AmorfoDesignlab. A graphic design studio, focused on experimental and commercial design, with a vision: to generate a global presence for his Mexican design team - to work with "turning heads" that combine Mexican culture with international design standards, creating a new graphic language while having an awful lot of fun in the process.

Meanwhile, Rick is in the process of successfully realising his visions. But no longer on his own: after its takeoff phase, his AmorfoDesignlab, together with other designers from Monterrey, founded UDS (United Design Brands). To work in teams has its advantages, Rick believes: with complex projects, each participant is able to bring in his or her own talents and use them to the fullest.

On the topic of the logo, Rick has some good advice on hand: "If you find new ways to communicate the right message, then you have also delivered your own design statement."

MUSIK

HOW MANY PEOPLE READY TO ROCK THE HOUSE?

fragen die Gorillaz. Die Antwort aus der Designerszene ist eindeutig: „Viele!" Denn die Zeichen der Zeit stehen wieder auf Rock 'n' Roll im Musikgeschäft. Die materiellen Tonträger sind obsolet. Techno ist müde. Electronica hat sich in versponnene Intellektuellennischen zurückgezogen. Konsequenz fürs Design? So laut wie der Sound, so radikal brutal die Logos. Was früher Heavy-Metal-typisch war, ist heute Mainstream.

VEREINNAHMUNG

Gestalter usurpieren die Zeichen.

Es geschieht friedlich, weil es keine Gegenwehr gibt: Viele auf tradierte konventionelle Inhalte verweisende Zeichen entziehen sich zwangsläufig ihren eigentlichen Bedeutungsmustern, weil sie von den Gestaltern in neue Kontexte gestellt werden - und dann, als Logos, plötzlich ganz neue Geschichten erzählen, denen der indifferente Zeitgeist gerne zuhört, weil sich aus diesen Geschichten beliebte Handlungsmuster ableiten lassen. Zum Beispiel Präferenzen für Produkte und Dienstleistungen. In der ästhetischen Theorie wird unter dem Motto The Pictorial Turn darüber räsoniert, ob das Bild noch immer eine repräsentative Abbildbeziehung zur Realität hat oder nicht mehr haben kann. Im Umfeld der Marktwirtschaft zwangsläufig auf Pragmatismus konditionierte Gestalter haben diese Frage längst beantwortet.

MONTERREY, MEXIKO

AMORFODESIGNLAB

I am a walking disaster

Nein, das ist keine Selbsteinschätzung des mexikanischen Designers Ricardo - Rick - Danilo Bracho. Es ist das Motiv eines seiner zahllosen T-Shirt-Kreationen, die international bekannte DJs, zusammen mit Flyern und Merchandise-Artikeln, in alle Ecken der Welt zu den angesagtesten Partys getragen haben. Ganz nach der Devise: irony first!

Rick selbst ist das Gegenteil von depressiv, was seine Lebens- und Arbeitsphilosophie bestätigt: „Meine Philosophie ist die Ausgeglichenheit, das mit sich selbst im Gleichgewicht sein. Warum? Es schafft Harmonie - und das ist ein gutes Gefühl. Du musst fähig sein, sowohl die guten wie die schlechten Dinge anzunehmen und damit umgehen. Die einfachsten, simplen Dinge im Leben sind die besten. Es sind die Basiskonzepte. Du nimmst es von dort, und alles läuft rund. Du musst hart arbeiten, klar, aber du musst relaxt bleiben, die Ideen in die richtige Richtung fließen lassen. Du musst geduldig sein, lernen, und auch Risiken eingehen. Arroganz? Bringt gar nichts! Bescheiden bleiben, aber die eigene Arbeit schätzen, Leuten helfen, die Hilfe benötigen, sie werden es zurückgeben, wenn du's mal nötig hast."

Rick ist in Monterrey zu Hause, der drittgrößten Stadt von Mexiko. Seine Karriere als Designer hat er in einigen bekannten Agenturen und Designbüros der Stadt begonnen: Danilo Black, Zona-Zero, 1:0:1. Apropos 1:0:1. Dort schaffte Rick bereits den Durchbruch: Zusammen mit seinen Kollegen hat er in diesem Studio „Domestica" in die Welt gestellt - ein cooles Magazin, das einen neuen Standard im mexikanischen Grafikdesign setzte. Besonders wichtig für Rick war natürlich in dieser Zeit „PastillaDigital": Eine ideale Plattform, um die eigenen Arbeiten in der internationalen Szene bekannt zu machen. Zum Beispiel die legendären T-Shirts (siehe oben).

Dann fand Rick, der sich neben Street Art, zeitgenössischer Kunst, Philosophie, Fast Food, Film und der Natur von der Musik in allen möglichen Stilarten und Ausdrucksformen inspirieren lässt, also dann fand es Rick irgendwann an der Zeit sich auf eigene Füße zu stellen. Das Resultat dieses Entschlusses heißt AmorfoDesignlab. Ein auf experimentelles u n d kommerzielles Design fokussiertes Grafikdesignstudio mit einer Vision: Präsenz für die mexikanische Designszene in der ganzen Welt zu generieren - mit „turning heads"-Arbeiten, welche die mexikanische Kultur mit internationalen Designstandards kombinieren, eine neue grafische Sprache zu kreieren und dabei, ja, jede Menge Spaß zu haben.

Mittlerweile ist Rick mit Erfolg dabei seine Vision umzusetzen. Aber nicht mehr allein: Nach der Anfangsphase hat sein AmorfoDesignlab zusammen mit anderen Designern aus Monterrey UDS (United Design Brands) gegründet. Im Team arbeiten bringt Vorteile, meint Rick: Jeder kann bei komplexen Projekten seine eigenen Talente einbringen und voll ausleben.

Zum Thema Logo hat Rick einen guten Rat auf Lager: „Wenn du neue Wege findest, die richtige Message zu kommunizieren, dann hast du soeben dein Statement im Design abgegeben."

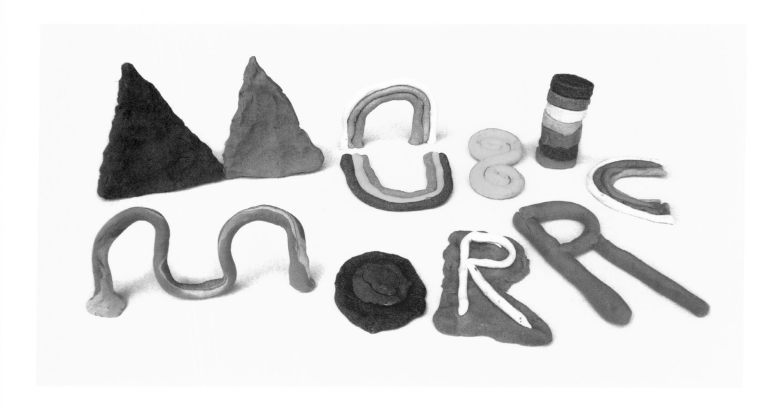

01 human empire

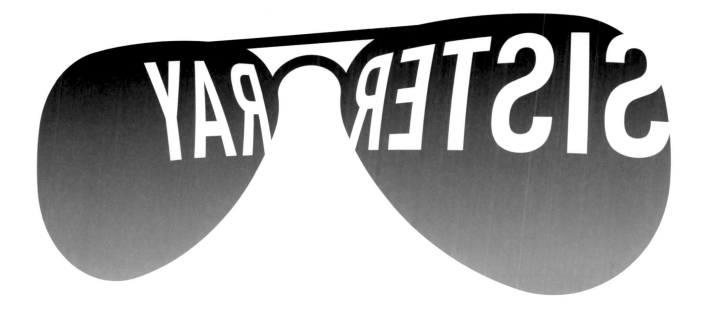

01 Sagmeister Inc.

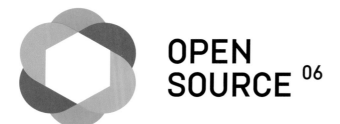

01 Bionic Systems

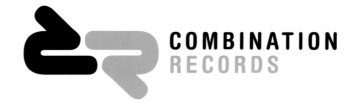

02 Zeek&Destroy

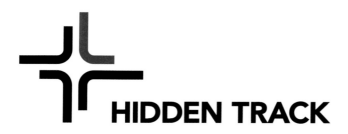

03 blackjune

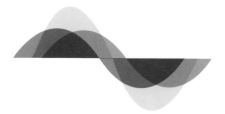

04 multifresh

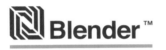

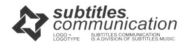

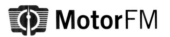

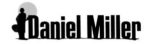

01 Engine   02 Engine   03 Dirk Rudolph   04 Jason Kochis

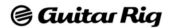

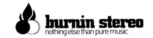

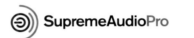

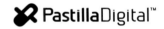

05 Pfadfinderei   06 Labooo   07 Studio Output   08 AmorfoDesignlab™

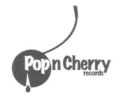

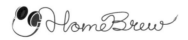

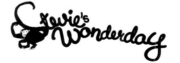

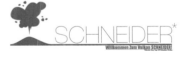

09 johnjayart.com   10 DTM_INC   11 Zeek&Destroy   12 Ketchup Arts

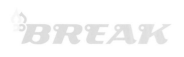

01 Pfadfinderei

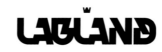

02 Attak

03 Pfadfinderei

04 Braveland Design

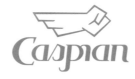

05 onrushdesign / front

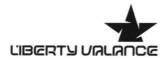

06 Attak

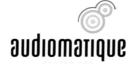

07 weissraum.de(sign)

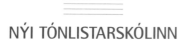

08 310k

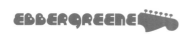

09 johnjayart.com

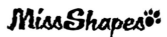

10 jl-prozess

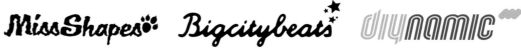

11 Borsellino & Co.

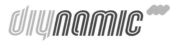

12 Axel Domke

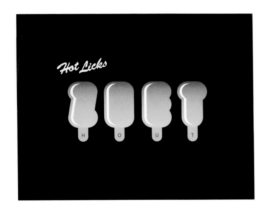

01 Niels Shoe Meulman

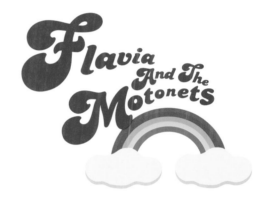

02 Gastón Caba

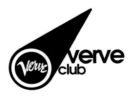

03 Dirk Rudolph

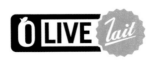

04 Blindresearch

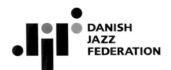

05 re-public

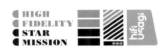

06 Ashi & office Greminger

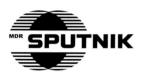

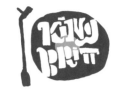

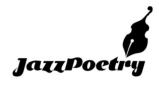

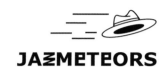

01 Pfadfinderei

02 struggle inc.

03 Attak

04 Ottograph

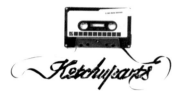

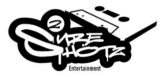

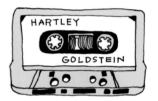

05 Ketchup Arts

06 Kosta Lazarevski / rdy

07 Ottograph

08 Keren Richter

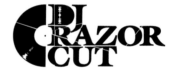

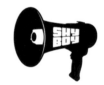

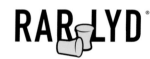

09 Emmi Salonen

10 Die Seiner

11 ZIP Design

12 Designbolaget

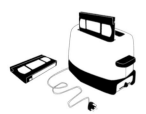

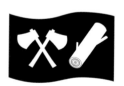

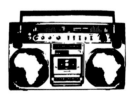

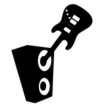

13 Plastic Kid

14 Jonas Vögeli

15 struggle inc.

16 Instant

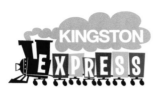

01 112 Ocean Drive

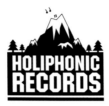

02 Tado

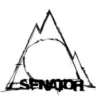

03 Jussi Jääskeläinen

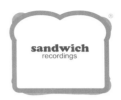

04 Mattisimo

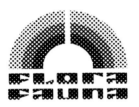

05 frans carlquist

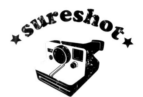

06 Annabelle Mehraein

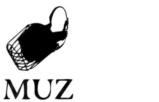

07 National Forest

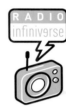

08 jum

09 Out Of Order

10 DTM_INC

11 luca Marchettoni

12 Kosta Lazarevski / rdy

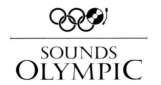

13 Visual Mind Rockets

14 Georg Schatz

15 Akira Sasaki

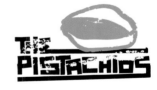
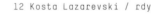

16 Jawa and Midwich

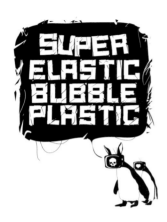

02 Kingsize

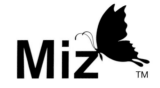

03 Laurent Fétis

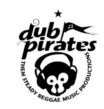

04 artless Inc

01 Superexpresso

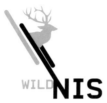

05 raum mannheim

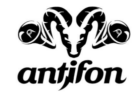

06 backyard 10

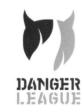

07 Floor Wesseling Ix Opus

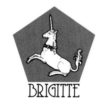

08 jl-prozess

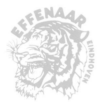

09 space3

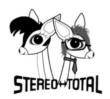

10 Cabine

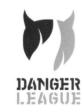

11 clandrei

12 Semisans

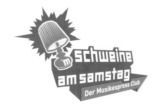

13 backyard 10

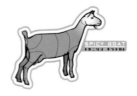

14 Ottograph

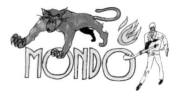

15 Dennis Eriksson

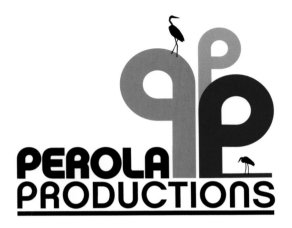

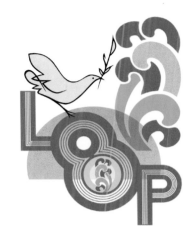

01 inkgraphix

02 Studio Oscar

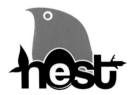

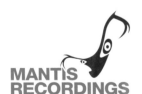

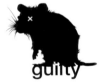

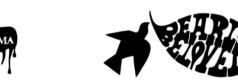

03 Povilas Utovka

04 Maya Hayuk

05 desres design group

06 radargraphics

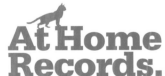

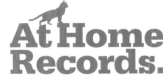

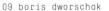

07 Ninjacruise

08 Studio Output

09 boris dworschak

10 Superexpresso

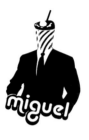

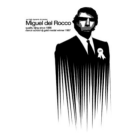

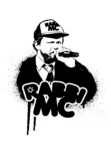

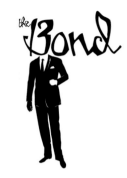

01 Labooo

02 Labooo

03 Fluid Creativity

04 Discodoener

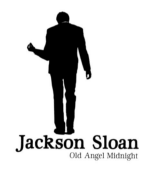

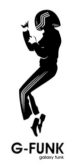

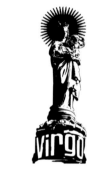

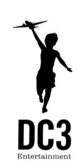

05 Gianni Rossi

06 Michaël Pinto

07 La Fusée

08 Supershapes

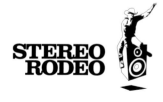

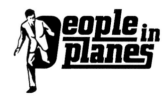

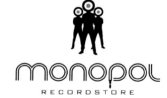

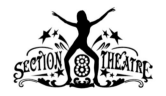

09 Kallegraphics

10 Airside

11 Studio Output

12 Labor für visuelles Wachstum™

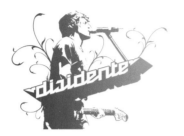

01 MH grafik

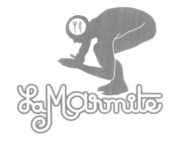

02 Atelier Télescopique

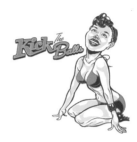

03 Ashi & office Greminger

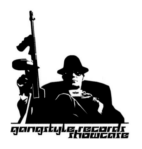

04 Attak

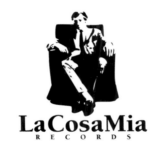

05 Zeek&Destroy

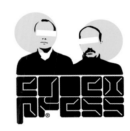

06 viagrafik

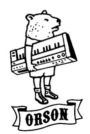

07 andrew rae

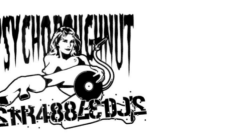
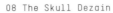

08 The Skull Dezain

09 Positron

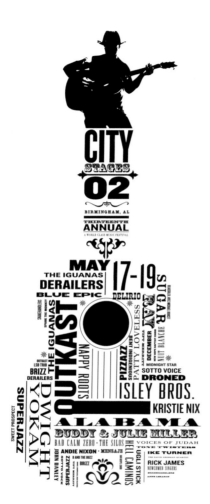

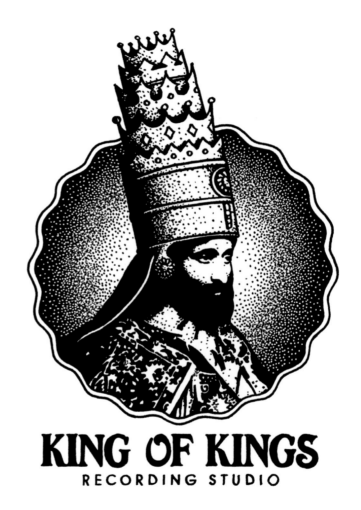

01 iaah

02 Finsta

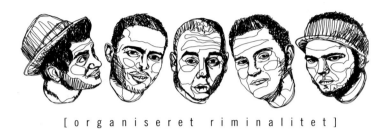

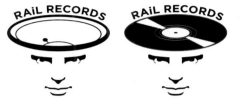

01 Mikkel Grafixico Westrup

02 Resin[sistem] design

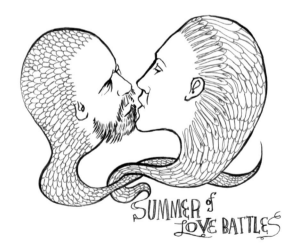

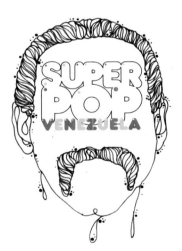

03 Maya Hayuk

04 Masa

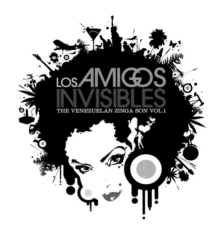

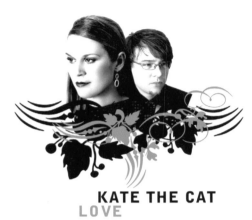

01 Masa

02 Le_Palmier Design

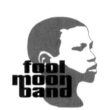

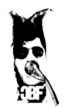

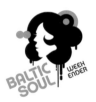

03 Emil Hartvig

04 Roya Hamburger

05 Konstantinos Gargaletsos

06 Le_Palmier Design

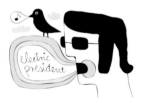

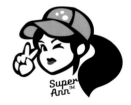

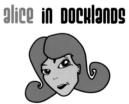

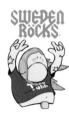

07 human empire

08 kame design

09 Ottograph

10 Raffaele Primitivo

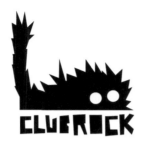

01 ZIP Design

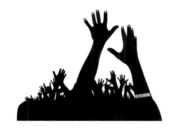

02 Stockbridge International

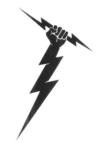

03 Attak

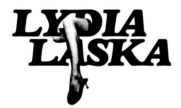

04 Norwegian Ink

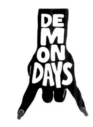

05 Parra

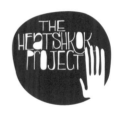

06 Alëxone

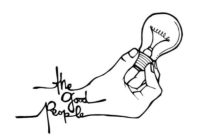

07 Sellout Industries

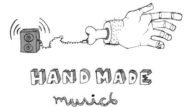

08 Tohyto

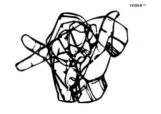

09 jewboy Corporation™

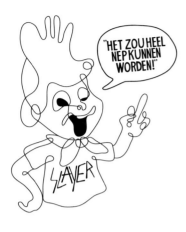

01 Parra

02 DTM_INC

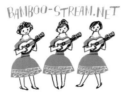

05 Naho Ogawa

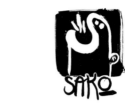

03 Dimaquina

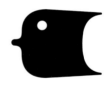

06 112 Ocean Drive

04 Alëxone

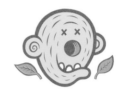

07 Dennis Worden

08 ZIP Design

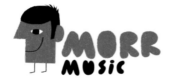

09 human empire

10 Crush Design

11 nem

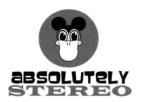

12 Ottograph

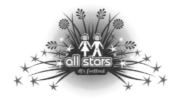

13 Catalina Estrada Uribe

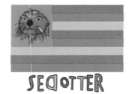

14 dynamo-ville

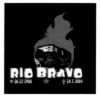

15 formdusche

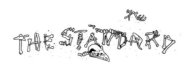

01 tstout inc.

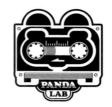

02 Form

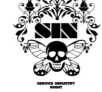

03 Fase

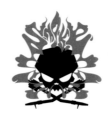

04 Raffaele Primitivo

05 Raffaele Primitivo

06 Studio Output

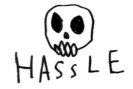

07 Supermundane

08 Chris Bolton

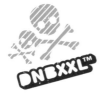

09 Engine

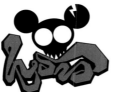

10 Raffaele Primitivo

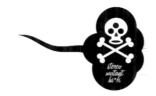

11 Dr. Alderete

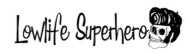

12 Jason Kochis

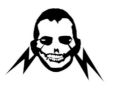

13 Positron

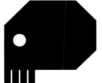

14 nem

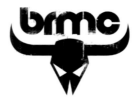

15 Attak

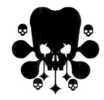

16 dzgnbio

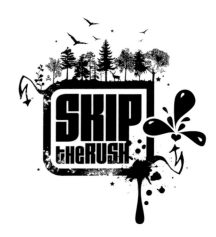

01 Hypnoteis

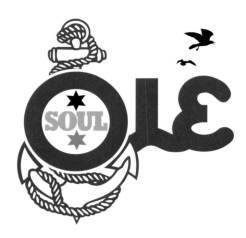

02 Discodoener

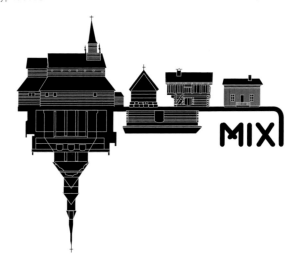

03 newoslo

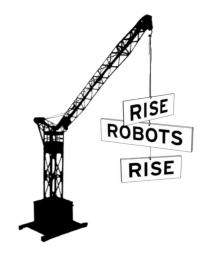

04 red design

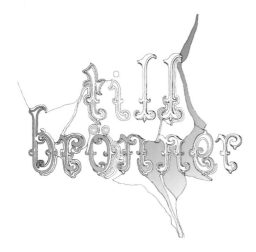

01 Dirk Rudolph

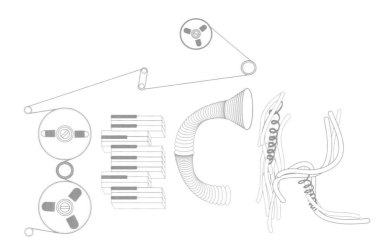

02 evaq studio

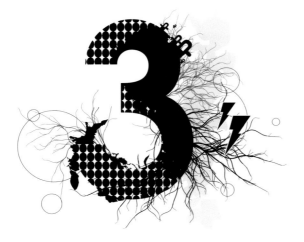

03 AmorfoDesignlab™

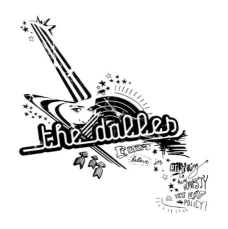

04 3 deluxe

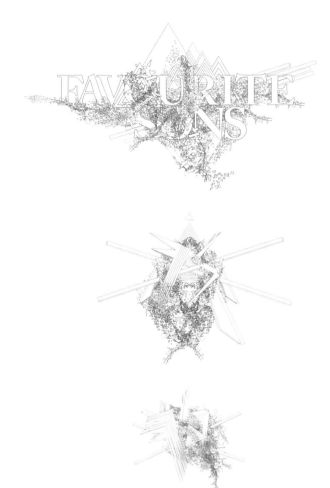

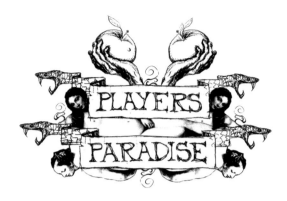

02 Jussi Jääskeläinen

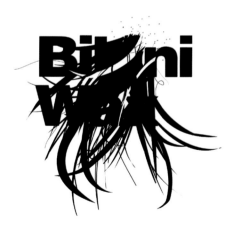

01 lifelong friendship society

03 Chris Bolton

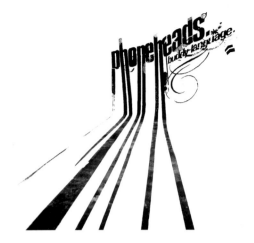

01 Zeek&Destroy

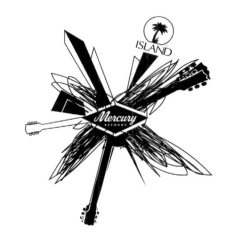

02 Le_Palmier Design

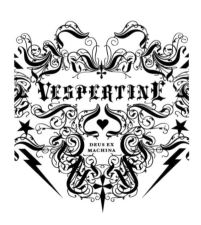

03 Stolen Inc.

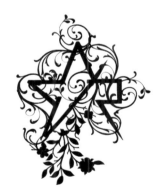

04 Dirk Rudolph

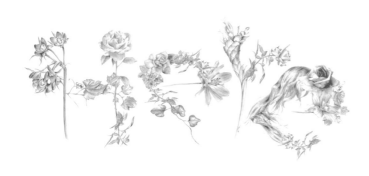

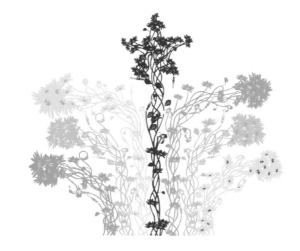

01 Adapter

02 ZIP Design

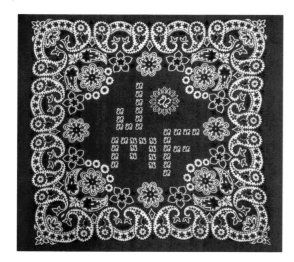

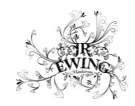

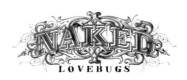

04 Martin Kvamme

05 Büro Destruct

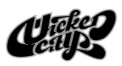

03 Maya Hayuk

06 Out Of Order

07 Yoshi Tajima

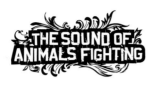

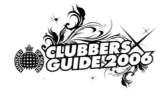

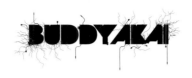

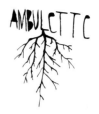

01 Cape Arcona Typefoundry

02 Engine

03 AmorfoDesignlab™

04 Ohio Girl Design

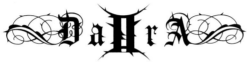

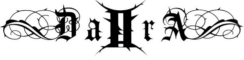

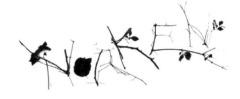

05 Miha Artnak

06 Zeek&Destroy

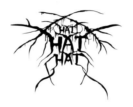

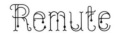

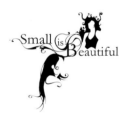

07 Martin Kvamme

08 Grandpeople

09 ROM studio

10 zookeeper

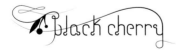

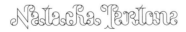

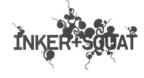

11 ROM studio

12 Atelier télescopique

13 zucker und pfeffer

14 Carlos Bêla

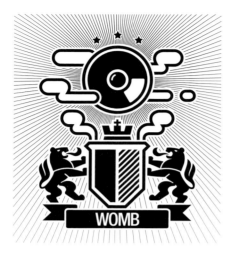

01 Power Graphixx

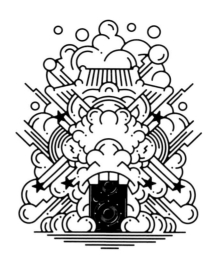

02 Tsuyoshi Hirooka

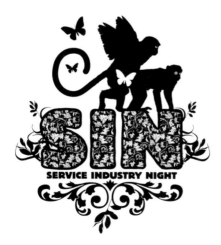

03 Studio Output

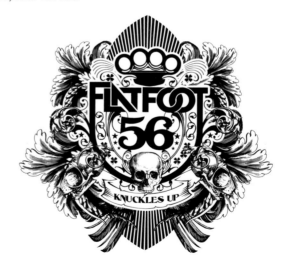

04 Hydro74

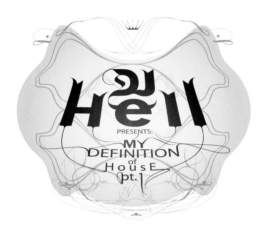

01 Herbert Baglione

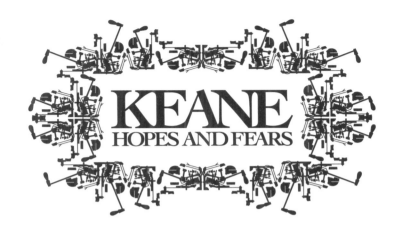

02 Moving Brands

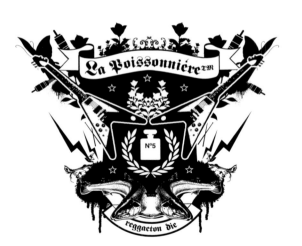

03 No-Domain

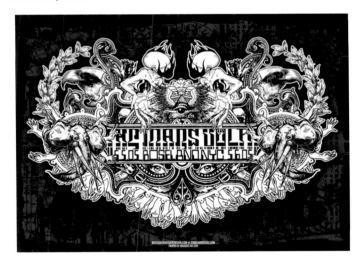

04 Jared Connor

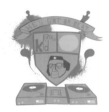

01 No-Domain

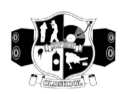

02 Anónimo Studio

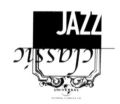

03 DTM_INC

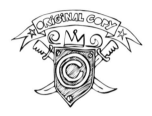

04 Karoly Kiralyfalvi

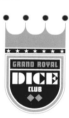

05 Braveland Design

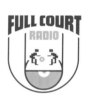

06 Braveland Design

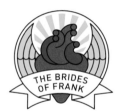

07 Rinzen

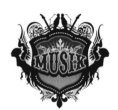

08 Le_Palmier Design

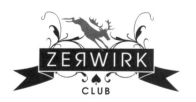

09 C100

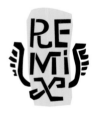

10 Hula Hula

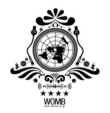

11 Hideaki Komiyama

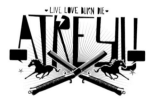

12 Plastic Kid

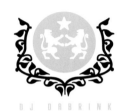

01 weissraum.de(sign)

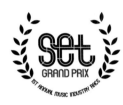

02 Yorgo Tloupas

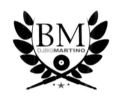

03 Dimomedia Lab

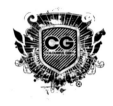

04 Salon Vektoria

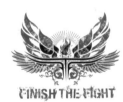

05 Keep Adding

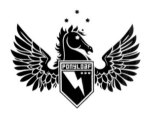

06 Rinzen

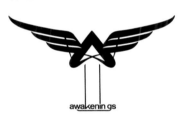

07 ehquestionmark

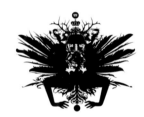

08 Joe A. Scerri

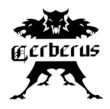

09 Barbara (Babsi) Lippe

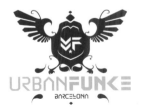

10 Inocuodesign

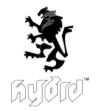

11 Raffaele Primitivo

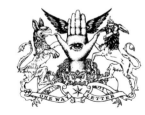

12 Jason Kochis

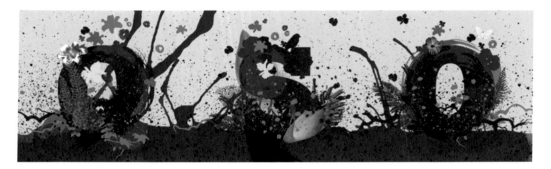

01 red design

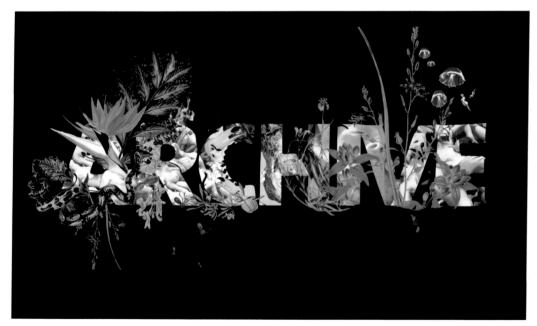

02 Insect Design

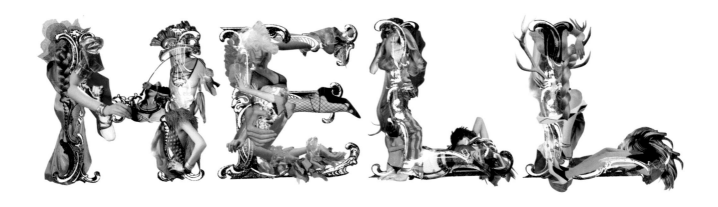

01 Yoshi Tajima

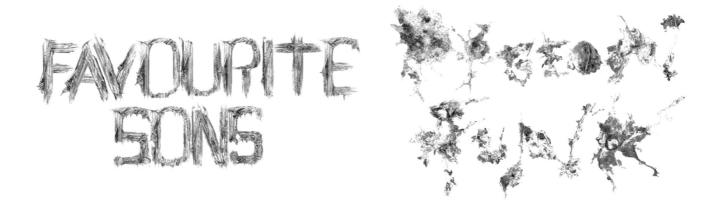

02 lifelong friendship society

03 Slang

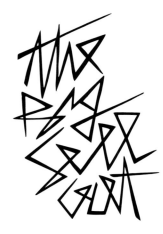

01 Parra

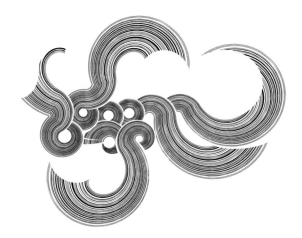

02 Inocuodesign

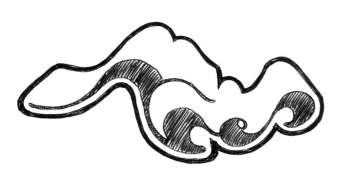

03 ehquestionmark

04 ehquestionmark

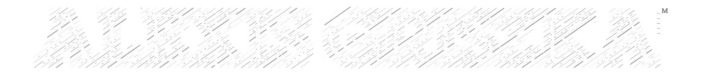

01 cabina

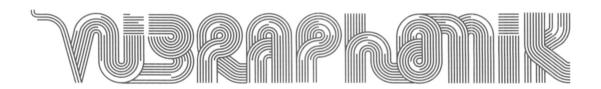

02 Tohyto

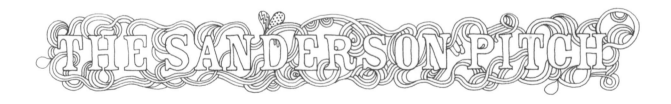

03 ZIP Design

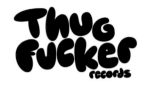

01 Laundry

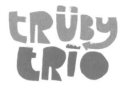

02 Nish

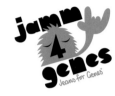

03 struggle inc.

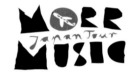

04 jeremyville

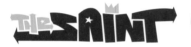

05 Sellout Industries

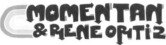

06 Sellout Industries

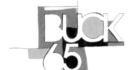

07 human empire

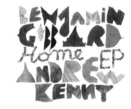

08 human empire

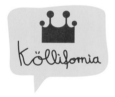

09 christian walden

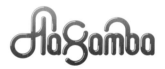

10 Hugh Morse

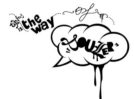

11 inkgraphix

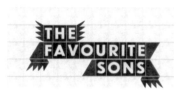

12 lifelong friendship society

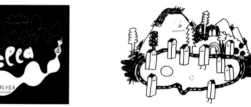
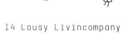

13 human empire

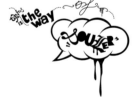

14 Lousy Livincompany

15 the red is love

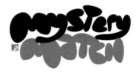

16 Grandpeople

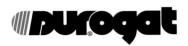

01 Hyl Design

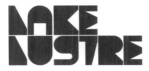

02 red design

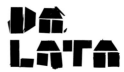

03 Joe A. Scerri

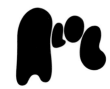

04 Crush Design

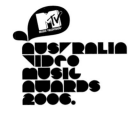

05 viagrafik

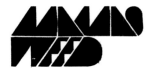

06 Neubau.

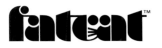

07 viagrafik

08 Grandpeople

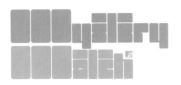

09 Umeric

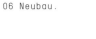

10 Engine

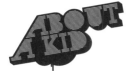

11 typotherapy+design inc.

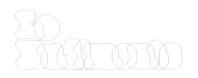

12 typotherapy+design inc.

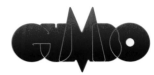

13 Laundry

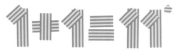

14 viagrafik

15 Miha Artnak

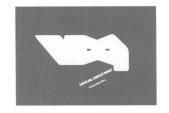

16 Ketchup Arts

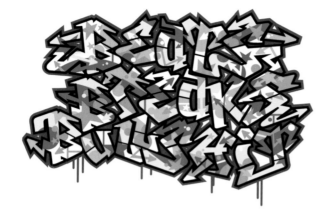

01 DTM_INC

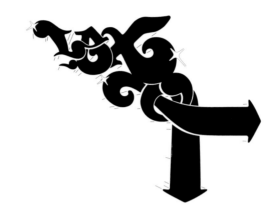

02 ehquestionmark

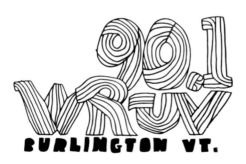

03 tstout inc.

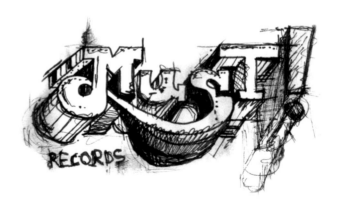

04 Jussi Jääskeläinen

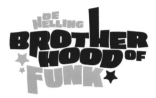

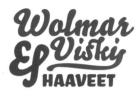

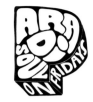

01 Out Of Order

02 Pietari Posti

03 Parra

04 Parra

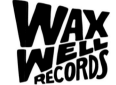

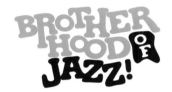

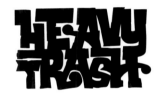

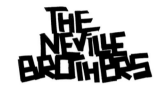

05 Parra

06 Out Of Order

07 Rinzen

08 JDK

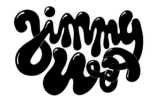

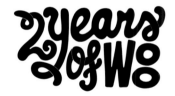

09 Parra

10 Parra

11 Parra

12 Nonstop

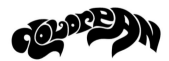

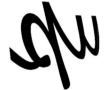

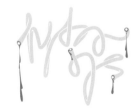

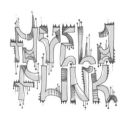

13 tstout inc.

14 Oliver Kartak

15 Raffaele Primitivo

16 struggle inc.

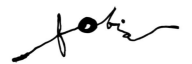

01 Hula Hula

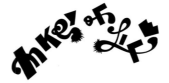

02 A-Side Studio

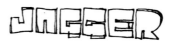

03 the red is love

clandrei

04 clandrei

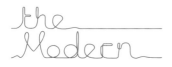

05 Form

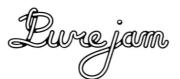

06 nem

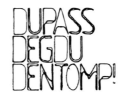

07 Kallegraphics

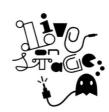

08 the red is love

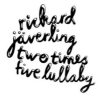

09 PMKFA

10 No-Domain

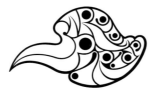

11 Hausgrafik

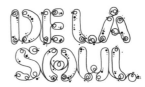

12 Masa

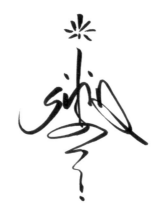

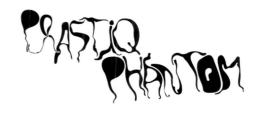

01 usugrow

02 Nando Costa

03 stylorouge

04 Akiza

05 Martin Kvamme

06 Akiza

07 Cape Arcona Typefoundry

08 derfaber

09 Nohemi Dicuru

10 Sammy Stein

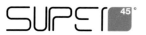

01 Flavio Bagioli

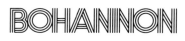

02 C100

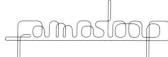

03 Keloide.net

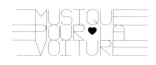

04 Codeluxe

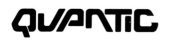

05 red design

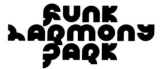

06 Systm

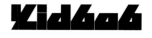

07 Slang

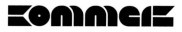

08 Pfadfinderei

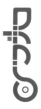

09 Magenta Creative Networks

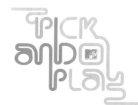

10 :phunk studio

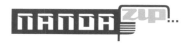
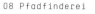
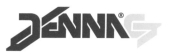

11 Axel Domke

12 Bionic Systems

13 viagrafik

14 Alexander Wise

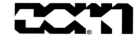

15 viagrafik

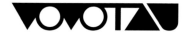

16 Positron

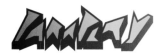

01 Grandpeople

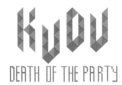

02 evaq studio

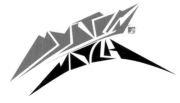

03 Laundry

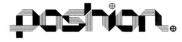

04 Creative Pride

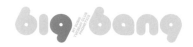

05 QuickHoney

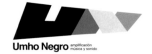

06 Flavio Bagioli

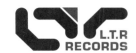

07 dzgnbio

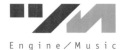

08 Engine

09 Hyl Design

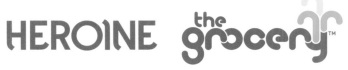

10 Mattisimo

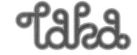

11 AmorfoDesignlab™

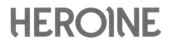

12 Yuu Imokawa

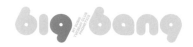

13 yippieyeah cooperative

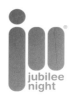

01 Tilt

02 Pep Karsten

03 Oliver Kartak

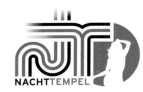

04 Out Of Order

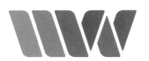

05 Maniackers Design

06 archetype : interactive

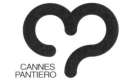

07 Tabas

08 Hyl Design

09 archetype : interactive

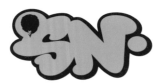

10 Out Of Order

11 desres design group

12 radargraphics

13 DesignChapel

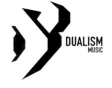

14 weissraum.de(sign)

15 Attak

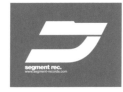

16 Pep Karsten

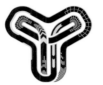

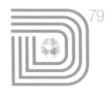

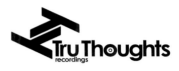

01 Magenta Creative Networks

02 CityDeep Music

03 weissraum.de(sign)

04 red design

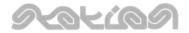

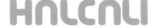

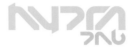

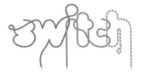

05 Hyl Design

06 Form

07 Raffaele Primitivo

08 Studio Output

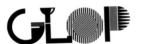

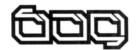

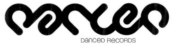
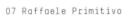
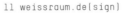

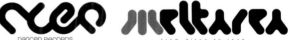

09 No-Domain

10 dzgnbio

11 weissraum.de(sign)

12 Ketchup Arts

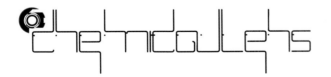

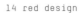

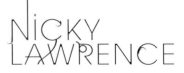

13 SignalStrong

14 red design

15 typotherapy+design inc.

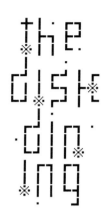

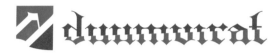

03 dzgnbio

01 ten_do_ten

02 ten_do_ten

04 the wilderness

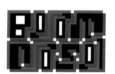

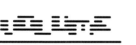

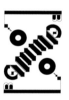

05 Floor Wesseling Ix Opus

06 resistro®

07 Syrup Helsinki

08 Resin[sistem] design

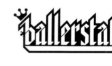

09 Tohyto

10 viagrafik

11 JDK

12 Raffaele Primitivo

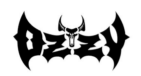

01 Jason Kochis

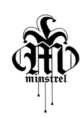

02 Floor Wesseling Ix Opus

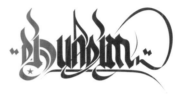

03 Inocuodesign

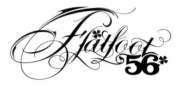

04 Hydro74

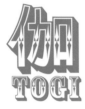

05 Yuu Imokawa

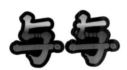

06 dainippon

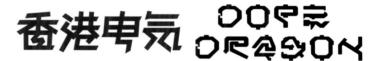

07 archetype : interactive

08 apishAngel

09 Ketchup Arts

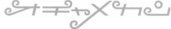

10 Raredrop

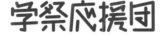

11 Raredrop

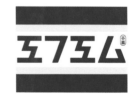

12 Raredrop

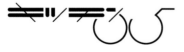

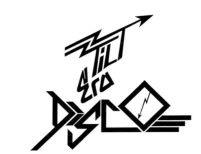

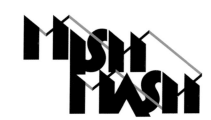

01 Raffaele Primitivo

02 Dan Sparkes

03 Insect

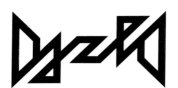

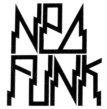

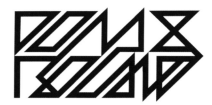

04 Atelier télescopique

05 Raffaele Primitivo

06 Raffaele Primitivo

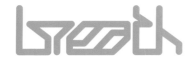

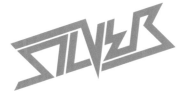

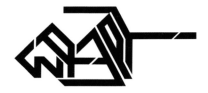

07 Raffaele Primitivo

08 Raffaele Primitivo

09 Dan Sparkes

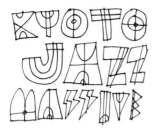

01 struggle inc.

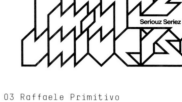

02 Hiroki Tsukuda

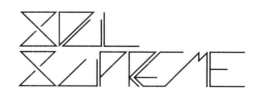

03 Raffaele Primitivo

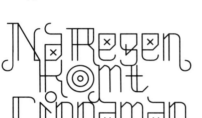

04 News

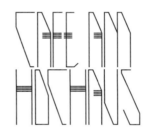

05 C100

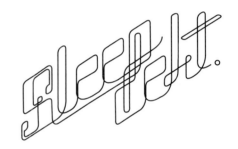

06 No-Domain

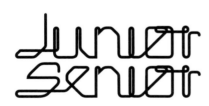

07 PMKFA

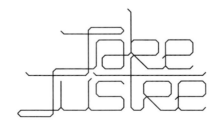

08 Joe A. Scerri

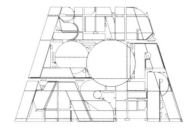

09 PMKFA

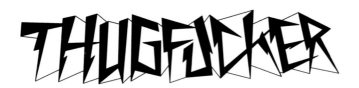

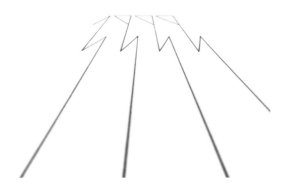

01 Nish

02 Vår

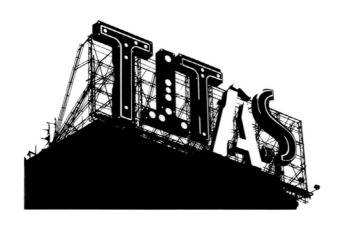

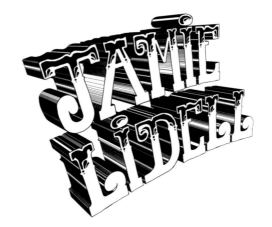

03 resistro®

04 Dan Sparkes

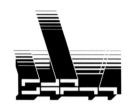

01 ehquestionmark

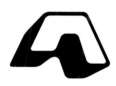

02 ehquestionmark

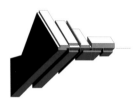

03 Laurent Fétis

04 Laurent Fétis

05 frans carlquist

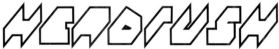

06 DTM_INC

07 PMKFA

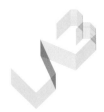

08 eduhirama

09 Studio Output

10 Nish

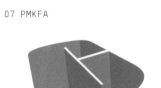

11 Sesame Studio

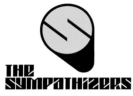

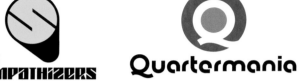

01 Attak

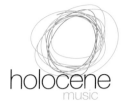

02 Cape Arcona Typefoundry

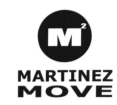

03 multifresh

04 Ottograph

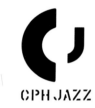

CPH JAZZ

05 Hellebek + Lemvig

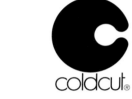

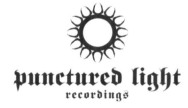

06 viagrafik

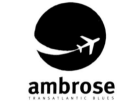

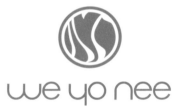

07 raum mannheim

08 Carsten Giese

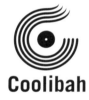

Coolibah

09 backyard 10

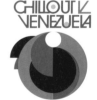

10 Engine

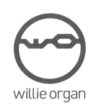

11 GrafficTraffic

12 Maniackers Design

IN FOCUS

13 weissraum.de(sign)

14 Kasia Korczak / SLAVS

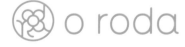

15 Masa

16 resistro®

01 Engine

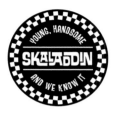

02 viagrafik

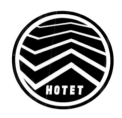

03 Station

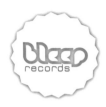

04 DigitalPlayground Studio

05 Axel Domke

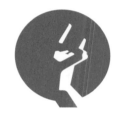

06 Tsuyoshi Kusano Design

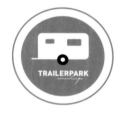

07 Rune Mortensen

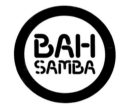

08 red design

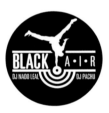

09 resistro®

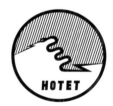

10 Station

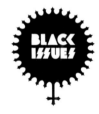

11 Grandpeople

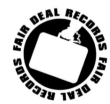

12 space3

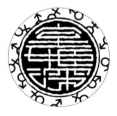

13 Jun Watanabe

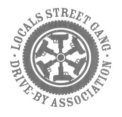

14 Mikkel Grafixico Westrup

15 Sagmeister Inc.

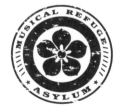

16 Engine

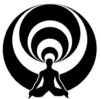

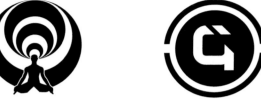

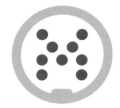

01 strange//attraktor: 02 Danny Franzreb   03 Engine   04 Studio Output

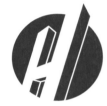

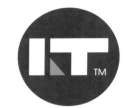

05 Semisans   06 onrushdesign / front   07 precursor   08 News

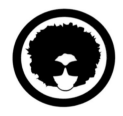

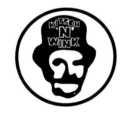

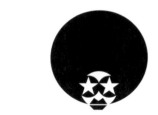

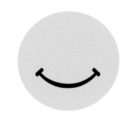

09 Salon Vektoria   10 Crush   11 Tilt   12 onrushdesign / front

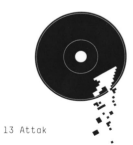

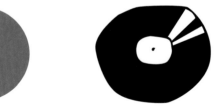

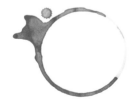

13 Attak   14 310k   15 No-Domain   16 ehquestionmark

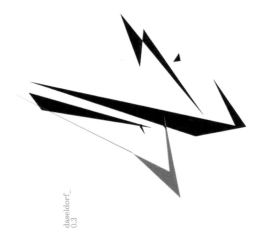

daseldorf_
0.3

01 Accept & Proceed

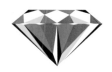

02 Team Manila

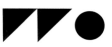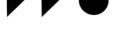

03 Paul Snowden

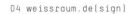

04 weissraum.de(sign)

05 News

06 Formgeber

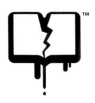

07 Labor f. visuelles Wachstum™

08 Le_Palmier Design

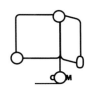

09 hintzegruppen

10 Nando Costa

11 GillespieFox

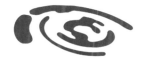

12 Labor f. visuelles Wachstum™   13 Lorenzo Geiger

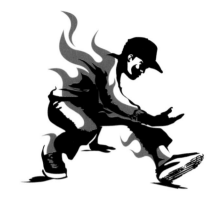

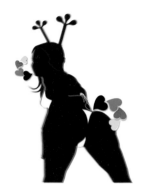

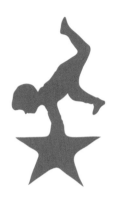

01 Michaël Pinto

02 Floor Wesseling Ix Opus

03 luca Marchettoni

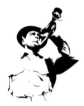

04 Attak

05 Gianni Rossi

06 Raffaele Primitivo

07 News

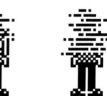
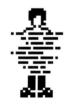
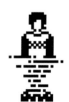
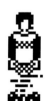
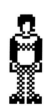

08 Tsuyoshi Hirooka

01 Miha Artnak

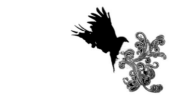

02 raum mannheim

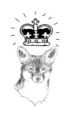

03 Sammy Stein

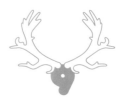

04 yippieyeah cooperative

05 clandrei

06 Miha Artnak

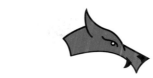

07 Kjetil Vatne

08 Le_Palmier Design

09 Zeek&Destroy

10 Raffaele Primitivo

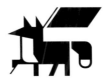

11 frans carlquist

12 AmorfoDesignlab™

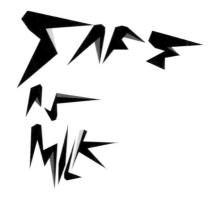

01 Grandpeople

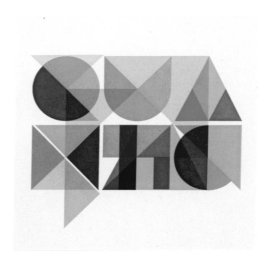

02 red design

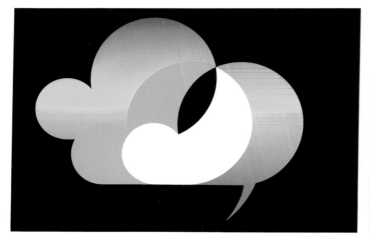

03 Pfadfinderei

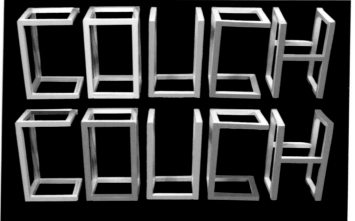

04 human empire

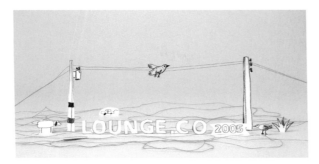

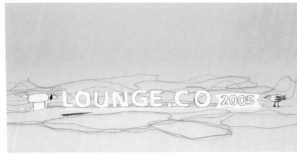

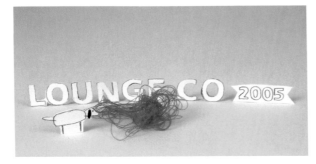

01 Cuartopiso

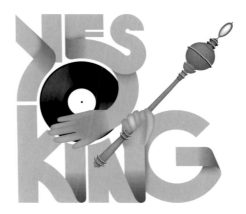

02 PMKFA

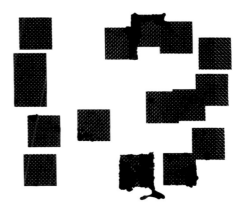

03 Tsuyoshi Hirooka

OTHER, ART, UNCLASSIFIABLE

CREATIVE SPACES HAVE NO BOUNDARIES

To arrange something, to manifest something where earlier there was nothing at all. To question the grammar of symbolic language and turn it on its head. To hazard experiments where the results may be without purpose – but never without meaning. 2,300 years ago, Plato wrote that "concealed deep within each object is the idea of that object, its essence."

"ANYTHING GOES" DOESN'T WORK

A ban on images.

By now, the "anything goes" discourse has gathered dust. Postmodernist arbitrariness is no longer in pristine condition. But what to do when the inventory of theory offers no new hats to wear? You just don the old one! You quote and recycle, help yourself to this or that, turning first this way, than that - until you stumble upon certain cultural limits that have suddenly become more distinct. The so-called new seriousness is cheerfully foiled - both formally and experimentally. Yet a political correctness rooted in a genuine social background can occasionally generate empty space, where symbols or images can no longer penetrate.

CARLOS BÊLA

Without design, there is no life at all.

São Paulo is Brazil's financial and cultural heart, and this is where Carlos Bêla lives and creates. A designer active in numerous disciplines, he has issued a statement that reads like a manifesto: "Design has become fundamental to our lives. There is no life any longer without design. There is no turning back from this fact. Design is everywhere, in everything we touch, see… or hear. Music is also design."

Carlos was born in 1974 and earned a diploma from the College of Fine Arts of the FAAP (Fundação Armando Alvares Penteado). In 1995, he began his professional career in motion graphics with the promo team of MTV Brazil. Alongside his work in video, animation and film, Carlos also created the program's logo. The logo is an important subject for him. Ever since his college days, he has enjoyed developing logos, sometimes even inventing visual identities for imaginary clients. "I believe that a logo is the soul of a graphic project. When I create a logo, I relate it to ideas that contribute to the visual identity and complement the overall concept."

After years of working in motion graphics, Carlos automatically perceives movement in every design: "When I design a logo, I already see how it would behave as an animation, even if it is intended for print media."

Since 2000, Carlos also entertains a professional association with the design and animation studios of Lobo, for whom he has realised numerous projects, among others Diesel, Panasonic, Nike, Nickelodeon, Coca-Cola, Cartoon Network, Budweiser, Volkswagen, Viva Channel and MTV International. Offering creative design solutions and animations for well-known agencies and television stations are among his current professional activities.

Which leaves his own projects. Provocative experiments that acknowledge no boundaries between design, art, and music, resonate strongly in the global art and design scenes, and have been featured in major publications. Among these are Shots, Stash, Flips, +81, Designplex (Japan), as well as numerous books published by Die Gestalten Verlag (Los Logos, 72 dpi Anime, Brazil Inspired, Disorder in Progress, Latino, On Air). Carlos' works were shown at ResFest and the Sundance Film Festival. He has received awards twice at the Bienal de Design Gráfico Brasileiro, as well as from One Show and BDA, among others. One highlight of his experimental works is the Projecto Golden Shower - an homage to 1980s pop culture.

And how does Carlos view his own creations? What matters to him in his own work? "I don't really have a personal philosophy that guides me when doing my projects. However, an issue which I consider to be of the utmost importance in the execution of my work is the concept - that is, the idea behind the design. I think that the concept is essential, and I always flee from "eye candy" projects where certain shapes or colours are selected purely for their effect and appearance."

ANDERE, KUNST, UNKLASSIFIZIERBAR

GESTALTERISCHE RÄUME SIND GRENZENLOS

Dort etwas arrangieren, manifestieren, wo vorher nichts war. Die Grammatik der Zeichensprache hinterfragen und ad absurdum führen. Experimente wagen, deren Resultate vielleicht zweck-, aber alles andere als sinn-los sind. „Tief in jedem Ding verborgen ist die Idee dieses Dings oder seine Essenz". Hat Plato gesagt. Vor 2300 Jahren.

ALLES GEHT GEHT NICHT

Bildverbot.

Der Anything-Goes-Diskurs ist mittlerweile etwas angestaubt. Die postmoderne Beliebigkeit nicht mehr in ganz taufrischem Zustand. Doch was tun, wenn es keinen neuen Hut im Laden der Theorien gibt? Man setzt sich prompt den alten auf! Man zitiert und recyclet, bedient sich hier und dort, wandelt um und wandelt ab - bis man an gewisse kulturelle Grenzen stößt, die plötzlich deutlicher geworden sind. Die sogenannte neue Ernsthaftigkeit wird gerne konterkariert - formal und experimentell. Doch die über einen realen gesellschaftlichen Hintergrund verfügende politische Korrektheit kann manchmal auch Leerräume generieren, in die keine Zeichen und Bilder mehr eindringen.

SAO PAULO, BRASILIEN

CARLOS BÊLA

Es gibt kein Leben ohne Design.

Sao Paulo, das wirtschaftliche und kulturelle Herz von Brasilien. Hier lebt und kreiert Carlos Bela. Ein in vielen Disziplinen arbeitender Gestalter mit einem Statement, das sich wie ein Manifest liest: „Design ist zu einem fundamentalen Element unseres Lebens geworden. Es gibt kein Leben mehr ohne Design. Das ist eine unumkehrbare Entwicklung. Design ist überall, in allem, was wir berühren, sehen ... oder hören. Musik ist ebenfalls Design."

Carlos, Jahrgang 1974, der ein Diplom am College of Fine Arts der FAAP (Fundação Armando Alvares Penteado) erworben hat, begann 1995 seine berufliche Laufbahn mit Motion Graphics im Promoteam von MTV Brazil. Neben seiner Arbeit mit Video, Animation und Film hat Carlos auch das Logo des Senders kreiert. Logos sind für ihn ein wichtiges Thema. Seit seiner Collegezeit entwickelt Carlos gerne Logos und dachte sich gelegentlich auch neue visuelle Identitäten für imaginäre Kunden aus. „Ich denke, das Logo ist die Seele eines grafischen Projekts. Wenn ich ein Logo kreiere, dann ordne ich ihm Ideen zu, die in die visuelle Identität einfließen können und dazu beitragen, das generelle Konzept zu vervollständigen." Nach zehn Jahren Motion Graphics sieht Carlos in jedem Design automatisch die Bewegung: „Während der Gestaltung eines Logos erkenne ich bereits, wie es sich in animierter Form verhält - selbst wenn es nur für den Printbereich bestimmt ist."

Seit 2000 ist Carlos mit den Design- und Animationsstudios von Lobo beruflich verbunden, mit denen er zahlreiche Projekte für u. a. Diesel, Panasonic, Nike, Nickelodeon, Coca Cola, Cartoon Network, Budweiser, Volkswagen, Viva Channel und MTV International realisierte. Kreative Designlösungen und Animationen für bekannte Agenturen und TV-Stationen gehören zu seinen beruflichen Aktivitäten.

Und da sind da noch die eigenen Projekte. Spannende Experimente, in denen es zwischen Design, Kunst und Musik keine Grenzen gibt, die in der globalen Kunst- und Designszene auf Resonanz stoßen und Thema in wichtigen Publikationen waren. Dazu gehören Shots, Stash, Flips, +81, Designplex (Japan), sowie zahlreiche Bücher des Gestalten Verlags (Los Logos, 72 dpi Anime, Brasil Inspired, Disorder in Progress, Latino, On Air). Die Arbeiten von Carlos waren am ResFest und auf Sundance Film Festivals vertreten und wurden zweimal an der Bienal de Design Gráfico Brasileiro sowie von der One Show, von BDA und anderen ausgezeichnet. Ein Highlight der experimentellen Arbeiten von Carlos bildet das Projecto Golden Shower - eine Hommage an die Popkultur der 80er.

Und wie sieht Carlos selbst sein Schaffen, was ist ihm bei seiner Arbeit wichtig? „Ich habe keine persönliche Philosophie, die mich bei meinen Projekten leitet. Doch ein Punkt ist bei meiner Arbeit von äußerster Wichtigkeit: Das Konzept. Damit meine ich, die Idee hinter dem Design. Ich glaube, ein Konzept ist essenziell, und ich flüchte immer vor ‚Eye-Candy'-Projekten, bei denen gewisse Formen oder Farben nur auf Basis ihres Erscheinens, ihrer Wirkung gewählt werden."

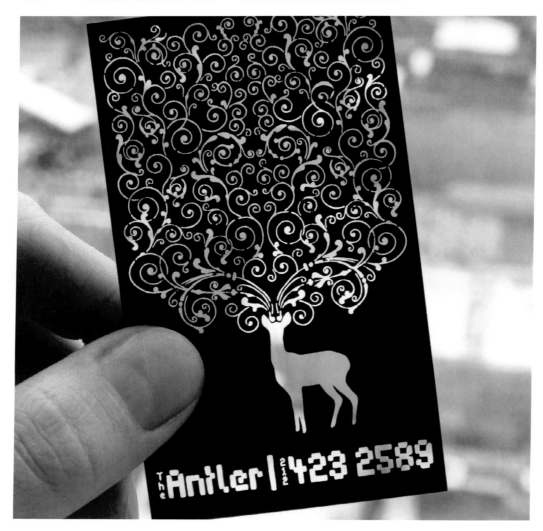

01 Sagmeister Inc.

reticulo endoplasmático

02 Carlos Bêla

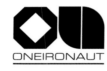

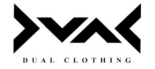

01 JDK

02 Muller

03 Manuel Musilli

04 Manuel Musilli

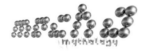

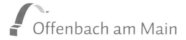

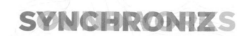

05 Formgeber

06 Typosition

07 iaah

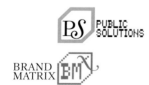

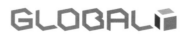

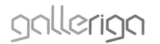

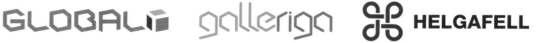

08 HardCase Design Dmitri

09 weissraum.de(sign)

10 Mikkel Grafixico Westrup

11 Analog.Systm

retículo endoplasmático

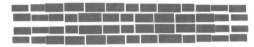

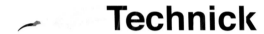

01 Carlos Bêla

02 TGB design

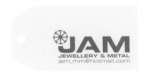

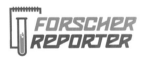

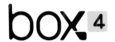

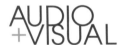

03 Resin[sistem] design

04 Visual Mind Rockets

05 Dimaquina

06 Engine

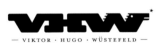

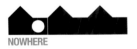

07 Carsten Raffel

08 Flavio Bagioli

09 Coldwater Graphiix

10 Canefantasma Studio

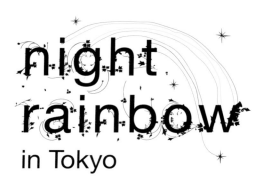

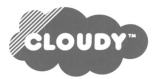

02 AKA

03 backyard 10

01 Coutworks

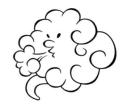

04 Jun Watanabe

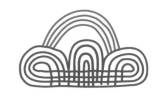

05 human empire

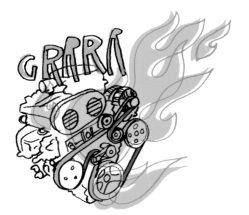

06 Hula Hula

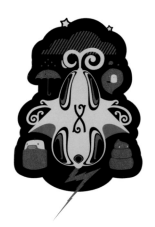

07 Nanospore

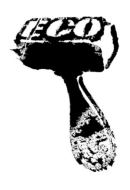

08 Dan Sparkes

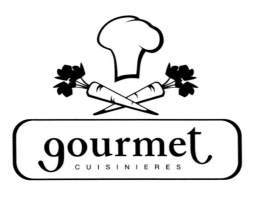

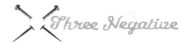

02 Three Negative

03 backyard 10

01 chemicalbox

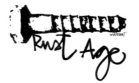

04 Stockbridge International

05 Mikkel Grafixico Westrup

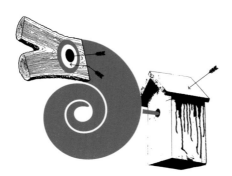

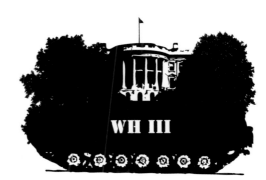

06 Dan Sparkes

07 actiondesigner

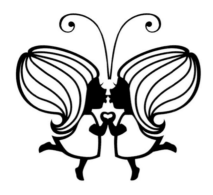

01 decoylab

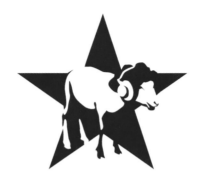

02 Gints Apsits

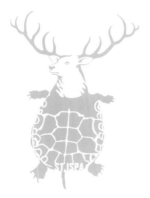

03 Gints Apsits

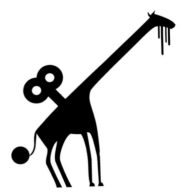

04 cubemen studio

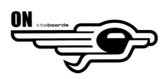

01 weissraum.de(sign)

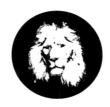

02 A-Side Studio

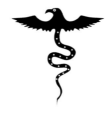

03 boris dworschak

04 J. Tuominen, Jukka Pylväs

05 Magnetofonica

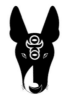

06 Makak Factory

07 Makak Factory

08 Miha Artnak

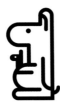

09 cubemen studio

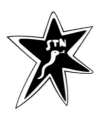

10 J. Tuominen, Jukka Pylväs

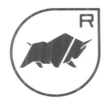

11 Shivamat

12 daniel neye / trb.

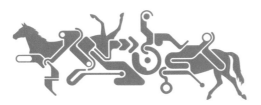

13 ASH

14 boris dworschak

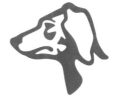

15 Draplin

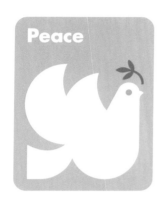

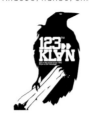

02 123klan

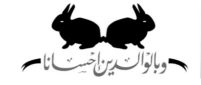

03 Fase

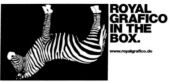

04 Accident Grotesk!

01 Draplin

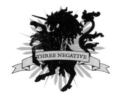

05 Three Negative

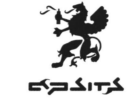

06 Gints Apsits

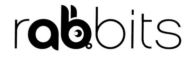

07 Carsten Raffel

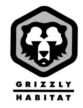

08 Draplin

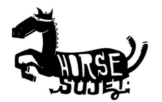

09 Alëxone

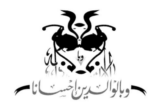

10 Fase

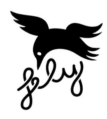

11 J. Tuominen, Jukka Pylväs

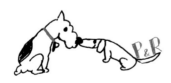

12 Naho Ogawa

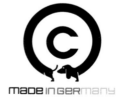

13 Shivamat

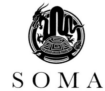

14 Sanjai Bhana

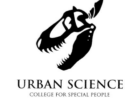

15 Microbot David Fuhrer

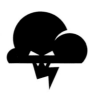

01 viagrafik

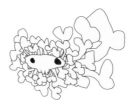

02 Sammy Stein

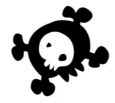

03 Sammy Stein

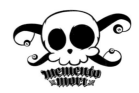

04 HelloBard.com

05 Mini Miniature Mouse

06 Nando Costa

07 Dimomedia Lab

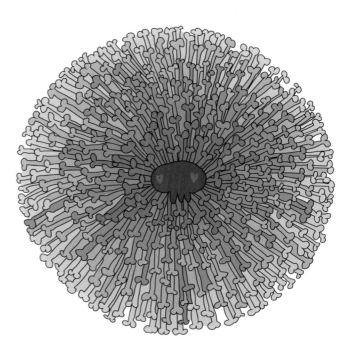

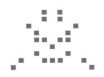

08 Attak

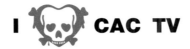

09 Povilas Utovka

10 Sammy Stein

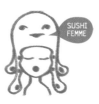

01 Lapin

02 bleed

03 Leon Vymenets

04 Steven Harrington

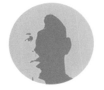

05 Superpopstudio

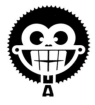

06 Carsten Raffel

07 Alëxone

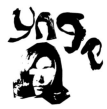

08 Positron

09 YOK

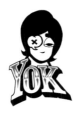

10 YOK

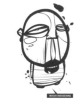

11 Inocuodesign

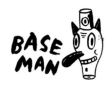

12 Critterbox LLC

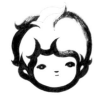

13 Lolo

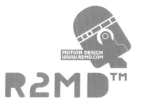

14 Adhemas

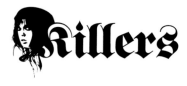

15 Salon Vektoria

16 Blindresearch

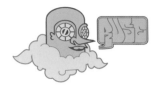

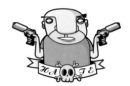

01 Critterbox LLC

02 Büro Brendel

03 ruse76

04 seacreative

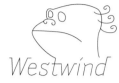

05 Lindedesign

06 Magnetofonica

07 Boris Hoppek

08 onrushdesign / front

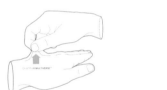

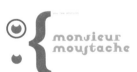

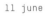

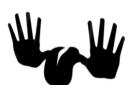

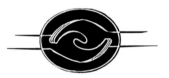

09 +ISM

10 Attak

11 june

12 Semisans

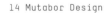

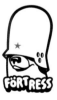

13 Alëxone

14 Mutabor Design

15 Flying Förtress

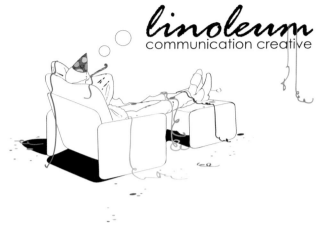

01 Linoleum

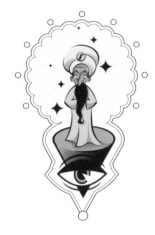

02 Fakir

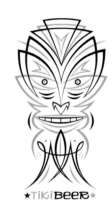

03 Dr. Alderete

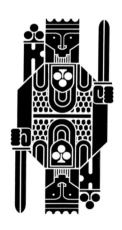

04 Keep Left Studio

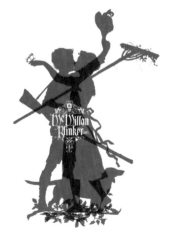

05 Graeme McMillan

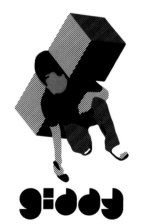

06 Tsuyoshi Hirooka

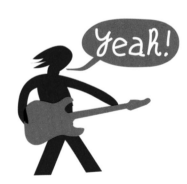

07 human empire

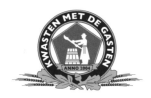

01 Ottograph

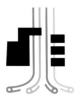

02 austrianillustration.

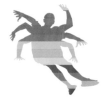

03 interspectacular

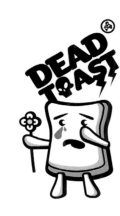

04 Ryohei Tanaka

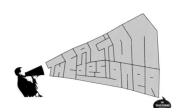

05 Naho Ogawa

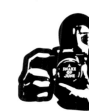

06 Gianni Rossi

07 Lapin

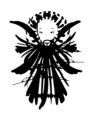

08 Stockbridge International

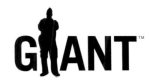

09 actiondesigner

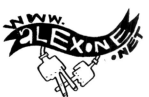

10 Blindresearch

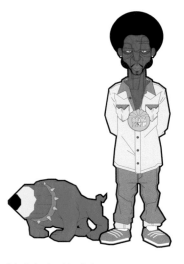

11 Akiza

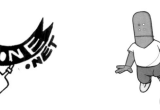

12 Alëxone

13 Onlyforthefuture

14 Onlyforthefuture

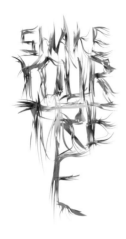

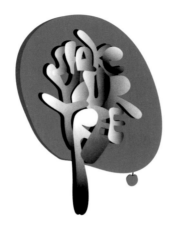

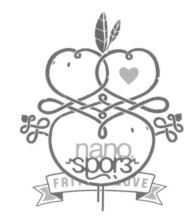

01 christian walden

02 christian walden

03 Nanospore, llc

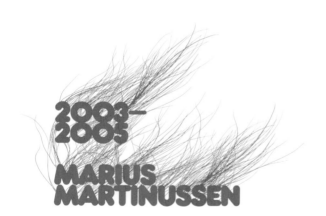

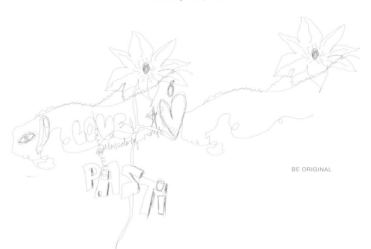

BE ORIGINAL

04 Kallegraphics

05 Thomas Nolfi

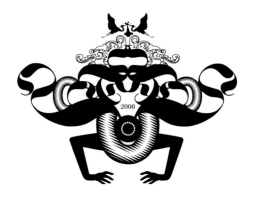

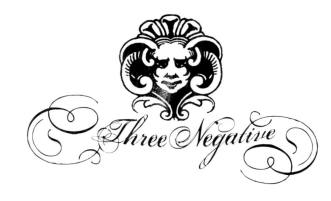

01 Joe A. Scerri

02 Three Negative

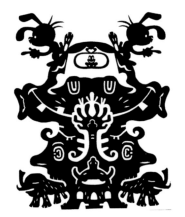

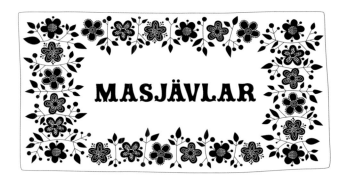

03 Ryohei Tanaka

04 Fellow Designers

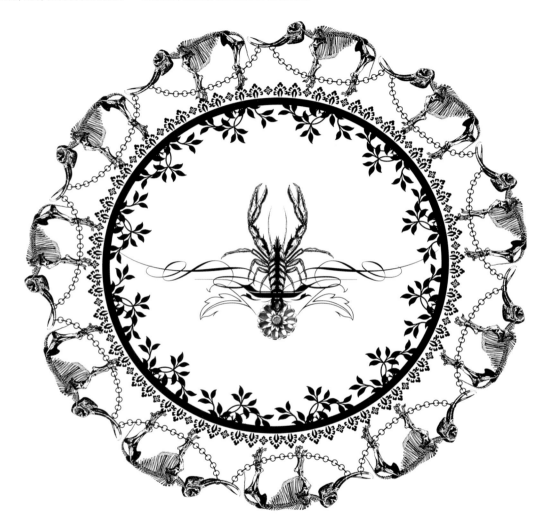

01 decoylab

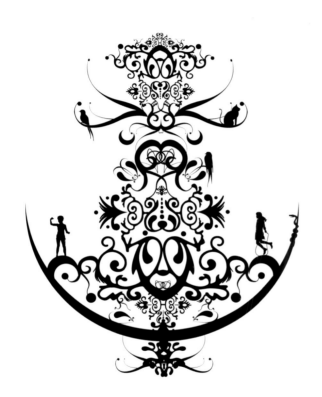

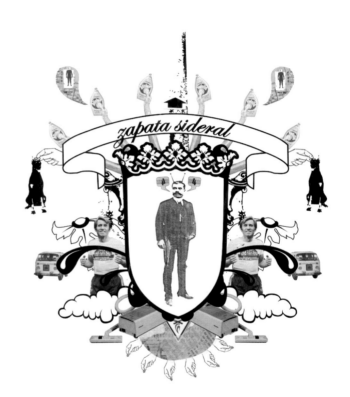

01 ROM studio   02 Tohyto

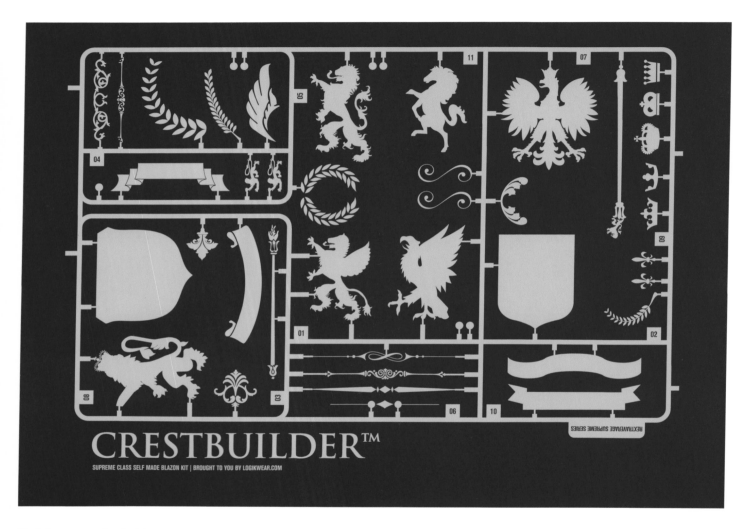

CRESTBUILDER™

SUPREME CLASS SELF MADE BLAZON KIT | BROUGHT TO YOU BY LOGIKWEAR.COM

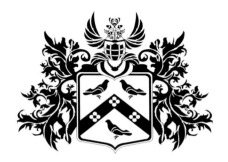

01 strange//attraktor:

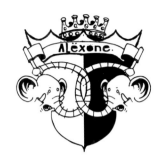

02 The Skull Dezain

03 Alëxone

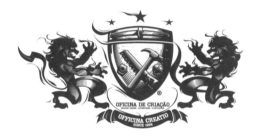

04 Adhemas

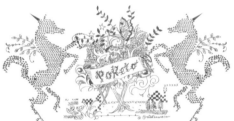

05 Miki Amano

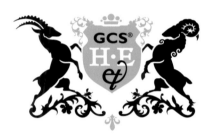

06 Bionic Systems

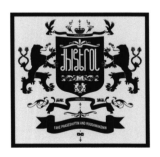

07 Karoly Kiralyfalvi

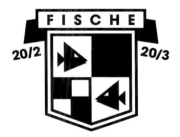

08 viagrafik

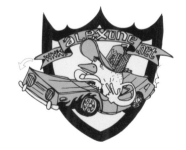

09 Alëxone

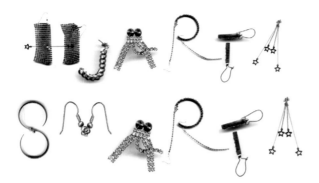

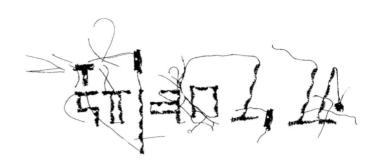

01 Hjärta Smärta

02 Laborator

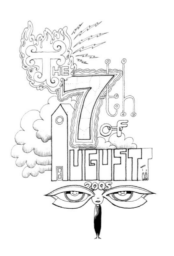

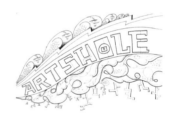

05 Dan Abbott

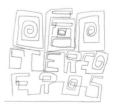

03 Frederique Daubal

04 Dan Abbott

06 Leon Vymenets

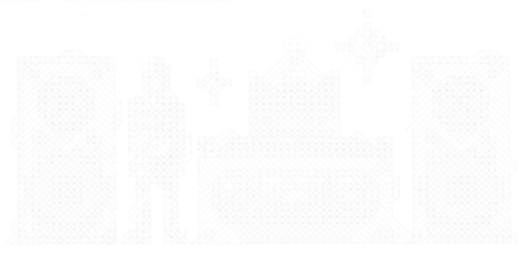

01 Tsuyoshi Hirooka

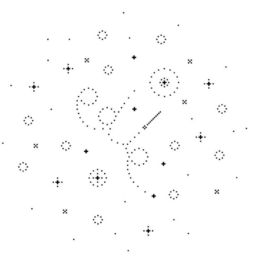

02 ten_do_ten

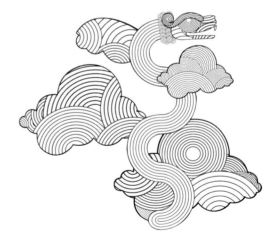

03 ROM studio

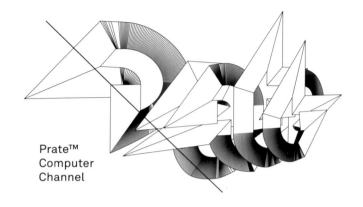

Prate™
Computer
Channel

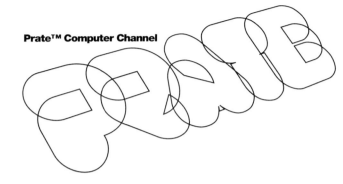

Prate™ Computer Channel

01 Studio Sans Nom

02 Studio Sans Nom

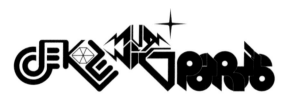

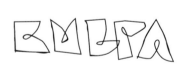

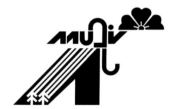

03 Dan Sparkes

04 cisma

05 Dan Sparkes

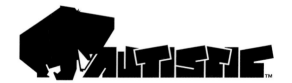

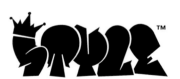

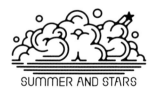

06 viagrafik

07 viagrafik

08 Tsuyoshi Hirooka

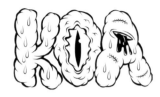

01 Koadzn

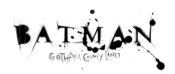

02 Jason Kochis

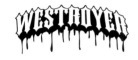

03 iaah

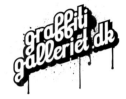

04 Mikkel Grafixico Westrup

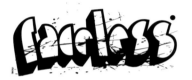

05 Karoly Kiralyfalvi

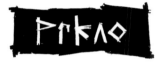

06 Laborator

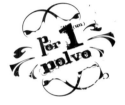

07 Magnetofonica

08 KesselsKramer

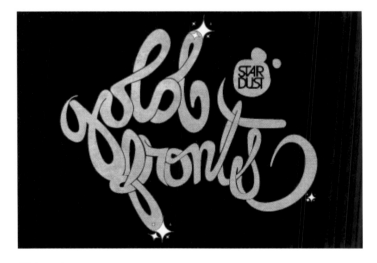

09 Laundry

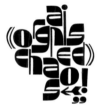

10 Keep Left Studio

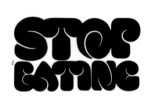

11 Keep Left Studio

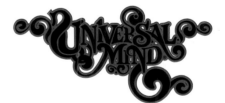

12 Keep Left Studio

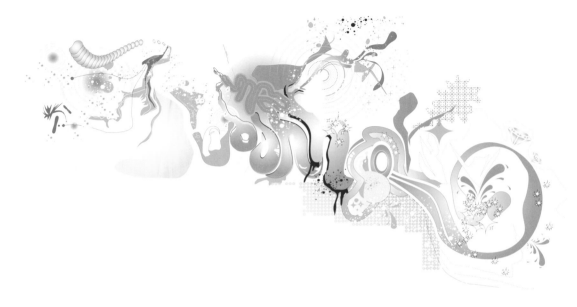

01 Laundry

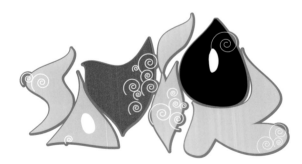

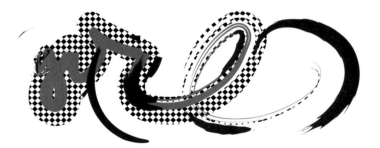

02 Ninjacruise

03 Laundry

01 Strukt Visual Network

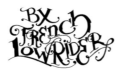

02 Alëxone

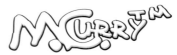

03 Ninjacruise

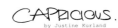
by Justine Kurland

by Camille Vivier

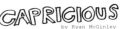
by Ryan McGinley

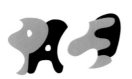

04 Hausgrafik

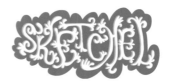

05 Laundry

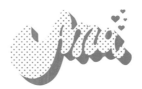

06 Hula Hula

CAPRICIOUS
by Vivian Joyner

by Miss Liz Wendelbo

Capricious.
by Sophie Mörner

by Louise Enhörning

by Hanna Liden

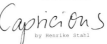

07 Karen Jane

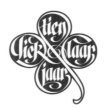

08 space3

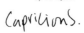

09 Razauno

Capricious
by Henrike Stahl

CAPRICIOUS
by Anti Color

CAPRICIOUS
by Ro Agents

Capricious.
by Caitlin Teal Price

10 Mikko Rantanen

Café Cyprus

11 archetype : interactive

12 Niels Shoe Meulman

13 KesselsKramer

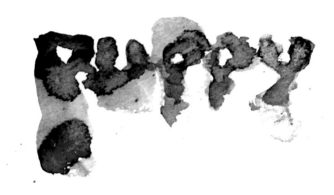

01 Keep Left Studio

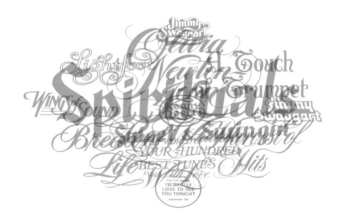

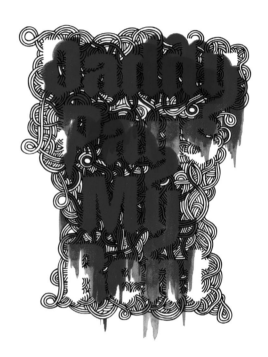

03 ZIP Design

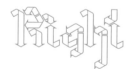

02 Graeme McMillan

04 DTM_INC   05 XYZ.CH

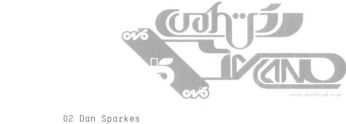

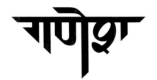

02 Dan Sparkes

03 The Skull Dezain

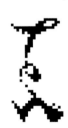

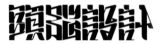

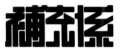

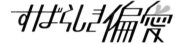

04 The Skull Dezain

05 The Skull Dezain

06 Studio Maverick

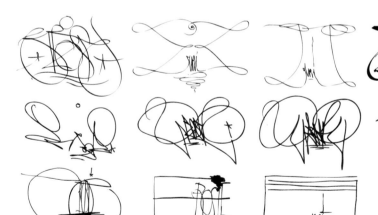

01 ten_do_ten

07 Studio Erosie

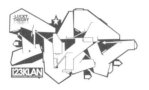

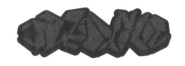

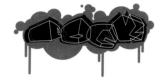

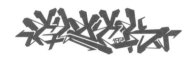

01 123klan

02 Regina

03 Salon Vektoria

04 Mikkel Grafixico Westrup

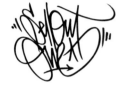

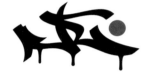

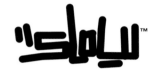

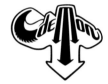

05 Sellout Industries

06 Resin[sistem] design

07 viagrafik

08 ehquestionmark

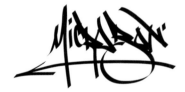

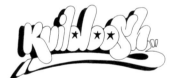

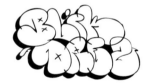

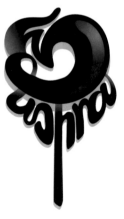

09 Microbot David Fuhrer

10 Dan Sparkes

11 Karoly Kiralyfalvi

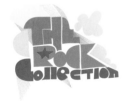

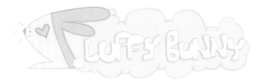

12 Laundry

13 Cherrybox Studios

14 ehquestionmark

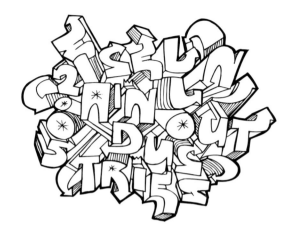

01 Sellout Industries

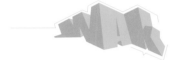

02 Salon Vektoria

04 Razauno

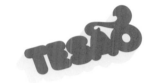

03 Dimaquina

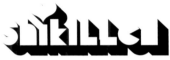

05 Jun Watanabe

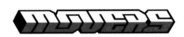

06 MvM / Maarten van Maanen

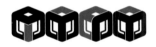

07 Tsuyoshi Hirooka

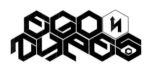

08 SHOK1

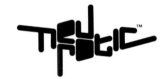

09 viagrafik

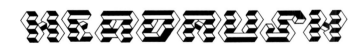

10 DTM_INC

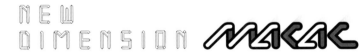

11 Tsuyoshi Hirooka

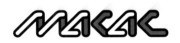

12 Makak Factory

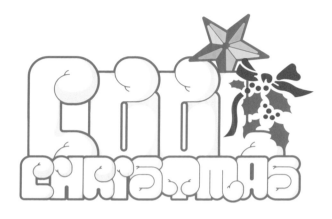

01 Tsuyoshi Hirooka

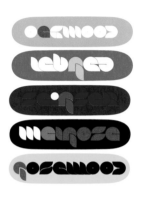

02 Laundry

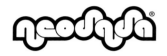

03 viagrafik

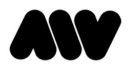

04 Labor f. visuelles Wachstum™

05 Konstantinos Gargaletsos

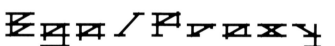

06 Tsuyoshi Hirooka

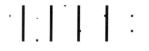

07 Power Graphixx

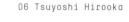

08 onrushdesign / front

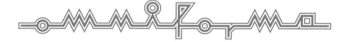

09 Lukatarina

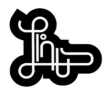

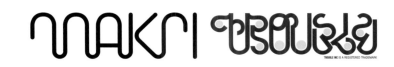

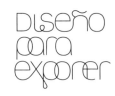

01 Plastic Kid

02 spin

03 Sellout Industries

04 Blu Design

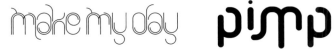

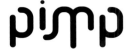

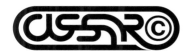

05 Kallegraphics

06 paulroberts.tv

07 Laurent Fétis

08 Dan Sparkes

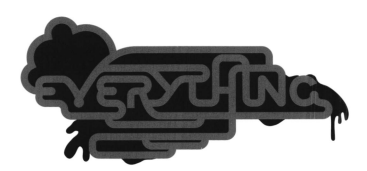

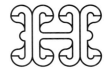

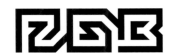

10 No-Domain

11 Power Graphixx

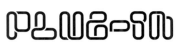

09 William Morrisey

12 Tsuyoshi Hirooka

13 zime SOL crew

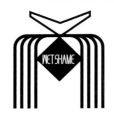

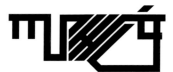

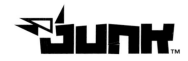

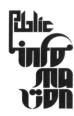

01 Dan Sparkes

02 viagrafik

03 Dan Sparkes

04 Dan Sparkes

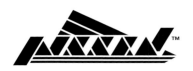

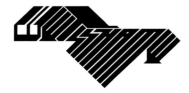

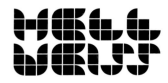

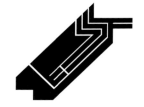

05 viagrafik

06 Dan Sparkes

07 Dan Sparkes

08 austrianillustration.com

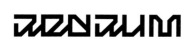

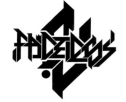

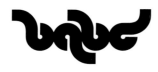

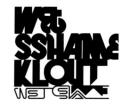

09 Power Graphixx

10 Extraverage Productions

11 Faith

12 Dan Sparkes

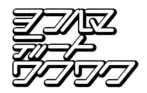

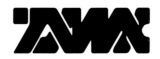

13 Omochi

14 Mikkel Grafixico Westrup

15 The Skull Dezain

16 cryogenicx.com

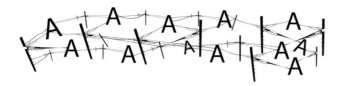

01 Dimomedia Lab

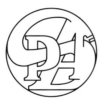

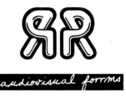

02 cubemen studio

03 Resin[sistem] design

04 MaMadesign AB

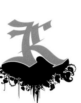

05 Mattisimo

06 Stockbridge International

07 Maak

08 Povilas Utovka

09 Tnop™ & ®bePOS|+|VE

10 derfaber

11 MH grafik

12 Airside

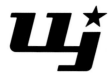

01 Klaus Wilhardt

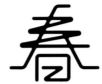

02 Jenni Tuominen, J. Pylväs

03 Polygraph

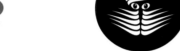

04 DTM_INC

05 Friends With You

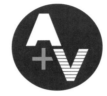

06 Station

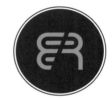

07 Engine

08 Mattisimo

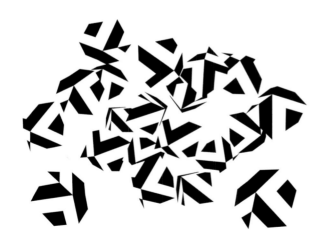

09 cubemen studio

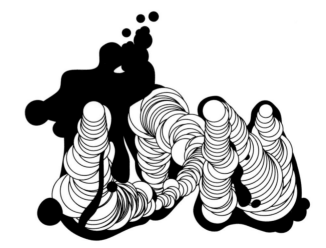

10 0c/0m/0y/0k

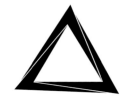

01 Nando Costa

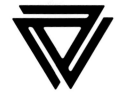

02 Nando Costa

03 Out Of Order

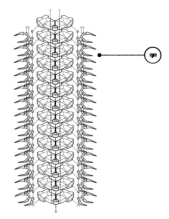

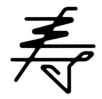

04 Omochi

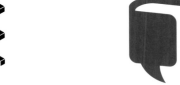

05 Tsuyoshi Hirooka

06 jl-prozess

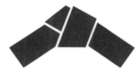

07 +ISM

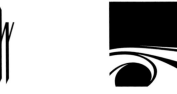

08 Polygraph

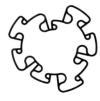

09 MaMadesign AB

10 Formikula

11 Tnop™ & ®bePOS|+|VE

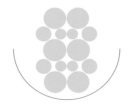

12 Omochi

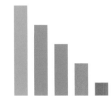

13 resistro®

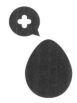

14 Carlos Bêla

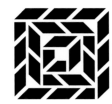

15 MaMadesign AB

POLITICAL

THE COMMUNICATION OF VALUES REPLACES POLITICAL SLOGANS

In retreat today are symbols that communicate in an explicitly political way. A response to a widely voiced disenchantment with politics? Emphasis has shifted to the social context and to a confrontation with society's criteria of value. This leads to a shift of visual metaphors, increasingly drawn from the reservoir of mythology.

CONSERVATISM

Rearguard action.

"All design is an embodiment of politics," claims Regula Stämpfli[1] and immediately supplies a rationale for this claim: "If politics are conceived as something shaped by time, space and perception, then design is also part of it." If we take the thesis of this political scientist further and apply it to the design of symbols, then an additional trend becomes conspicuous, and one that manifests itself in Tres Logos: retrogression. Conservatism is enjoying a heyday. Design supports the zeitgeist in its rearguard action. Well-established codes, methods and principles are retrieved from the back drawers, remixed, and fashionable creations pieced together. Experimental? To be sure - but the tried-and-tested serves as safe raw material.

1.   Regula Stämpfli, "Wie politisch ist denn Design," lecture delivered at the "Colloquium on Design & Democracy," Hochschule für Gestaltung und Kunst Zürich, Nov 2005.

PARIS, FRANCE
LOÏC SATTLER

A densely metaphorical story.

When positively overwhelmed by ingenious, blatant, playful, dreamy, politically correct and incorrect, provocative, neo-romantic and many other visual impressions on his platform lysergid.com, which are perpetually joined by new ones; when checking out the latest trends in design, fashion, media, art, advertising, theory and more on the blog attached to his platform and moderated by him; and when reading his interviews with designers from every corner of the globe in the virtual community Uailab, at some point you have to ask yourself: How does he manage all of this, and what is it that actually drives him? Enthusiasm, says Loïc Sattler. And he elaborates: "Let's just say I'm always interested and enthusiastic. Inspired by everything, everywhere, I'm the type of guy who is totally in love with visual creation, who needs to share it under any circumstances. My aim is to be understood as an individual who wishes to take things further by empowering my profession as best as I can."

Loïc was born in Strasbourg in 1980. In 1998, he decided to get serious about his design career and began to study multimedia and art. Seven years of hard work followed. During his study years, Loïc worked in a variety of fields: print, 3D, motion design, fashion styling and others. He completed his studies at Stuttgart with a Master's Degree in New Media Theory and a thesis formulated by his curator, Russian net.art artist Olia Lialina. In 2003, he launched his platform lysergid.com (see above) into virtual orbit. Today, Loïc is an art director at a well-known Paris agency. A brief selection from his client list for web, CD-ROM, print and video projects: Mercedes Group (Publicis), Porsche Group (Freelance), Warner Brothers (Blackmountain), IBM (Blackmountain), Design Council London (Projektriangle), L'Oreal (Fullsix), Azur Assurances (Publicis), Grand Optical (Fullsix), Procter & Gamble (Fullsix UK). Loïc is also active as a journalist in various media. His "XS OBJECTS" projects were displayed at the design biennale at St. Etienne and Toulon.

Loïc and the logo: "Logo design is a visual stimulus. A dense metaphorical narrative that, in my opinion, combines four different forces: beauty, sensuality, compatibility (meaning serving representative functions) and uniqueness. As a picture, a sign, a font or a combination of the three, a logo must express these forces. Then it is only a matter of striking a balance between experimentation, concept and continuity, in accordance with the client's demands. But don't forget that the logo is a distilled catalyst, that each sign has its very own meaning."

POLITIK

WERTVERMITTLUNG ERSETZT POLITPAROLEN

Die explizit politisch kommunizierenden Zeichen sind auf dem Rückzug. Reaktion auf eine allgemein konstatierte Politikverdrossenheit? Das Hauptgewicht hat sich auf den sozialen Kontext und die Auseinandersetzung mit den Wertemaßstäben der Gesellschaft verlagert. Dies führt zu einer Verschiebung der bildlichen Metaphern, die sich vermehrt aus dem Fundus der Mythologie bedienen.

KONSERVATISMUS

Rückzugsgefechte.

„Alles Design ist inkarnierte Politik", behauptet Regula Stämpfli[1], und liefert gleich die Begründung nach: „Wenn Politik als etwas von Zeit, Raum und Wahrnehmung Geformtes verstanden wird, so gehört auch Design dazu." Wenn man die These der Politikwissenschaftlerin weiterführt und auf das Design von Zeichen appliziert, dann wird ein weiterer, in Tres Logos manifestierter Trend deutlich: Die Rückbesinnung. Konservatismus hat Konjunktur. Die Gestaltung beteiligt sich an der Seite des Zeitgeistes am Rückzugsgefecht: Sichere, gut etablierte Kodierungen, Methoden und Prinzipien werden aus der Schublade hervorgeholt, neu aufgemischt und modischen Kreationen aufgepfropft. Experimente? Ja schon, aber: Bewährtes ist ein sichererer Rohstoff.

1.   Regula Stämpfli, „Wie politisch ist denn Design", Vortrag, gehalten anlässlich des Kolloquiums zu Design & Demokratie, Hochschule für Gestaltung und Kunst Zürich, Nov. 2005.

PARIS, FRANKREICH
LOIC SATTLER

Eine dichte metaphorische Geschichte.

Wenn man auf seiner Plattform lysergid.com (abgekürzt LSD, wie eine bewusstseinserweiternde Droge) von genialen, krassen, verspielten, verträumten, politisch korrekten und inkorrekten, provokanten, neuromantischen und vielen anderen visuellen Impressionen, zu denen sich ständig neue gesellen, geradezu überflutet wird; wenn man sich auf dem der Plattform angedockten und von ihm selbst moderierten Blog die aktuellsten Trends in Design, Mode, Medien, Kunst, Werbung, Theorie und mehr reinzieht; und wenn man dann auch noch seine Interviews mit Gestaltern aus allen Ecken der Welt in der virtuellen Community Uailab liest, ja dann fragt man sich schon irgendwann: Wie schafft der das eigentlich alles, und was treibt ihn überhaupt an? Enthusiasmus, meint Loic Sattler. Um den geht es hier nämlich: „Ich bin nun mal enthusiastisch und interessiert. Inspiriert überall von allem. Ich bin der Typ, der in totaler Liebe mit visuellen Kreationen verbunden ist und dieses Gefühl gerne mit anderen teilen will. Ich möchte als ein Mensch verstanden werden, der will, dass sich die Dinge weiterentwickeln, indem er sein Metier mit neuen Impulsen verstärkt, so gut er kann."

Loic stammt aus Straßburg, wo er 1980 geboren wurde. 1998 beschloss er, mit seiner Designerkarriere ernst zu machen: Er begann ein Studium in Multimedia und Kunst. Sieben Jahre harte Arbeit folgten. Während seiner Studienzeit arbeitete Loic in verschiedenen Bereichen: Print, 3D, Motion Design, Modestyling und anderen. Er schloss sein Studium mit einem Master in New Media Theory in Stuttgart ab, mit einer Thesis seiner Kuratorin, der russischen net.art-Künstlerin Olia Lialina. 2003 schoss er seine Plattform lysergid.com (siehe oben) in den virtuellen Orbit. Heute arbeitet Loic in einer bekannten Pariser Agentur als Art Director. Ein kleiner Auszug aus seiner Kundenliste für Web-, CD-ROM-Print- und Videoprojekte: Mercedes Group (Publicis), Porsche Group (Freelance), Warner Brothers (Blackmountain), IBM (Blackmountain), Design Council London (Projektriangle), L'Oreal (Fullsix), Azur Assurances (Publicis), Grand Optical (Fullsix), Procter & Gamble (Fullsix UK). Loic ist auch publizistisch für verschiedene Medien aktiv. Sein „XS OBJECTS"-Projekt wurde an den Design Biennalen von St. Etienne und Toulon gezeigt.

Loic und das Logo: „Logodesign ist ein visueller Stimulus, eine dichte metaphorische Geschichte, die meiner Meinung nach vier Kraftfelder verbindet: Schönheit, Sinnlichkeit, Kompatibilität (im Sinne von repräsentativ) und Einzigartigkeit. Diese Kräfte muss das Logo ausdrücken - als ein Bild, ein Zeichen, eine Schrift oder eine Kombination dieser drei. Dann ist alles nur noch eine Frage der Balance zwischen Experimentierfreudigkeit und Konzeptualität, gemäß den Anforderungen des Kunden. Man sollte nie vergessen, dass das Logo ein konzentrierter Katalysator ist, dass jedes Zeichen seine ureigene Bedeutung hat."

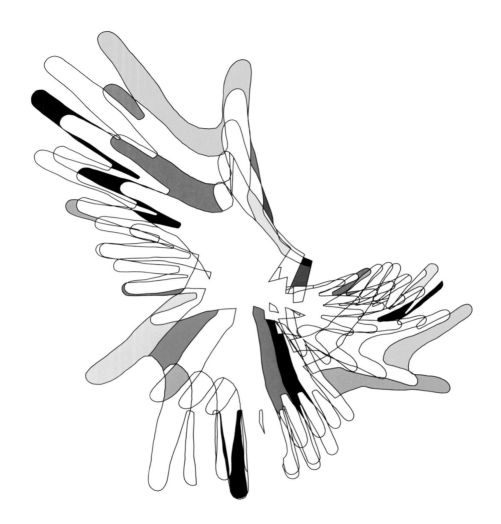

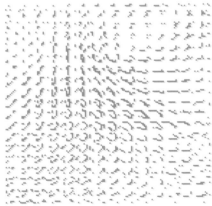

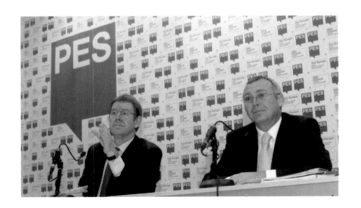

01 29 degres

02 Floor Wesseling Ix Opus Ada

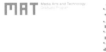

13 03 projekttriangle

15 04 base

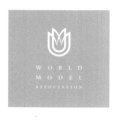

01 Simon & Goetz Design

02 Kontrapunkt

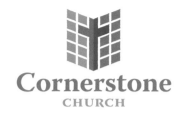

Cornerstone
CHURCH

03 David Maloney

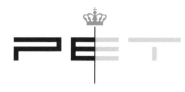

04 Kontrapunkt

marxsistas

05 Designunion

ROSENROT

06 3 deluxe

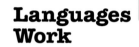 **Languages
Work**

07 Brighten the corners

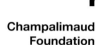 **Champalimaud
Foundation**

08 STUDIO DUMBAR

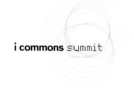 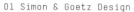 i commons summit

09 Moniteurs

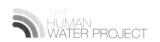 THE
HUMAN
WATER PROJECT

10 sunrise studios

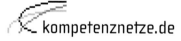 kompetenznetze.de

11 HardCase

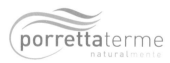 porrettaterme
naturalmente

12 ABC&Z

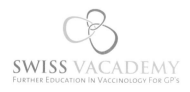 SWISS VACADEMY
FURTHER EDUCATION IN VACCINOLOGY FOR GP's

13 29 degres

PFADI KANTON SOLOTHURN

14 Klauser Weibel Design

Pastoralkreis Frauenfeld Gachnang Uesslingen

15 Atelier Mühlberg

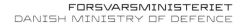

FORSVARSMINISTERIET
DANISH MINISTRY OF DEFENCE

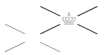

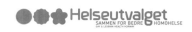 Helseutvalget
SAMMEN FOR BEDRE HOMOHELSE
GAY & LESBIAN HEALTH NORWAY

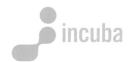 incuba

01 Kontrapunkt

02 Superlow

03 cabina

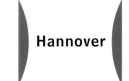 Hannover

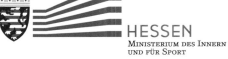 HESSEN
MINISTERIUM DES INNERN
UND FÜR SPORT
Zentrale für Datenverarbeitung

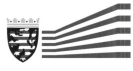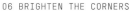 T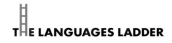E LANGUAGES LADDER

04 HardCase

05 HardCase

06 BRIGHTEN THE CORNERS

HumboldtStiftung

National Kidney
Foundation™

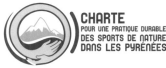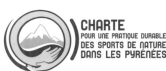 CHARTE
POUR UNE PRATIQUE DURABLE
DES SPORTS DE NATURE
DANS LES PYRÉNÉES

DEMOCRACIA
Popular

07 MWK - Zimmermann und Hähnel

08 Mark Sloan

09 zookeeper

10 Magnetofonica

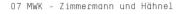 *Quarzo* della **Porretta**

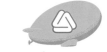

CIDADE SUSTENTÁVEL

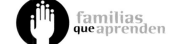 familias
que aprenden

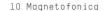 MAGDALENA   BAYKEEPERS

11 ABC&Z

12 Dimaquina

13 Kimera

14 Hula Hula

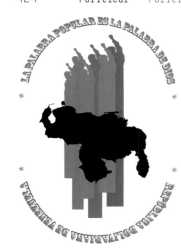

02 Fupete Studio

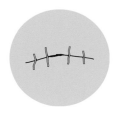

03 granit di Lioba Wackernell

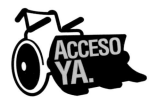

04 Floor Wesseling Ix Opus

01 Magnetofonica

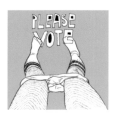

05 the red is love

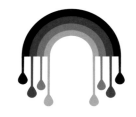

06 Emmi Salonen

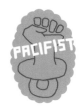

07 Fase

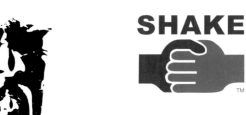

09 derek johnson

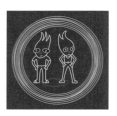

10 Maya Hayuk

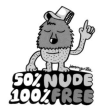

11 Maya Hayuk

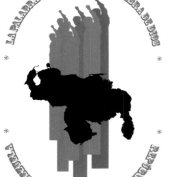

08 Gints Apsits

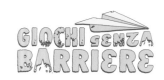

12 ABC&Z

13 Judith Zaugg

14 jeremyville

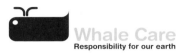

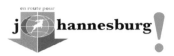

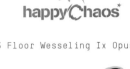

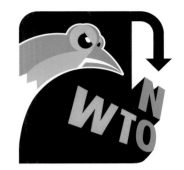

01 sunrise studios

02 Superpopstudio

03 Floor Wesseling Ix Opus

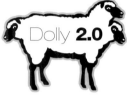

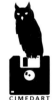

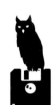

05 MIKEL MIKEL

06 HandGun

07 HandGun

04 Shivamat

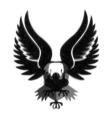

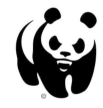

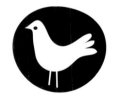

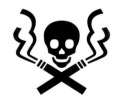

08 Floor Wesseling Ix Opus

09 Emil Hartvig

10 human empire

11 Floor Wesseling Ix Opus

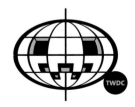

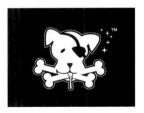

12 anna-OM-line.com

13 Carsten Raffel

14 Labor f. visuelles Wachstum™   15 Salon Vektoria

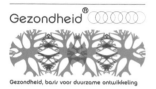

01 Superpopstudio

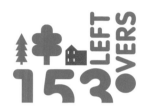

02 Grandpeople

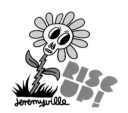

03 jeremyville

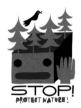

04 human empire

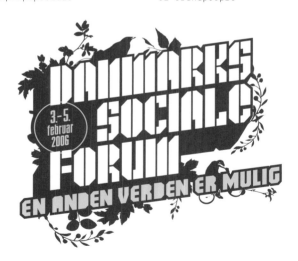

05 the Legalizer ApS

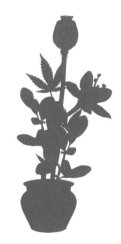

06 310k

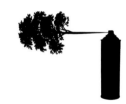

07 Out Of Order

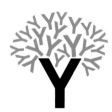

08 Pentagram

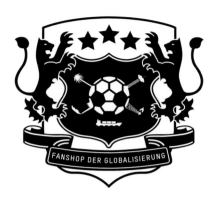

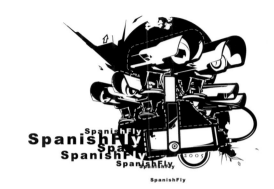

01 onlab

02 44 flavours

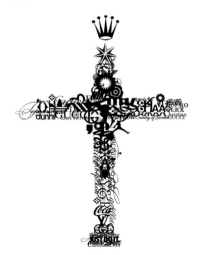

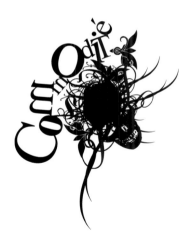

03 The KDU

04 Loic Sattler

05 Inocuodesign

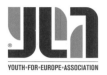

01 Karoly Kiralyfalvi

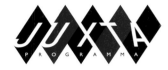

02 Niels Shoe Meulman

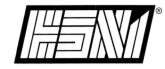

03 viagrafik

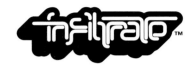

04 viagrafik

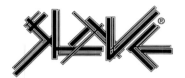

05 viagrafik

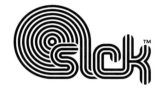

06 viagrafik

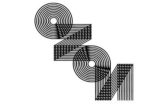

07 Floor Wesseling Ix Opus

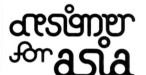

08 june

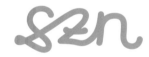

09 Atelier Mühlberg

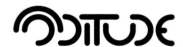

10 The Vacuum Design

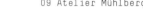
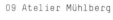

11 Bringolf Irion Vögeli

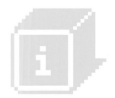

12 cabina

13 Parra

14 Loic Sattler

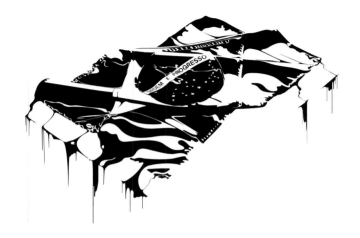

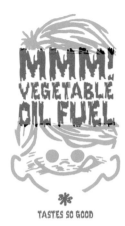

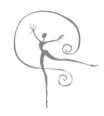

03 a+morph

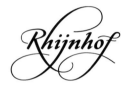

01 Nando Costa

02 JDK

04 MvM

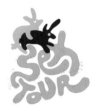

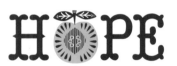

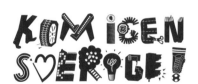

05 Studio Output

06 Chris Rubino

07 BankerWessel

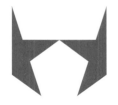

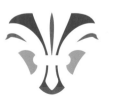

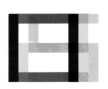

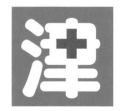

08 Kosta Lazarevski / rdy

09 Kontrapunkt

10 Kontrapunkt

11 dainippon

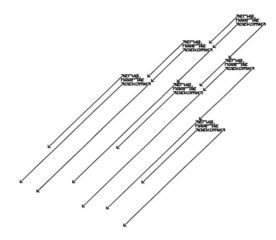

01 Floor Wesseling Ix Opus Ada

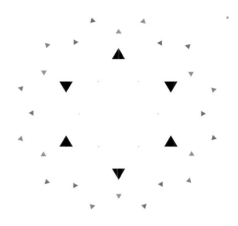

02 Alexander Fuchs

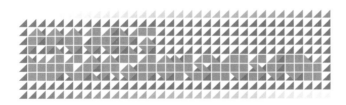

03 Bodara

04 MaMadesign AB

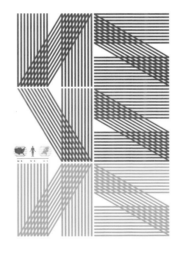

05 Floor Wesseling Ix Opus

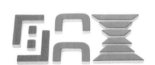

06 dainippon

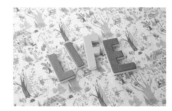

07 dainippon

SPORTS

SAVAGELY GOOD

Populating today's logos are creatures (animal beings löschen) from the world of traditional fables, for example those of La Fontaine, but also real ones from the wild, embedded in fashionable shapes and colours. They symbolise power and courage, purity and strength. And the noble (and occasionally forgotten) goals of Monsieur de Coubertin, who translated the Olympic spirit from Antiquity to the modern world.

ESSENCE

Attention: Heavy load.

Clearly, the claim (supported by textbook communication theory) that the logo constitutes the essence of the message has lost its relevance. Is being systematically undermined. Designers cram in everything they consider aesthetic - especially images and still more images. Reductions are replaced by pictorial, illustrative, ornamental, almost holistic compositions. A panoramic view with complex scenery instead of close-ups focused on essentials. Now it is not just the lead actor, but all of the walk-ons and extras who have to fit into the picture. Of course, this is not least of all due to new computer technologies and tools which "let you to do everything."

MASA, MIGUEL VASQUES

The Fusion of urbanity and folklore.

"My work strongly emphasises references to Latin American pop culture and to ideas drawn from global contemporary street culture. The fusion of tendencies drawn from both urban and folkloric sources generates results that are powerful and distinctive - which is what I'm trying to create in my own work." Illustrations signed "MASA" - standing for Miguel Vasquez - have already appeared in more than 30 books produced by international publishers. Among them are Victionary, PIE Books and Laurence King in London, Idn, not to mention Die Gestalten Verlag. The list of international magazines that have featured illustrations by MASA is no less impressive: Xlr8r, Tokion (USA), POUND (Canada), VOGUE Brasil, Tómalá, Platanoverde and Etecé Magazine (Spain).

An important source of inspiration for MASA has been the work of Venezuelan designers from the 1950s, 60s and late 70s. Among them are Gerd Leufert and M. F. Nedo. "I am drawn to bold, black images that are simple in form and capable of becoming simple logos." As a child Miguel Vasquez, an illustrator and designer who lives in Venezuela's largest metropolis, was already interested in typography and symbols in their manifold forms. "They reveal names and meanings and were the first of the forms around me that I explored."

Branding is an important topic for this designer from Caracas, who is active as an art director in addition to his work in illustration. He is also involved in motion graphics, a field that constantly grows in importance alongside parallel developments in media and technology.

Brands, says Miguel, strive to present their clients as unique, strong, and easily recognisable. "To draw attention to themselves and beat the competition," is Miguel's client-oriented summary. And with his work in the areas of brand identity and logos, this is precisely his objective. "I use different materials and techniques to create bold images. My sources of inspiration are not found in the design field, but elsewhere. I tend to cross over in my search for meanings and forms." MASA's clients come principally from the areas of sport, entertainment, music, fashion, and youth-oriented culture. Among them are Nike, Volkswagen, Sony Entertainment, Television Latin America, AXN Channel Latin America, HBO Group Latin America, Die Gestalten Verlag, Upper Playground, Fifty24SF and KONG.

MASA on the logo? "With the logo, presence is everything. The first impression! For me, designing a logo is always FUN. It's like playing with a puzzle, finding the individual parts, adjusting and modifying them in every conceivable way in order to get the result I'm striving for, the one I really like."

SPORT

TIERISCH GUT

Tierische Wesen aus überlieferten Fabelwelten wie derjenigen von La Fontaine, aber auch ganz reale Tiere aus der Wildbahn bevölkern, eingebettet in modische Farben- und Formenkontexte, die Logos. Sie symbolisieren Kraft und Mut, Reinheit und Stärke. Sie stehen für die hehren (gelegentlich in Vergessenheit geratenen) Ziele des Monsieur de Coubertin, der die antike Idee von Olympia in die Neuzeit transportiert hat.

ESSENZ

Achtung Schwertransport.

Die lehrbuchhafte, kommunikationswissenschaftlich untermauerte These vom Logo als Essenz einer Botschaft hat ganz offensichtlich an Relevanz eingebüßt. Wird systematisch unterlaufen. Die Designer packen alles rein, was sie für ästhetisch halten - vor allem Bilder und nochmals Bilder. Reduktionen werden von bildhaften, illustrativen, ornamentalen, eigentlich fast ganzheitlichen Kompositionen abgelöst. Totale mit komplexer Szenerie statt aufs Wesentliche fokussiertes Close-up. Nicht mehr nur der Hauptdarsteller, sondern alle Statisten und Komparsen müssen ins Bild. Das liegt, klarer Fall, natürlich nicht zuletzt an den neuen Computertechnologien und -werkzeugen, mit denen sich „alles machen lässt".

CARACAS, VENEZUELA
MASA, MIGUEL VASQUES

Die Fusion von Urbanität und Folklore.

„Meine Arbeiten haben einen starken Bezug zum lateinamerikanischen Pop und zu globalen Street-Culture-Ideen. Aus der Fusion urbaner und folkloristischer Tendenzen resultieren starke, eigenständige Resultate - und genau solche Resultate versuche ich mit meinen Arbeiten zu erreichen." Mit MASA, das für Miguel Vasquez steht, wurden bereits Illustrationen in über dreißig Büchern renommierter internationaler Verlage signiert. Darunter Victionary, PIE Books und Laurence King in London, Idn und auch der Gestalten Verlag gehört dazu. Die Liste der internationalen Magazine, in denen MASA-Illustrationen schon zu sehen waren, ist nicht weniger beeindruckend: Xlr8r, Tokion (USA), POUND (Kanada),VOGUE Brasil, Tómalá, Platanoverde and Etecé Magazine (Spanien).

Eine wichtige Inspirationsquelle für MASA sind auch die Arbeiten venezolanischer Designer aus den 50er, 60er und den späten 70er Jahren des letzten Jahrhunderts. Dazu gehören unter anderem Gerd Leufert und M. F. Nedo. „Kräftige schwarze Bilder, die eine simple Form oder ein einfaches Logo sein können - das fasziniert mich." Miguel Vasquez, der in der venezolanischen Metropole lebende Designer und Illustrator, hat sich jedoch bereits in seiner Kindheit für Typografie und Zeichen in ihren mannigfaltigen Formen interessiert. „Sie offenbaren Namen und Meinungen und waren die ersten uns umgebenden visuellen Formen, die ich entdeckt habe."

Branding ist ein wichtiges Thema für den Gestalter aus Caracas, der neben der Illustration auch in der Art Direction tätig ist und sich auf dem analog zu den technologischen und medialen Entwicklungen ständig wichtiger werdenden Gebiet der Motion Graphics engagiert.

Marken, meint Miguel, sind nach wie vor bestrebt, sich ihren Kunden als einzigartig, potent und leicht wiedererkennbar zu präsentieren: „Auf sich aufmerksam machen und die Konkurrenz schlagen", bringt er es echt kundenorientiert auf den Punkt - und strebt mit seiner Arbeit in den Bereichen Brand Identity und Logo genau dieses Ziel an. „Dabei setze ich verschiedene Materialien und Techniken ein. Meine Inspirationen beziehe ich nicht aus dem Design, sondern ‚crossover', aus anderen Quellen, Meinungen und Formen." MASA's Kunden kommen hauptsächlich aus den Bereichen Sport, Entertainment, Musik, Mode und jugendorientierter Kultur: Nike, Volkswagen, Sony Entertainment, Television Latin America, AXN Channel Latin America, HBO Group Latin America, Die Gestalten Verlag, Upper Playground, Fifty24SF, KONG gehören dazu.

MASA und die Logos? „Präsenz ist alles bei einem Logo. Der erste Eindruck! Wenn ich ein Logo gestalte, dann ist das immer ‚fun'. Es ist wie ein Puzzle - Einzelteile finden, auf alle möglichen Arten aufeinander abstimmen, modulieren. Bis ich das erreicht habe, was ich angestrebt habe und was mir am besten gefällt."

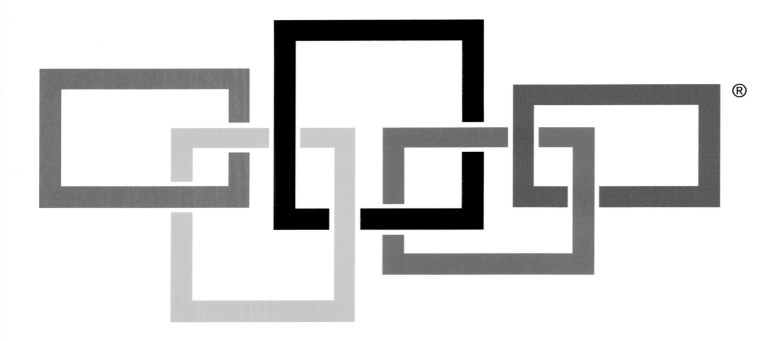

01 Futro

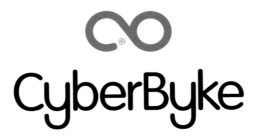

01 stylodesign

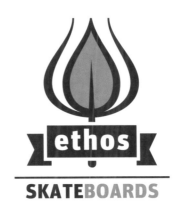

02 jum

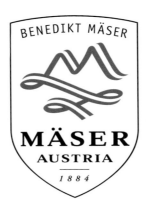

03 Simon & Goetz Design

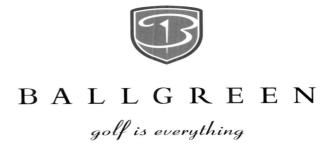

04 Simon & Goetz Design

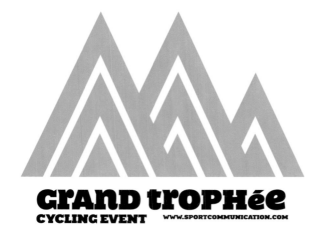

01 Trafik

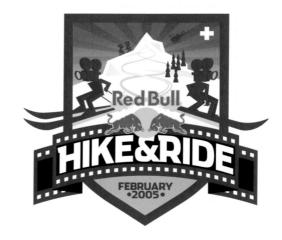

02 Büro Destruct

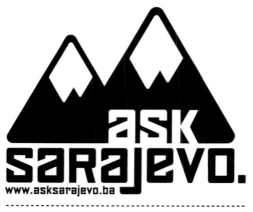

03 Skin Design

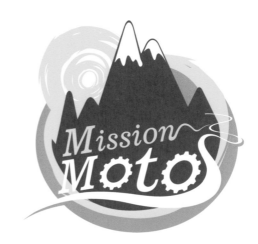

04 zookeeper

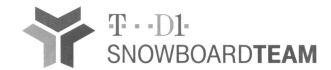

01 AKA

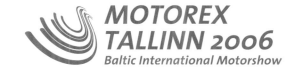

02 Velvet

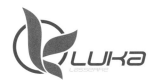

03 zookeeper

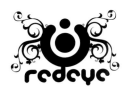

04 Draplin

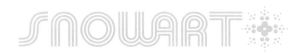

05 cabina

06 JDK

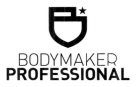

07 zookeeper

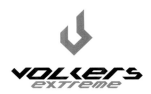

08 GWG

09 Toxic design

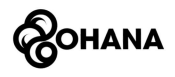

10 Salon Vektoria

11 Yorgo Tloupas

12 viagrafik

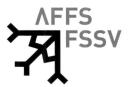

13 29 degres

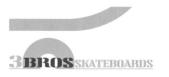

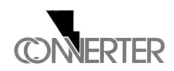

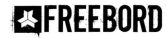

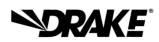

01 Christian Rothenhagen

02 3 deluxe

03 viagrafik

04 The Vacuum Design

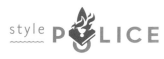

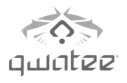

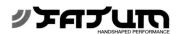

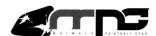

05 Carsten Raffel

06 bleed

07 viagrafik

08 I&EYE

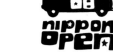

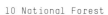

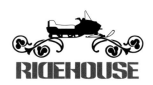

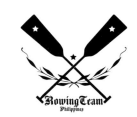

09 JDK

10 National Forest

11 Karoly Kiralyfalvi

12 Team Manila

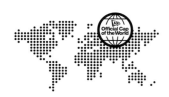

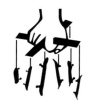

13 JDK

14 National Forest

15 Ketchup Arts

16 Carsten Raffel

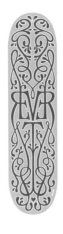

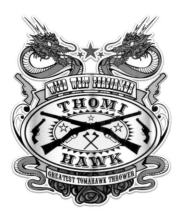

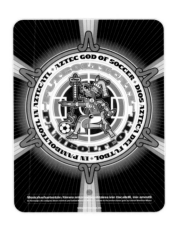

01 Niels Shoe Meulman

02 J6Studios

03 Kimera

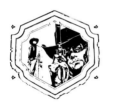

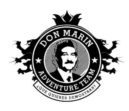

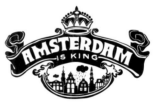

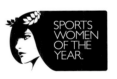

04 3 deluxe

05 AmorfoDesignlab™

06 Parra

07 Konstantinos Gargaletsos

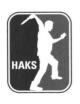

08 J6Studios

09 Systm

10 chemicalbox

11 viagrafik

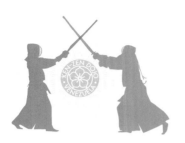

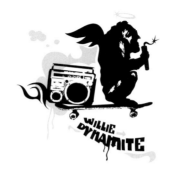

01 Ariel Pintos

02 Michaël Pinto

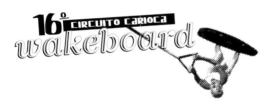

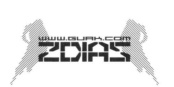

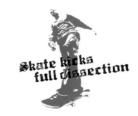

03 Transittus

04 Ketchup Arts

05 Coutworks

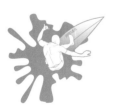

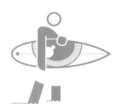

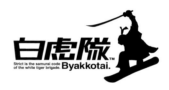

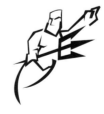

06 Shivamat

07 Carsten Raffel

08 GUAK

09 Attak

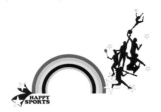

01 anna-OM-line.com

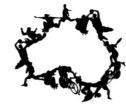

02 Digart Graphics

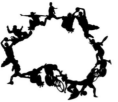

03 Studio Maverick

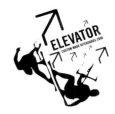

04 weissraum.de(sign)

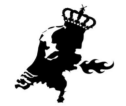

05 Floor Wesseling Ix Opus

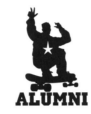

06 J6Studios

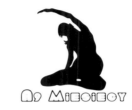

07 Guadamur

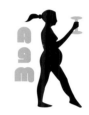

08 Guadamur

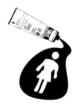

09 Ohio Girl Design

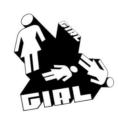

10 Ohio Girl Design

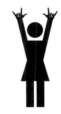

11 Ohio Girl Design

12 Kosta Lazarevski / rdy

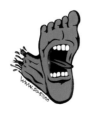

13 Christian Albriktsen

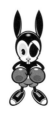

14 Carsten Raffel

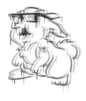

15 Carsten Raffel

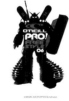

16 Marcar/kindness

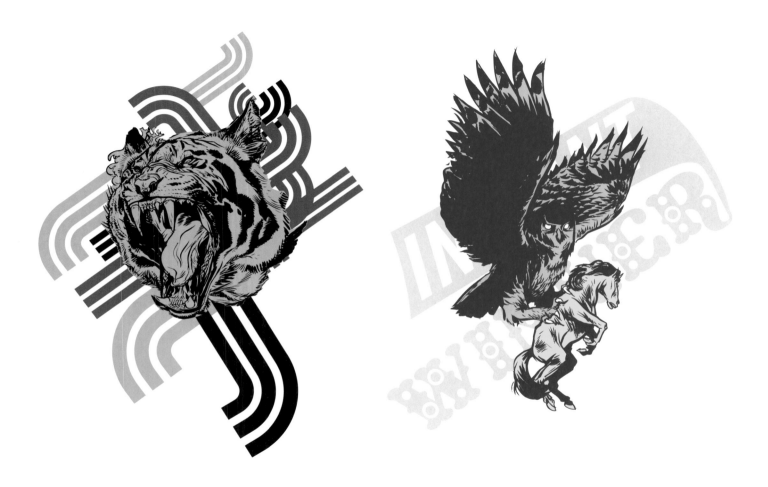

01 enginesystem   02 enginesystem

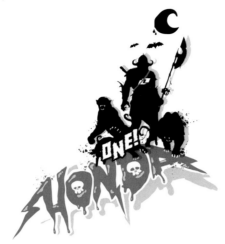

01 Bionic Systems

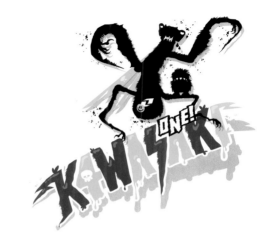

02 Bionic Systems

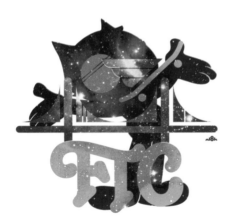

03 Nish

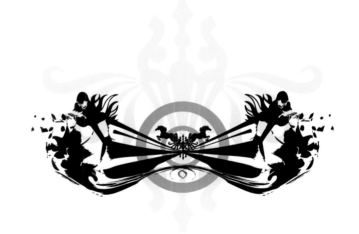

04 ROM studio

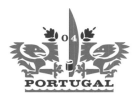

01 jum

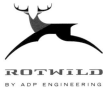

02 asmallpercent

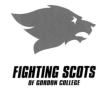

03 Simon & Goetz Design

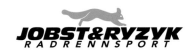

04 jl-prozess

05 Ashi & office Greminger

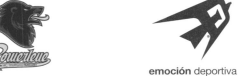

06 Paco Aguayo

07 viagrafik

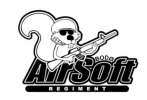

08 Christian Albriktsen

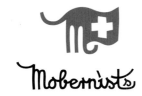

09 Flying Förtress

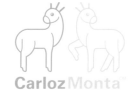

10 Onlyforthefuture

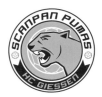

11 seventysix

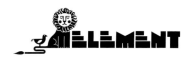

12 National Forest

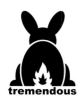

13 Formgeber

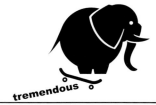

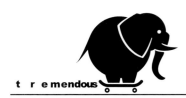

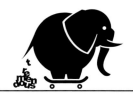

14 Formgeber

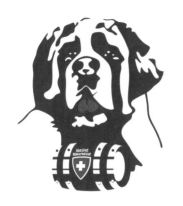

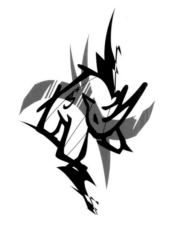

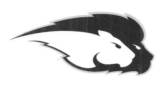
03 Mark Sloan

04 David Maloney

05 bleed

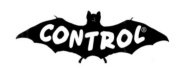
06 Yo Freeman

01 Lunatiq

02 Michaël Pinto

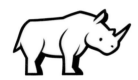

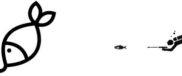

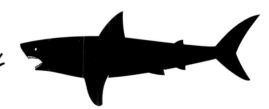

07 jum

08 the red is love

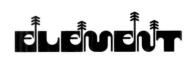
09 jum

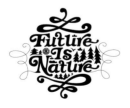

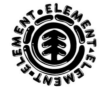

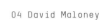

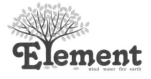

10 National Forest

11 National Forest

12 National Forest

13 National Forest

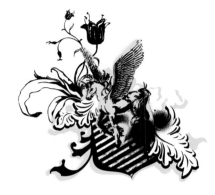

01 3 deluxe

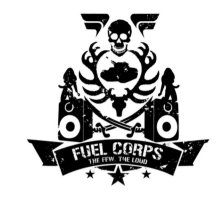

02 Engine

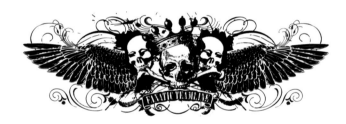

03 3 deluxe

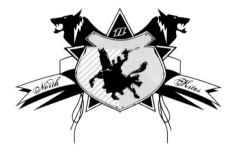

04 C100

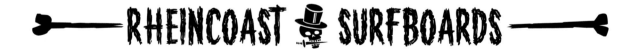

05 leBeat

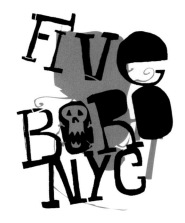

01 A-Side Studio

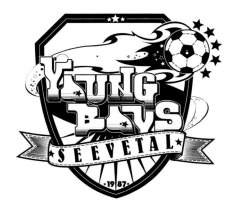

02 44 flavours

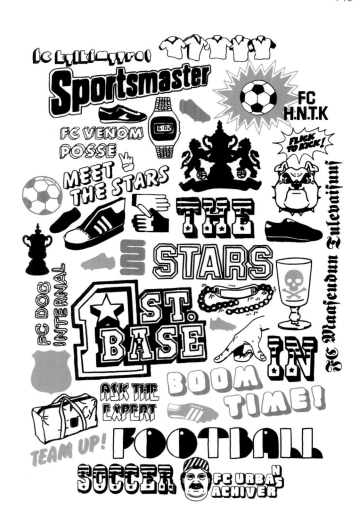

03 Jenni Tuominen, Jukka Pylväs

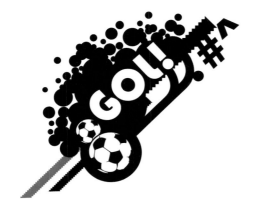

01 Fase

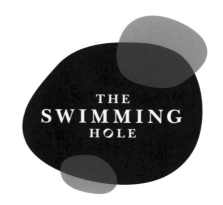

02 JDK

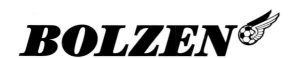

03 Jürgen und ich

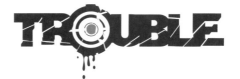

04 dzgnbio

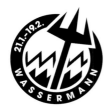

05 viagrafik

06 weissraum.de(sign)

07 Floor Wesseling Ix Opus

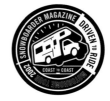

08 Draplin

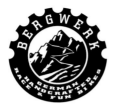

01 Magma

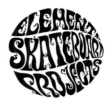

02 Emil Kozak

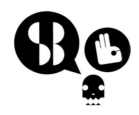

03 National Forest

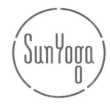

04 Raredrop

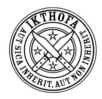

05 viagrafik

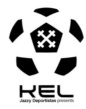

06 Hideaki Komiyama

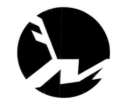

07 Lukatarina

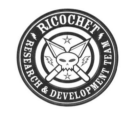

08 J6Studios

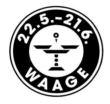

09 J6Studios

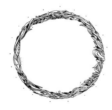

10 Michael Genovese

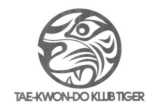

11 VIA01

12 leBeat

13 Emil Kozak

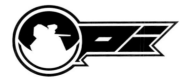

14 I&EYE

15 I&EYE

16 Ariel Pintos

NUMERO
HELSINKI
CUP

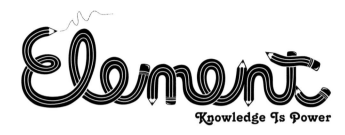

01 Jenni Tuominen, Jukka Pylväs

02 National Forest

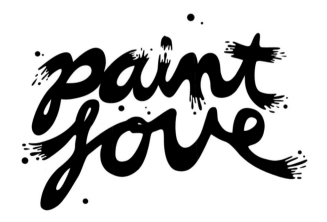

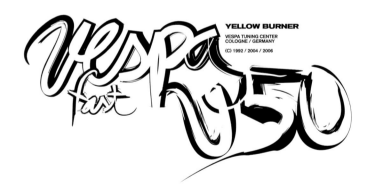

03 National Forest

04 Accident Grotesk!

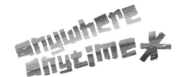

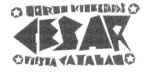

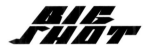

01 3 deluxe

02 3 deluxe

03 3 deluxe

04 3 deluxe

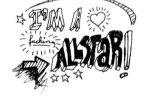

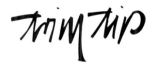

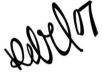

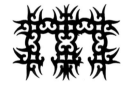

05 3 deluxe

06 3 deluxe

07 3 deluxe

08 Magma

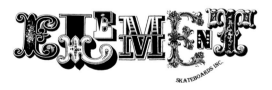

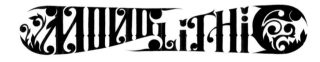

09 National Forest

10 WGD

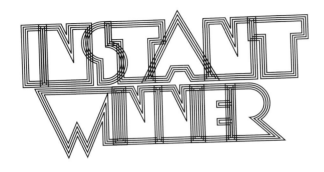

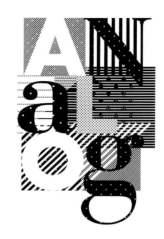

01 Emil Kozak

02 Nish

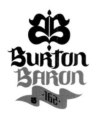

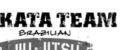

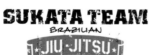

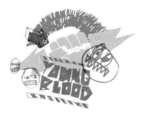

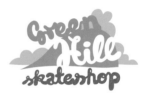

03 JDK

04 NeoDG

05 3 deluxe

06 Flying Förtress

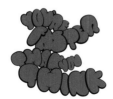

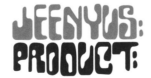

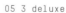

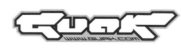

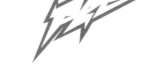

07 Adam Cruickshank

08 struggle inc.

09 GUAK

10 Axel Peemöller

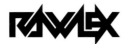

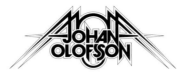

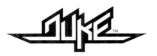

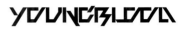

01 Büro Destruct

02 JDK

03 viagrafik

04 C100

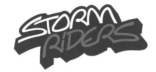

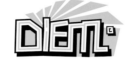

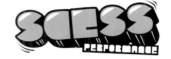

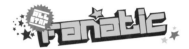

05 Flying Förtress

06 Flying Förtress

07 inkgraphix

08 3 deluxe

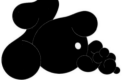

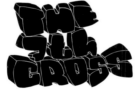

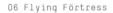

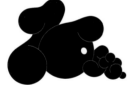

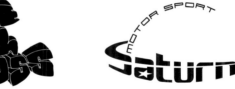

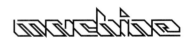

09 Shinpei Yamamori

10 3 deluxe

11 GUAK

12 Alexander Wise

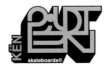

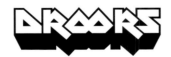

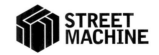

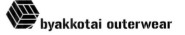

13 Dan Sparkes

14 Supermundane

15 Alexander Wise

16 Coutworks

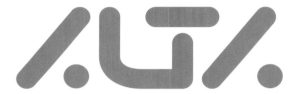

01 bleed

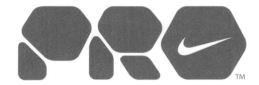

02 Tnop™ & ®bePOS|+|VE

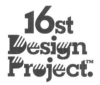

03 Shinpei Yamamori

04 Draplin

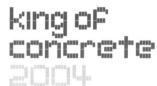

05 Intercity

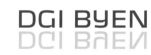

06 Kontrapunkt

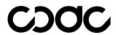

07 JDK

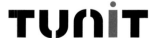

08 Kontrapunkt

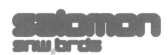

09 A-Side Studio

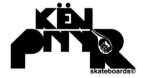

10 Dan Sparkes

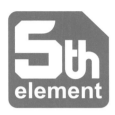

01 backyard 10

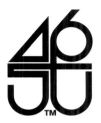

02 Shinpei Yamamori

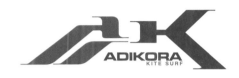

03 Keloide.net

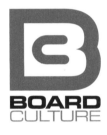

04 Sesame Studio

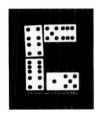

05 Yo Freeman

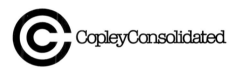

06 JDK

07 Yorgo Tloupas

08 3 deluxe

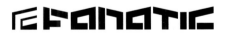

09 viagrafik

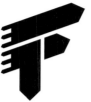

01 viagrafik

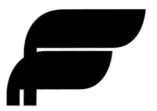

02 A-Side Studio

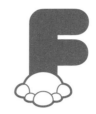

03 Sesame Studio

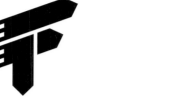

04 Nish

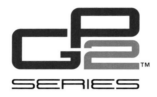

05 Scott Duke

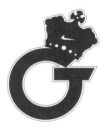

06 Mattisimo

07 typotherapy+design inc.

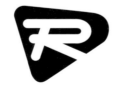

08 Yorgo Tloupas

09 Yorgo Tloupas

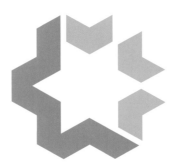

01 Draplin

02 bleed

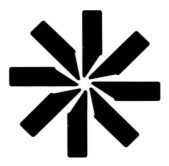

03 Resin[sistem] design

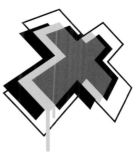

04 Michaël Pinto

ADDRESS INDEX

#

2098 Germany
30, 207, 312
info@2098.org
www.2098.org

:g / studio-gpop UK
149, 175, 209, 275, 281
info@studio-gpop.com
www.studio-gpop.com

:phunk studio Singapore
31, 60, 62, 205, 271, 358
info@phunkstudio.com
www.phunkstudio.com

+ISM UK
391, 415
info@plusism.com
www.plusism.com

0c/0m/0y/0k Germany
173, 188, 265, 268, 283, 414
Daniel Adolph
daniel@0c0m0y0k.de
www.0c0m0y0k.de

112 Ocean Drive Sweden
77, 327, 336
gustav@112oceandrive.com
www.112oceandrive.com

123Buero Germany
60, 125, 140
Timo Gaessner
hello@123buero.com
www.123buero.com

123klan France
230, 261, 388, 408
scien-klor@123klan.com
www.123KLAN.com

1508 Denmark
59
info@1508.dk
www.1508.dk

29 degres Switzerland
32, 47, 48, 75, 102, 122,
127, 187, 294, 297, 421,
422, 429, 439
Nathalie Oswald
info@29-degres.com
www.29-degres.com

2Advanced Studios USA
144, 157, 195, 209
Baz Pringle
info@2advanced.com
www.2advanced.com

3 deluxe Germany
91, 119, 124, 172, 181, 280,
339, 422, 440, 441, 448,
453, 454, 455, 457
graphics@3deluxe.de
www.3deluxe.de

310k Netherlands
24, 30, 79, 95, 100, 119,
190, 262, 281, 294, 324,
370, 426
310k
info@310k.nl
www.310k.nl

344 Design USA
42, 278, 309
Stefan G. Bucher
logos@344design.com
www.344design.com

3volt Design Germany
128, 198
NeNAD Lalos
nenad@3volt.de
www.3volt.de

44 flavours Germany
37, 58, 59, 62, 65, 91, 98,
124, 145, 147, 150, 158,
172, 204, 206, 208, 270,
272, 282, 427, 449
info@44flavours.de
www.44flavours.de

A

a+morph Germany
73, 115, 430
Irene Marx
info@a-morph.de
www.a-morph.de

ABC&Z Italy
422, 423, 424, 429
Matteo Carboni
grafica@abcz.it
www.abcz.it

Dan Abbott UK
400
mister.dan@virgin.net
www.axelburger.com

Abraka France
187, 222
Carine Abraham
carine.abraham@free.fr
www.abraka.com

Accept & Proceed UK
371
David Johnston
info@acceptandproceed.com
www.acceptandproceed.com

Accident Grotesk! Germany
54, 61, 76, 128, 190, 206,
388, 452
Alex Klug, Timothy Santore
welovedesign@
accidentgrotesk.com
www.accidentgrotesk.com

Katrin Acklin Germany
74, 75, 81, 312
katrin@katrinacklin.com
www.katrinacklin.com

actiondesigner Norway
61, 117, 143, 158, 190, 385,
393
the@actiondesigner.com
www.actiondesigner.com

Adapter Japan
187, 313, 342
info@adapter.jp
www.adapter.jp/

Adhemas Brazil
52, 263, 307, 390, 399
Adhemas Batista
abs@adhemas.com
www.adhemas.com

Paco Aguayo Mexico
37, 65, 67, 68, 78, 80, 122,
271, 446
www.haiku.com.mx

Martin Aigner Austria
68, 70, 80
office@martinaigner.com
www.martinaigner.com

Airside UK
66, 330, 413
info@airside.co.uk
www.airside.co.uk

AKA Germany
384, 439
Annika Kaltenthaler
annika.kaltenthaler@gmx.de
www.annikakaltenthaler.de

Akiza France
240, 241, 357, 393
Robinson, Akiza
contact@akiza.net
www.akiza.net

Christian Albriktsen Norway
282, 443
albriks@gmail.com

Dr. Alderete Mexico
39, 57, 141, 151, 159, 337,
392
Jorge Alderete
contacto@jorgealderete.com
www.jorgealderete.com

Alëxone France
52, 58, 93, 116, 335, 336,
388, 390, 391, 393, 399, 405
info@alexone.net
www.alexone.net

Alphabetical Order® Sweden
41, 306
everyone@
alphabeticalorder.com
www.alphabeticalorder.com

Miki Amano Japan
36, 102, 170, 224, 238, 399
mikiamano@mikiamano.com
www.mikiamano.com

Amen Germany
46, 55, 75, 191, 205
Michaela Mansch, Claudio
Prisco
amen@soseies.com
www.soseies.com

AmorfoDesignlab™ Mexico
28, 32, 58, 65, 66, 149,
163, 189, 230, 251, 253,
277, 323, 339, 343, 359,
373, 429, 441
Rik Davila Bracho
rik@amorfodesignlab.com
www.amorfodesignlab.com

Mai-Britt Amsler Denmark
89
Mai-Britt Amsler,
Lene Sørensen
mail@lenesoerensen.dk
93
mail@maibrittamsler.dk
www.maibrittamsler.dk

Analog.Systm Iceland
185, 38
Oscar Bjarnason
analog@sys.is
analog.sys.is

And Switzerland
47, 69
Jean-Benoit Lévy
www.and.ch
www.and.ch

Peter Anderson UK
168, 183, 298, 306
peter@
idesign2.gotadsl.co.uk
www.interfield-design.com

anna-OM-line.com Spain
55, 311, 425, 443
Anna Maria López López
hello@anna-OM-line.com
www.anna-OM-line.com

Anónimo Studio Venezuela
295, 308, 346
Hector Do Nascimento
anonimo@anonimostudio.com
www.anonimostudio.com

apishAngel UK
144, 363
Nick Walker
nick@apishangel.com
www.apishangel.com

Gints Apsits Latvia
47, 296, 310, 386, 388, 424
apsits@apsits.com
www.apsits.com

archetype : interactive
China
26, 69, 118, 123, 208, 311,
360, 363, 405
John Wu
john@a-i.com.hk
www.a-i.com.hk

Annella Armas Venezuela
47, 129
tierrachiquire@cantv.net

Tatiana Arocha Colombia
161, 190
tatiana@
servicio-ejecutivo.com
www.tatianaarocha.com

artless Japan
44, 118, 122, 223, 328
Anan Keigo
info@artless.gr.jp
www.artless.gr.jp

Miha Artnak Slovenia
28, 43, 45, 56, 58, 90, 99,
179, 196, 197, 200, 201,
343, 353, 373, 387
miha@artnak.net
www.artnak.net

Ash Denmark
196, 387
Victor Ash
va@victorash.net
www.victorash.net

Ashi & office Greminger
Switzerland
60, 64, 76, 153, 171, 204,
238, 325, 331, 446
Achilles Greminger
info@ashi.ch
www.ashi.ch

A-Side Studio UK
48, 64, 68, 70, 75, 105,
117, 147, 193, 219, 236,
245, 252, 260, 270, 275,
296, 305, 306, 356, 387,
449, 456, 458
contact@a-sidestudio.co.uk
www.a-sidestudio.co.uk

asmallpercent USA
33, 90, 200, 223, 311, 446
Grant Hanna
Tim Ferguson Sauder
info@asmallpercent.com
www.asmallpercent.com

Atelier Mühlberg Switzerland
42
Claude Borer
mail@atelier-muehlberg.ch
www.atelier-muehlberg.ch

Atelier Télescopique France
20, 36, 49, 100, 129, 269,
331, 343, 364
atelier-telescopique@
wanadoo.fr
www.ateliertelescopique.com

Atomic Attack Hong Kong
30, 65, 123, 153, 280
Calvin Ho
chairmancal@
atomicattack.com
www.atomicattack.com

Marc Atlan USA
34, 265, 276, 282
info@marcatlan.com
www.marcatlan.com

Attaboy USA
114, 187
Attaboy
info@yumfactory.com
www.yumfactory.com

Attak Netherlands
28, 31, 40, 43, 70, 71, 99,
100, 127, 147, 148, 152,
154, 156, 157, 190, 193,
204, 206, 208, 271, 284,
324, 326, 331, 335, 337,
360, 368, 370, 372, 389,
391, 429, 442
attak@attakweb.com
www.attakweb.com

austrianillustration.com
Austria
39, 48, 75, 227, 228, 393,
412
Fabienne Feltus
office@
austrianillustraion.com
www.austrianillustration.com

automatic USA
117, 234, 235, 271, 312
Charles Wilkin/Automatic
info@automatic-iam.com
www.automatic-iam.com

B

backyard 10 Germany
50, 120, 225, 253, 261, 272,
281, 328, 368, 384, 385, 457
Harold Lazaro
lazaro@backyard10.com
www.backyard10.com

Flavio Bagioli Chile
158, 279, 358, 359, 383
info@desorg.cl
www.desorg.cl

Herbert Baglione Brazil
345
herbert@herbert.ind.br
www.herbert.ind.br

Balsi Grafik Switzerland
25, 38, 129, 281
www.balsi.li

Bandage Denmark
36, 262, 274
info@bandage.dk
www.bandage.dk

BankerWessel Sweden
57, 114, 430
Ida Wessel, Jonas Banker
info@bankerwessel.com
www.bankerwessel.com

Base USA
105, 421
infos@basedesign.com
www.basedesign.com

BEK03 Venezuela
97, 142, 144, 149, 157, 164,
173, 180, 199, 213
info@bek03.com
www.bek03.com

Carlos Bêla Brazil
264, 308, 343, 381, 383, 415
cb@carlosbela.com
www.goldenshower.gs

Benwar Home Design France
95, 99
Benoit Matrion
ben@tvwar.org
www.tvwar.org

Thomas Beyer Germany
33, 56, 91
tb@thomasbeyer.de
www.thomasbeyer.de

Sanjai Bhana Canada
33, 295, 388
info@sanjaibhana.com
www.sanjaibhana.com

Bianca Strauch Germany
151
bianca@biancastrauch.de

Binatural Brazil
252, 264
Sung Hean
info@binatural.com.br
www.binatural.com.br

Bionic Systems Germany
23, 42, 294, 295, 304, 322,
358, 399, 445
info@bionic-systems.com
www.bionic-systems.com

Bionyc Industries UK
189, 302, 305
info@bionyc.com
www.bionyc.com

bisdixit Spain
100
Alex Gifreu+Pere
Alvaro+Carles Murillo
bis@bisdixit.com
www.bisdixit.com

Tim Bjørn Denmark
59
info@madebytim.com
www.madebytim.com

blackjune Germany
28, 52, 63, 67, 69, 77, 78,
218, 219, 222, 223, 224,
233, 238, 247, 260, 271,
275, 276, 278, 311, 322
info@blackjune.com
www.blackjune.com

bleed Norway
23, 45, 59, 65, 89, 113,
126, 226, 242, 299, 390,
440, 447, 456, 459
Dag Solhaug
bleed@bleed.no
www.bleed.no

Blindresearch Germany
325, 390, 393
Sven Zuege
sven@blindresearch.com
www.blindresearch.com

Blink Blink Brazil
161
paula@blinkblink.com.br
www.blinkblink.com.br

Blu Design Mexico
143, 161, 211, 411
Carolina Rodriguez
carolina@blu-studio.com
www.blu-studio.com

Bodara Switzerland
188, 431
Ivo Runggaldier
bodara@bodara.ch
www.bodara.ch

Chris Bolton Finland
69, 121, 130, 337, 340
chris@chrisbolton.org
www.chrisbolton.org

Imma Bordell | La Mirona
Spain
221
immab@santamagdalena.net

Petra Börner UK
170, 287
petraborner@beeb.net
www.borner.se

Borsellino & Co. Germany
23, 26, 64, 138, 206, 222,
294, 324
Piero Borsellino
mail@borsellino.net
www.borsellino.net

Felix Braden Germany
27, 28, 32, 35, 44, 45, 142,
150, 159, 161, 186
info@felixbraden.de
www.floodfonts.com

brandigloo Germany
139
Daniel Goddemeyer
dgo@brandigloo.com
www.brandigloo.com

Braveland Design USA
159, 206, 324, 346
Dave Bravenec
braveland@earthlink.net
www.bravelanddesign.com

Brighten the corners UK
59, 118, 126, 422, 423
Billy Kiossoglou,
Frank Philippin
contact@
brightenthecorners.com
www.brightenthecorners.com

Bringolf Irion Vögeli
Switzerland
61, 78, 428
Alexandra Noth
mail@bivgrafik.ch
www.bivgrafik.ch

Maik Brummundt Germany
60
mail@maikbrummundt.de
www.maikbrummundt.de

Jon Burgerman UK
39, 100, 152, 234
fries@jonburgerman.com
www.jonburgerman.com

Büro Brendel Germany
186, 391
info@buerobrendel.de
www.buerobrendel.de

Büro Destruct Switzerland
35, 62, 65, 75, 277, 311,
342, 438, 455
Hlreber
hl@burodestruct.net
www.burodestruct.net

Büro Otto Sauhaus Germany
274
Sarah Lamparter
angebot@ottosauhaus.de
www.ottosauhaus.de

büro uebele Germany
48, 59, 80, 125
Prof. Andreas Uebele
info@uebele.com
www.uebele.com

C

C100 Germany
346, 358, 365, 448, 455
hello@c100studio.com
www.c100studio.com

Clrqa Venezuela
116, 156, 189, 195, 271
Alec Méndez
clrqa@clrqa.com
www.clrqa.com

cabina Argentina
67, 95, 228, 245, 270, 295,
351, 423, 428, 429, 439
info@espaciocabina.com.ar
www.espaciocabina.com.ar

Cabine Germany
328
info@cabine.co.uk
www.cabine.co.uk

Calliope Studios USA
158, 227, 234, 294
JD Boujnah
jdb@calliopestudios.com
www.calliopestudios.com

Canefantasma Studio Italy
100, 113, 114, 117, 144,
226, 383
Mimmo Manes
m@canefantasma.com
www.canefantasma.com

Caótica Brazil
55, 107, 122, 124, 156, 199,
265
Christiano Calvet and Leonardo Eyer
caotica@caotica.com.br
www.caotica.com.br

Cape Arcona Typefoundry
Germany
27, 42, 163
Stefan Claudius
general@cape-arcona.com
www.cape-arcona.com

Frans Carlquist Sweden
327, 367, 373
frans@brilliant.nu
www.brilliant.nu/frans.html

Catalogtree Netherlands
56, 115, 128, 310
mail@catalogtree.net
www.catalogtree.net

Chapter3 USA
28, 42
Jens Karlsson
jens@chapter3.net
www.chapter3.net

chemicalbox Switzerland
44, 225, 244, 385, 441
mario buholzer
bureau@chemicalbox.com
www.chemicalbox.com

Cherrybox Studios USA
153, 408
Jessica Knapp
jessica@thecherrybox.com
www.thecherrybox.com

Deanne Cheuk USA
161, 176, 178, 179, 242,
243, 275
neomuworld@aol.com
www.neomu.com

Rob Chiu UK
23, 140, 299
info@theronin.co.uk
www.theronin.co.uk

Cisma Brazil
201, 203, 210, 271, 304,
305, 402
muitoprazer@cisma.com.br
www.cisma.com.br

CityDeep Music
361
mitzilla
mitzilla@citydeepmusic.com
www.citydeepmusic.com

clandrei Germany
68, 95, 328, 356, 373
Kai Brunning
clan@clandrei.de
www.clandrei.de

Stefan Claudius Germany
343, 357, 368
general@cape-arcona.com
www.cape-arcona.com

David Clavadetscher
Switzerland
204
david@clavadetscher.org
www.clavadetscher.org

Codeluxe Germany
277, 358
Hugo Goeldner
buero@codeluxe.com
www.codeluxe.com

Coldwater Graphiix Japan
82, 207, 269, 383
Tabito Mizuo
tabito@xenn.com

Colletivo Design Brazil
50, 140, 302
Colletivo
contato@colletivo.com
www.colletivo.com

Colourmovie USA
299, 311
michelle@colourmovie.com
www.colourmovie.com

Jared Connor USA
345
Jared Connor and Jermaine
Rogers
jared@
mexicanchocolatedesign.com
mexicanchocolatedesign.com

**Mariana de Vasconcellos
Lameiro da Costa** Brazil
101
mariana costa
marianavasc@hotmail.com

Nando Costa Brazil
151, 169, 186, 209, 212,
357, 371, 389, 415, 430
nando@nandocosta.com
www.nandocosta.com

Coutworks Japan
161, 199, 384, 442, 455
Daisuke Sato
info@coutworks.com
www.coutworks.com

Creative Pride UK
39, 166, 310, 359
Matt Kenyon
matt.kenyon@
creativepride.com
www.creativepride.com

Creative Review UK
131
Art direction: Nathan Gale
nathan.gale@centaur.co.uk
www.creativereview.co.uk

Critterbox LLC USA
390, 391
Gary Baseman
info@critterbox.com
www.critterbox.com

Adam Cruickshank Australia
103, 172, 294, 454
adam@regularproduct.com
www.regularproduct.com

Crush UK
23, 30, 66, 78, 158, 186,
336, 353, 370
Carl Rush
contact@crushed.co.uk
www.crushed.co.uk

Cruz Creative New Zealand
140
Darren D'Cruz
cruzcreative@xtra.co.nz

cryogenicx.com Japan
412
Jun Awano
jun@cryogenicx.com
www.cryogenicx.com

Cuartopiso Colombia
33, 65, 147, 151, 167, 375
Alejandro Posada
info@cuartopiso.com
www.cuartopiso.com

Cuban Council USA
151
Joe Kral
fidel@cubancouncil.com
www.cubancouncil.com

cubegrafik Switzerland
141
Steve Henseler
info@cubegrafik.com
www.cubegrafik.com

cubemen studio China
187, 199, 386, 387, 413, 414
Toby Yeung
toby@cubemen.com
www.cubemen.com

Cupco! Australia
144, 146, 150, 157, 175
Lucas Temby
momo@cupco.net
www.cupco.net

Cyklon Denmark
47, 99
Gytz
cyklon@cyklon.dk
www.cyklongrafik.net

D

Dainippon Japan
127, 312, 363, 430, 431
dainippon@type.org
dainippon.type.org

Frederique Daubal France
141, 177, 400
frederique@daubal.com
www.daubal.com

Decoylab USA
105, 209, 211, 228, 386, 396
Maiko Kuzunishi
info@decoylab.com
www.decoylab.com

DED Associates UK
43, 227
info@dedass.com
www.dedass.com

derfaber Switzerland
246, 247, 357, 413
mail@derfaber.ch
www.derfaber.ch

Designanorak / DSNRK UK
192, 201
Si Billam
si@designanorak.com
www.designanorak.com

Designbolaget Denmark
149, 276, 326
Claus Due
due@designbolaget.dk
www.designbolaget.dk

DesignChapel Sweden
144, 235, 360
Robert Lindström
info@designchapel.com
www.designchapel.com

Designkitchen Austria
48, 150, 165
arno@designkitchen.at
www.designkitchen.at

Designunion Germany
52, 59, 77, 422
Barbara Dechant
info@designunion-berlin.de
www.designunion-berlin.de

desres Germany
91, 329, 360
contact@www.desres.de
www.desres.de

dextro Austria
80, 210
dextro@dextro.org
www.dextro.org

diamond Germany
81
Kathrin Jachmann
info@diamond-gestaltung.de
www.diamond-gestaltung.de

Nohemi Dicuru-fashiongraphic
Venezuela
31, 48, 174, 247, 252, 259,
357
Nohemi Dicuru
ndicuru@cantv.net
www.fashiongraphic.com

Die Seiner Switzerland
226, 326
Lain
lain@sein.se
www.sein.se

Digart Graphics Australia
116, 186, 443
Marc Lynch
digart@bigpond.com
www.digart.com.au

DigitalPlayground Studio
Germany
31, 45, 99, 140, 148, 151,
153, 156, 163, 167, 198,
282, 369
Michael Fuchs
studio@digitalplayground.de
www.digitalplayground.de

Dimaquina Brazil
97, 104, 308, 336, 383, 409,
423
info@dimaquina.com
www.dimaquina.com

Dimomedia Lab Italy
31, 61, 78, 91, 96, 125,
139, 165, 196, 204, 236,
263, 305, 347, 389, 413
info@dimomedia.com
www.dimomedia.com

Glauco Diogenes Brazil
61, 145, 302
info@glaucodiogenes.com.br
www.glaucodiogenes.com.br

Discodoener Germany
21, 35, 48, 52, 330, 338
Marcus Fischer, Peter Palec,
Pit Lederle
info@discodoener.de
www.discodoener.de

Doma Argentina
50, 75
inflo@doma.tv
www.doma.tv

Axel Domke Germany
26, 36, 42, 52, 67, 120,
223, 324, 358, 369
axeldomke@mac.com
www.axeldomke.com

Donat Raetzo Union
Switzerland
31, 139
donat@ruthchristen.ch
www.ruthchristen.ch

dopepope USA
226
dope@dopepope.com
www.dopepope.com

Double Standards Germany
30, 83, 118
Barbara Krimm, Chris Reh-
berger
contact@doublestandards.net
www.doublestandards.net

Dr. Morbito & 1000Changos
Mexico
152, 153
1000changos/Omar Mijangos
drmorbito@yahoo.com.mx,
rudo71@yahoo.com.mx

dragon Japan
238
www.dragon76.net

Draplin USA
143, 206, 387, 388, 439,
450, 456, 459
Aaron James Draplin
draplin@draplin.com
www.draplin.com

Judith Drews Germany
99
post@judithdrews.de
www.judithdrews.de

DTM_INC Netherlands
45, 47, 60, 61, 71, 73, 78,
101, 120, 226, 272, 323,
327, 336, 346, 354, 367,
406, 409, 414
DTM INC
dtm_inc@hotmail.com

Scott Duke
458
Formula One Management in-
house design team

dynamo-ville USA
336
keith rocka
dynamo@dynamo-ville.com
www.dynamo-ville.com

Boris Dworschak Germany
187, 329, 387
Boris Dworschak
info@borisdworschak.de
www.borisdworschak.de

dzgnbio France
181, 187, 194, 211, 241,
252, 337, 359, 361, 362, 450
dzgnbio@gmail.com
www.dzgnbio.com

E

eduhirama Brazil
24, 40, 95, 367
Edu Hirama
eduhirama@yahoo.com.br

ehquestionmark UK
184, 252, 347, 350, 354,
367, 370, 408
bhatoptics
enquirehere@
ehquestionmark.com
www.ehquestionmark.com

Engine UK
38, 76, 93, 209, 302, 303,
307, 323, 337, 343, 353,
359, 368, 369, 370, 383,
414, 448
Dan Smith
info@engine-design.co.uk
www.engine-design.co.uk

enginesystem USA
444
Craig Metzger
Nathan Fox
www.enginesystem.com

env-design Germany
125
jonas grossmann
we@env-design.com
www.env-design.com

eP_ Brazil
211
Pipa and Carolina Aboarrage
pipa@epwww.com
www.epwww.com

Dennis Eriksson Sweden
114, 115, 158, 186, 328
dennis@woo.se

Matthias Ernstberger USA
229
m.ernstberger@gmx.de

Escobas Mexico
58, 74, 99, 102, 103, 152,
201
Corazon Diseño
escobas@escobas.com.mx
www.escobas.com.mx

e-Types Denmark
90, 206
info@e-types.com
www.e-types.com

Euro RSCG Fuel Worldwide UK
80
www.eurorscg.com

evaq studio USA
77, 265, 267, 339, 359
Asif Mian
asif@evaq.com
www.evaq.com

everyday icons Japan
82
Shinya Inamura
shinya@everydayicons.jp
portfolio.everydayicons.jp

Extraverage Productions
Hungary
42, 44, 47, 48, 52, 62, 63,
66, 73, 74, 79, 110, 114,
118, 120, 124, 125, 140,
142, 143, 144, 148, 151,
160, 161, 165, 168, 172,
175, 181, 194, 197, 198,
200, 201, 203, 206, 222,
231, 244, 251, 252, 261,
280, 346, 398, 399, 403,
408, 412, 428, 440
blikdsgn, Karoly Kiralyfalvi
drez@extraverage.net
www.extraverage.net

F

Faith Canada
199, 242, 246, 258, 305,
311, 412
Paul Sych
info@faith.ca
www.faith.ca

Fakir Mexico
176, 298, 313, 392
Diana Patricia González
fakirl@prodigy.net.mx, revi-
stafakir@gmail.com

Fase Argentina
151, 205, 224, 281, 304,
312, 337, 388, 424, 450
info@mundofase.com
www.mundofase.com

fatbob New Zealand
37, 207, 270
Klaus Kremer
klaus@fatbob.co.nz
www.fatbob.co.nz

Fellow Designers Sweden
152, 208, 237, 395
Paul Kühlhorn
Eva Liljefors
paul@fellowdesigners.com
www.fellowdesigners.com

Laurent Fétis France
91, 116, 122, 125, 328, 367,
411
info@laurentfetis.com
www.laurentfetis.com

feurer network Switzerland
33
Richard Feurer
richard.feurer@
feurer-network.ch
www.feurer-network.ch

Derek Johnson USA
38, 127, 191, 234, 424
derek@blueshape.com
www.blueshape.com

Julie Joliat Switzerland
118, 191, 254
julie@joliat.net
www.joliat.net

Juju's Delivery Germany
42
mail@jujus-delivery.com
www.jujus-delivery.com

Jules UK
230
jules@jules.net
www.jules.net

jum Germany
43, 75, 90, 142, 198, 234,
252, 295, 327, 437, 446, 447
jum@
unitedstatesofheart.com
www.unitedstatesofheart.com

june France
35, 63, 188, 191, 207, 226,
296, 391, 428
Julien Crouigneau
june@designjune.com
www.designjune.com

Jürgen und ich Germany
101, 122, 312, 450
Jürgen Frost
wir@juergenundich.de
www.juergenundich.de

K

Kallegraphics Norway
63, 66, 172, 176, 186, 204,
271, 307, 330, 356, 394, 411
email@kallegraphics.com
www.kallegraphics.com

Jeffrey Kalmikoff USA
24, 36, 37, 58, 73, 78
jeffrey@skinnycorp.com
www.ifd-lab.com

Hayato Kamono Japan
37, 42, 61, 188, 198
hayato@designurge.com
www.designurge.com

kame design USA
82, 334
Joachim Müller-Lancé
joachim@kamedesign.com
www.kamedesign.com

Kanardo France
32, 151
contact@kanardo.com
www.kanardo.com

Pep Karsten France
81, 207, 360
info@pepkarsten.com
www.pepkarsten.com

karlssonwilker USA
101
karlssonwilker
131
Emmi Salonen,
Art Director: Jan Wilker
www.karlssonwilker.com

K-Berg Projects Sweden
228, 250
info@k-berg.se
www.k-berg.se

Keep Adding USA
98, 347
mitzilla
info@keepadding.com
www.keepadding.com

Keep Left Studio Australia
30, 45, 51, 63, 66, 104,
110, 127, 136, 142, 184,
187, 195, 197, 230, 231,
242, 255, 256, 258, 259,
260, 261, 263, 267, 269,
286, 392, 403, 406
Luca Ionescu, Kevin Vo
kls@keepleftstudio.com
www.keepleftstudio.com

Keloide.net Spain
140, 160, 161, 182, 184,
197, 200, 201, 358, 457
Alvaro E. León R.
alvaro@keloide.net
www.keloide.net

KesselsKramer Netherlands
39, 58, 60, 77, 223, 240,
403, 405
ACNE
church@kesselskramer.nl
www.kesselskramer.com

Ketchup Arts Japan
71, 193, 197, 204, 207, 211,
280, 295, 297, 309, 323,
326, 353, 361, 363, 440, 442
Daisuke Miyamoto
info@ketchuparts.com
www.ketchuparts.com

Kimera Mexico
25, 150, 183, 423, 441
Gabriel Martínez Meave
gabriel@kimera.com.mx
www.kimera.com.mx

Kingsize Sweden
45, 235, 305, 328
Mika Pollack
mika@woo.se

Kiralyfalvi see Extraverage

Klauser Weibel Switzerland
92, 422
info@kwdesign.ch
www.kwdesign.ch

KMS Team Germany
23, 25, 59, 93
CD: Knut Maierhofer,
Design: Bruno Marek,
Bernhard Zölch
info@kms-team.de
www.kms-team.de

Koadzn France
65, 100, 175, 186, 253, 260,
261, 262, 279, 280, 403
Koa
koa@koadzn.com
www.koadzn.com

Jason Kochis USA
65, 102, 227, 230, 238, 247,
323, 337, 347, 363, 403
jason@jasonkochis.com
www.jasonkochis.com

kong Switzerland
45
wir@kong.ch
www.kong.ch

Kontrapunkt Denmark
22, 42, 119, 190, 295, 420,
422, 423, 430, 456
mail@kontrapunkt.com
www.kontrapunkt.com

Kasia Korczak / Slavs UK
368
kasia@theslavs.com
www.theslavs.com

Oliver Kartak Austria
355, 360
office@oliverkartak.com
www.oliverkartak.com

Emil Kozak Spain
61, 143, 201, 267, 271, 451, 454
info@emilkozak.com
www.emilkozak.com

Kummer & Herrman Netherlands
93
studio@kummer-herrman.nl
www.kummer-herrman.nl

Krv Kurva Portugal
191
Helder Araújo + Krv Kurva
info@krvkurva.org
www.krvkurva.org

Tsuyoshi Kusano Japan
131, 285, 292, 296, 311, 369
tsuyos-k@momo.so-net.ne.jp
www.kusano-design.com

Martin Kvamme Norway
32, 33, 59, 114, 123, 306,
342, 343, 357
info@unitdeltaplus.com
www.unitdeltaplus.com

kw43 Germany
24, 68, 74, 76, 158, 159
Christian Vöttiner
contact@kw43.de
www.kw43.de

L

La Fusée France
297, 330
Clément Perrotte
cp@fusee.com
www.fusee.com

La Superagencia ® Venezuela
96, 124
Luis E. Montenegro Lafont,
Art Director: Maria Alexandra Salamanqués
31, 79, 147, 196, 199, 208
Luis E. Montenegro Lafont
central@lasuperagencia.com
www.lasuperagencia.com

Labooo Germany
42, 79, 323, 330
Thomas Andritschke
office@labooo.de
www.labooo.de

Labor für visuelles Wachstum
Germany
28, 38, 45, 80, 81, 138,
150, 163, 165, 198, 264,
330, 371, 410, 425
Jens Lausenmeyer
jens@lausenmeyer.com
www.lausenmeyer.com

Laborator Czech Republic
56, 77, 205, 276, 278, 285,
400, 403
Petr Babák
info@laboratory.cz
www.laboratotry.cz

Lapin Spain
40, 141, 147, 150, 153, 159,
184, 390, 393
Jorge Navarro Herradon
lapin@lapinstudio.com
www.lapinstudio.com

Läufer + Keichel Germany
60
Marcus Keichel
info@laeuferkeichel.de
www.laeuferkeichel.de

Laundry USA
58, 111, 129, 180, 185, 309,
314, 315, 352, 353, 359,
403, 404, 405, 408, 410
PJ Richardson
pj@laundrymot.tv
www.laundrymot.tv

Kosta Lazarevski / rdy
138, 157, 185, 200, 282,
297, 312, 326, 327, 430, 443
rushersdieyoung@gmail.com
rushersdieyoung@gmail.com

Le_Palmier Design Germany
52, 70, 126, 334, 341, 346,
371, 373
Andreas Palm
design@lepalmier.de
www.lepalmier.de

leBeat Germany
148, 448, 451
a.kniepkamp@lebeat.de
www.lebeat.de

Cassie Leedham UK
55, 95, 97, 151
cassie@cassieleedham.com
www.cassieleedham.com

Urs Lehni Switzerland
63, 72
urs@our-magazine.ch
www.our-magazine.ch

less rain UK
30, 143
Lars Eberle
lars@lessrain.com
www.lessrain.com

Katharina Leuzinger UK
35, 53, 57
mail@katleuzinger.com
www.katleuzinger.com

Lifelong Friendship Society
USA
112, 179, 340, 349, 352
info@lifelongfriendshipso-
ciety.com
www.lifelongfriendshipso-
ciety.com

Lindedesign Germany
139, 148, 185, 204, 391
Christian Lindemann
info@lindedesign.de
www.lindedesign.de

Linoleum France
392
Ludovic Bondu
info@linoleum.fr
www.linoleum.fr

Jan-Kristof Lipp Germany
198
j.lipp@die-gestalten.de
www.die-gestalten.de

Barbara Lippe Austria
347
babsi@lippe.at
www.lippe.at

Lloyd & Associates Germany
228, 248, 252, 278
Kimberly Lloyd,
Annika Kaltenthaler
kl@qompendium.com
www.lloyd-associates.de

Lollek und Bollek Germany
117
hallo@lollekundbollek.de
www.lollekundbollek.de

Lolo Spain
390
lolo2077@yahoo.com
lolo2077@yahoo.com

Oscar Salinas Losada Mexico
43, 45, 82, 100, 172
oscar@manodelrey.com
www.manodelrey.com/oscar

Lousy Livincompany Germany
39, 172, 258, 264, 285, 286,
352
Stefan Marx
stefan@livincompany.de
www.livincompany.com

loyalkaspar USA
306, 307
Beat Baudenbacher
info@loyalkaspar.com
www.loyalkaspar.com

Lukatarina Slovenia
33, 47, 63, 114, 148, 301,
410, 451
Luka Mancini,
Katarina Mrvar
info@lukatarina.net
www.lukatarina.net

Lunatiq Canada
45, 63, 121, 142, 147, 240,
268, 447
Bogdan Truta
info@lunatiqwear.com
www.lunatiqwear.com

Bo Lundberg Sweden
68, 114
Bo Lundberg,
Jessica Disbrow
bo@bolundberg.com
www.bolundberg.com

M

Maak UK
200, 209, 250, 413
Mark Lewis Hodgson
www.maak.co.uk

Made Norway
190
info@madebymade.no
www.madebymade.no

Magenta Creative Networks
Venezuela
92, 118, 358, 361
Johana Ertl
info@magentanetworks.com
www.magentanetworks.com

Magma Germany
55, 76
Lars Harmsen
107
Maurice Redmond
157, 227, 240, 249, 263,
285, 451, 453
André Rösler
magma@magma-ka.de
www.magma-ka.de

Magnetofonica Venezuela
98, 173, 189, 296, 387, 391,
403, 423, 424
Laura González, Alvaro León
lorette@magnetofonica.net
www.magnetofonica.net

Makak Factory Belgium
387, 409
MAKAK
makak@netcourrier.com

makelike USA
24, 69, 81, 128
Rob Halverson
studio@makelike.com
www.makelike.com

David Maloney USA
22, 24, 27, 48, 139, 205,
295, 422, 447
david@david-maloney.com
www.david-maloney.com

MaMadesign AB Sweden
70, 90, 413, 415, 431
Marcus Gärde
info@mamadesign.se
www.mamadesign.se

Maniackers Design Japan
42, 61, 75, 82, 207, 234,
309, 311, 360, 368
Masayuki Sato
sato@mks.jp.org
www.mks.jp.org

Marcar/kindness UK
443
David Marcar, Oli Pepper
dave@lacegroup.com

Luca Marchettoni Italy
295, 327, 372
luca@w3d.it
www.w3d.it

Masa Venezuela
111, 141, 156, 159, 171,
230, 231, 233, 239, 240,
258, 261, 282, 295, 296,
304, 333, 334, 356, 368
info@masa.com.ve
www.masa.com.ve

mateuniverse Germany
27, 149, 153, 194
Derya Öztürk
info@mateuniverse.com
www.mateuniverse.com

Mattisimo USA
25, 34, 35, 43, 48, 59, 62,
68, 75, 141, 185, 197, 206,
208, 281, 285, 327, 359,
413, 414, 458
mattisimo.com

Mone Maurer Germany
177
mail@monemaurer.com
www.monemaurer.com

Graeme McMillan Canada
229, 392, 406
graememcmillan@t-online.de
www.graememcmillan.com

Me, Me USA
105
Peter Vattanatham,
Fiel Valdez
love@grafuck.com
www.grafuck.com

Rob Meek Germany
63
Rob Meek
logo@robmeek.com
www.robmeek.com

Annabelle Mehraein Germany
23, 69, 128, 327
a.mehraein@swsp.de
www.swsp.de

Meomi Design Canada
114, 233
info@meomi.com
www.meomi.com

Niels Shoe Meulman
Netherlands
30, 57, 77, 115, 122, 123,
163, 256, 258, 266, 275,
325, 405, 428, 441
info@unruly.nl
www.unruly.nl

MH grafik Switzerland
204, 277, 331, 413
Max Henschel
www.mhg.ch

PMKFA Japan
74, 172, 195, 273
Micke Thorsby
micke@pmkfa.com
www.pmkfa.com

Microbot Switzerland
145, 165, 198, 199, 281,
308, 388, 408
David Fuhrer
shell@microbot.ch
www.microbot.ch

Mikel Mikel UK
425
Miguel Angel Leyva
touch@mikelmikel.com
www.mikelmikel.com

milchhof : atelier Germany
42, 43, 94, 115, 266
Hans Baltzer
post@milchhof.net
www.milchhof.net

Mini Miniature Mouse USA
389
Fumi Nakamura
contact@
miniminiaturemouse.com
www.miniminiaturemouse.com

Mission Design Agency Norway
67
Karl Martin Saetren
www.mission.no

Mitch Paone USA
193, 204, 259, 309
mitch@
dreamersinkaesthetics.net
www.dreamersinkaesthetics.
net

Mode UK
189, 195
Ian Styles, Phil Costin
info@mode-mail.co.uk
www.mode-online.co.uk

modo Venezuela
188
alexander wright
alex@modovisual.com
www.modovisual.com

Molho Brazil
105, 113, 125, 171
Marcelo Garcia
marcelo@molho.tv
www.molho.tv

Moniteurs Germany
73, 42
info@moniteurs.de
www.moniteurs.de

morphor Switzerland
31, 34, 79
info@morphor.ch
www.morphor.ch

William Morrisey USA
24, 56, 126, 183, 236, 312,
411
hello@wmwmwm.com
www.wmwmwm.com

Hugh Morse UK
301, 35
info@hughmorse.com
www.hughmorse.com

Rune Mortensen Norway
97, 369, 429
post@runemortensen.no
www.runemortensen.no

Moving Brands UK
32, 69, 71, 345
info@movingbrands.com
www.movingbrands.com

moxi Switzerland
139, 196
mail@moxi.ch
www.moxi.ch

Mule Industry UK
197
Shaharzad Khan
info@muleindustry.com
www.muleindustry.com

Muller UK
34, 60, 70, 74, 172, 189,
211, 382
Tom Muller
tomm@hellomuller.com
www.hellomuller.com

Manuel Musilli Italy
382
manuel@digitalultras.com
www.digitalultras.com

multifresh USA
322, 368
David Nakamoto
david@multifresh.com
www.multifresh.com

Mutabor Design Germany
28, 69, 104, 119, 294, 391
info@mutabor.de
www.mutabor.de

MvM / Maarten van Maanen
Netherlands
56, 115, 194, 409, 430
contact@maartenvanmaanen.nl
www.maartenvanmaanen.nl

MWK - Zimmermann und Hähnel
Germany
59, 423, 429
Ben Wozniak
info@mwk-koeln.de
www.mwk-koeln.de

Mwmcreative UK
68, 206, 211
Maria da Gandra,
Maaike van Neck
info@mwmcreative.co.uk
www.mwmcreative.co.uk

Mytton Williams UK
429
Bob Mytton, Matt Judge
design@myttonwilliams.co.uk
www.myttonwilliams.co.uk

N

Nanospore, llc USA
384, 394
Paul Hwang
info@nanospore.org
nanospore.org

National Forest USA
51, 327, 440, 446, 447, 451,
452, 453
contact@
nationalforestdesign.com
www.nationalforest.com

Neasden Control Centre UK
186
steve@
neasdencontrolcentre.com
www.neasdencontrolcentre.com

Neeser & Müller Switzerland
59, 74, 91, 117, 118, 224,
278
info@neesermueller.ch
www.neesermueller.ch

nem Japan
336, 337, 356
Shinji Nemoto
s@nneemm.com
www.nneemm.com

NeoDG Argentina
36, 240, 253, 304, 454
neodg
info@neodg.com.ar
www.neodg.com.ar

Neubau Germany
62, 193, 200, 269, 353
Stefan Gandl
Stefan@NeubauBerlin.com
www.neubauberlin.com

newoslo USA
137, 264, 338
Live Huse
yo@newoslo.com
www.newoslo.com

News Netherlands
33, 100, 120, 128, 221, 365,
370, 371, 372
us@newsnewsnewsnews.net
www.newsnewsnewsnews.net

Daniel Neye / trb. Germany
387
mail@
jointransformberlin.com
www.jointransformberlin.com

Ninjacruise USA
141, 187, 231, 257, 329,
404, 405
Matthew Curry
matt@ninjacruise.com
www.ninjacruise.com

Nish USA
119, 123, 143, 144, 228,
352, 366, 367, 445, 454, 458
Steve Nishimoto
info@nish.net
www.nish.net

No-Domain Spain
82, 122, 123, 145, 153, 155,
211, 228, 271, 301, 303,
305, 345, 346, 356, 361,
365, 370, 411
ese@no-domain.com
www.no-domain.com

Thomas Nolfi Denmark
34, 38, 55, 74, 276, 394
nolfi@grafisk.dk
www.nolfi.dk

Nonstop Finland
57, 60, 355
Miika Saksi
nonstop@non-stops.com
www.non-stops.com

Norwegian Ink Norway
26, 56, 63, 102, 117, 141,
148, 151, 153, 157, 161,
175, 185, 188, 308, 335
post@norwegianink.com
www.norwegianink.com

nothing from outer space
Switzerland
25, 27, 28, 80
spacefox [matias krebs]
info@nothing.ch
www.nothing.ch

Timo Novotny Austria
307
Logo: Power Graphixx, Font:
Nik Thoenen, Font&Logo
Combination: Timo Novotny
filmremix@lifeinloops.com
www.lifeinloops.com

Nuuro Venezuela
160, 186, 196, 212
Alejandro Ghersi
alex@nuuro.net
www.nuuro.net

NYK Hungary
195, 196, 198, 209
Ágnes Koska
info@nyk.hu
www.nyk.hu

O

Naho Ogawa Japan
36, 234, 336, 388, 393
mail@naho.com
www.naho.com

Ohio Girl Design USA
284, 343, 443
Andy Mueller
info@ohiogirl.com
www.thequietlife.com

Akinori Oishi Japan
175
aki98@iamas.ac.jp
aki-air.com

Richard Øiestad Norway
204, 264
contact@retron.info
www.retron.info

Omochi Japan
64, 65, 66, 80, 82, 412, 415
omochigraphics@mac.com
homepage.mac.com/omochi-
graphics

onlab Switzerland
427
in@onlab.ch
www.onlab.ch

Onlyforthefuture Germany
393, 446
info@onlyforthefuture.com
www.onlyforthefuture.com

onrushdesign / front Iceland
31, 33, 160, 186, 324, 370,
391, 410
Ragnar Freyr Pálsson
ragnar@onrushdesign.com
www.onrushdesign.com

Alexandre Orion Brazil
97, 141
arte@tela.tv
www.tela.tv

Otherways 5th Floor Studio
Netherlands
126, 165
Donald Roos
donald.roos@otherways.nl
www.otherways.nl

Ottograph Netherlands
45, 63, 74, 284, 326, 328,
334, 336, 368, 393
ottograph3000
otto@ottograph.com
www.ottograph.com

Out Of Order Netherlands
69, 70, 125, 163, 195, 237,
239, 260, 327, 342, 355,
360, 415, 426
info@outoforder.nl
www.outoforder.nl

P

Pandarosa Australia
103, 150, 276
info@pandarosa.net
www.pandarosa.net

Pantiestudio Mexico
89, 129, 138, 429
Cejas
contacto@pantiestudio.com
www.pantiestudio.com

Parra Netherlands
115, 173, 226, 260, 270,
335, 336, 350, 355, 428, 441
parra@rockwellclothing.com
www.bigactive.com

Axel Peemöller Australia
78, 83, 149, 187, 197, 201,
209, 261, 271, 272, 275, 454
axel@de-war.de
www.de-war.de

Pentagram Germany
73, 91, 119, 127, 426
Justus Oehler
info@pentagram.de
www.pentagram.com

Perndl+Co Austria
90
Regula Widmer,
Josef Perndl,
Aleksandra Domanovic
office@perndl.at
www.perndl.at

Pfadfinderei Germany
25, 62, 323, 324, 326, 358,
374
critzla
zelt@pfadfinderei.com
www.pfadfinderei.com

Michaël Pinto France
330, 372, 442, 447, 459
michael.pinto@orange.fr

Ariel Pintos Venezuela
93, 109, 442, 451
arielpintos@cantv.net

Pixel Storm Switzerland
429
Andres Wanner
andres_wanner@yahoo.de
www.pixelstorm.ch

Plastic Kid Denmark
123, 157, 185, 232, 308,
326, 346, 411
Jakob Printzlau
jakob@plastickid.dk
www.plastickid.dk

Plasticbag Germany
194, 211
Philipp Körber
inquiries@plasticbag.de
www.plasticbag.de

PMKFA Japan
356, 365, 367, 375
Micke Thorsby
micke@pmkfa.com
www.pmkfa.com

Polygraph Japan
100, 210, 230, 237, 280,
295, 297, 306, 308, 414, 415
suwa@nyon-nyon.com
www.polygraph.jp

Positron Japan
43, 57, 205, 231, 236, 331,
337, 358, 390
info@the-positron.com
www.the-positron.com

Pietari Posti Spain
57, 355
info@pietariposti.com
www.pietariposti.com

Power Graphixx Japan
42, 55, 71, 82, 123, 253,
273, 283, 294, 295, 308,
344, 410, 411, 412, 429
Junya Saito
support@power-graphixx.com
www.power-graphixx.com

Precursor UK
69, 370
mail@precursorstudio.com
www.precursorstudio.com

Friederike Preuschen Germany
28

Raffaele Primitivo Italy
152, 188, 192, 193, 194,
224, 225, 226, 263, 270,
272, 275, 276, 334, 337,
347, 355, 361, 362, 364,
365, 372, 373
rapa@primitivodesign.com
www.primitivodesign.com

Projekttriangle Germany
188, 194, 226, 421
mail@projekttriangle.com
www.projekttriangle.com

propella Germany
61, 120
albanese@propella-design.de
www.propella-design.de

Q

Mathilde Quartier
Switzerland
28, 69, 73, 91
info@quartier-design.ch
www.quartier-design.ch

QuickHoney USA
82, 99, 143, 156, 359
Nana Rausch
me@quickhoney.com
www.quickhoney.com

R

radargraphics Netherlands
60, 68, 163, 329, 360
Henk van het Nederend
info@radargraphics.com
www.radargraphics.com

Andrew Rae UK
331
a@andrewrae.org.uk
www.andrewrae.org.uk

Carsten Raffel Germany
26, 35, 64, 142, 152, 172,
181, 228, 229, 268, 277,
308, 312, 383, 388, 390,
425, 440, 442, 443
carsten@
unitedstatesoftheart.com
www.unitedstatesoftheart.com

Axel Raidt Germany
24, 42, 129
www.raidt.com

Mikko Rantanen UK
243, 405
mikko@mikkorantanen.com
www.mikkorantanen.com

Raphazen Japan
176, 184, 210, 262
Hamadaya
info@raphazen.com
www.raphazen.com

Raredrop Japan
23, 24, 25, 37, 82, 95, 123,
200, 294, 309, 363, 451
Quentaro "ANI" Fujimoto
coffer@raredrop.jp
www.raredrop.jp

raum mannheim Germany
44, 52, 66, 79, 81, 93, 97,
98, 107, 108, 115, 127, 232,
328, 368, 373
Frank Hoffmann
www.raum-mannheim.com

Palle Bruun Rasmussen
Denmark
251
www.rvlt.com

Razauno Venezuela
126, 161, 245, 260, 405, 409
Max Vogel
info@razauno.com
razauno.com

red design UK
41, 63, 66, 78, 122, 213,
243, 338, 348, 353, 358,
361, 369, 374
info@red-design.co.uk
www.red-design.co.uk

redaktion »echtzeit« Germany
146, 151, 162, 166
Steffen Wierer, Svenja von
Döhlen (formdusche)
redaktion@echtzeit.org
www.echtzeit.org

Regina Japan
148, 408
ryo mastuura
republicofregina@
hotmail.com
www.republicofregina.com

re-p Austria
117
Nik Thoenen, Maia Gusberti
re-p@re-p.org
www.re-p.org

re-public Denmark
93, 277, 325
Louise Hessellund
info@re-public.com
re-public.com

Seth Rementer USA
44
info@commonplayer.com
www.commonplayer.com

Research Studios Berlin
Germany
26
berlin@researchstudios.com
www.researchstudios.com

Resin[sistem] Australia
33, 57, 75, 102, 140, 161,
184, 186, 201, 204, 252,
280, 333, 362, 383, 408,
413, 459
info@resindesign.com.au
www.resindesign.com.au

resistro Brazil
101, 139, 205, 362, 366,
368, 369, 415
Christiano Calvet
resistro@resistro.net
www.resistro.net

Resopal-Schallware Germany
77
eikes grafischer hort
yeah@resopal-schallware.com
www.resopal-schallware.com

Cybu Richli Switzerland
177, 210
i@cybu.ch
www.cybu.ch

Keren Richter USA
240, 282, 285, 326
keren@
bloodisthenewblack.com
www.notkeren.com

Rinzen Australia
39, 61, 63, 306, 309, 346,
347, 355
they@rinzen.com
www.rinzen.com

Paul Roberts UK
124, 189, 411
hello@paulroberts.tv
www.paulroberts.tv

Rocholl Selected Designs
Germany
22, 70, 190, 191, 292, 293
Frank Rocholl
www.rocholl.cc

Maria elena Velasco Rojas
Mexico
43

Rolitoland France
146, 147
Rolito
rolito@rolitoland.com
www.rolitoland.com

ROM studio Mexico
55, 101, 145, 162, 343, 397,
401, 445
Rodrigo Maceda del Rio
rom@romstudio.com.mx
www.romstudio.com.mx

Rosendahl Grafikdesign
Germany
25, 32, 44, 55, 91
Lars Borngräber
info@rosendahlgrafik.de
www.rosendahlgrafik.de

Gianni Rossi Italy
88, 152, 234, 330, 372, 393
contact@giannirossi.net
www.giannirossi.net

Christian Rothenhagen
Germany
30, 39, 160, 225, 228, 229,
240, 440
moin@
christianrothenhagen.com
www.christianrothenhagen.com

Chris Rubino USA
149, 206, 207, 208, 299,
312, 430
crubino@studio18hundred.com
www.chrisrubino.com

Dirk Rudolph Germany
323, 325, 339, 341
contact@dirkrudolph.de
www.dirkrudolph.de

ruse76 UK
124, 391
ruse
ruse76@hotmail.co.uk
www.ruse76.com

S

Sagmeister Inc. USA
321, 369, 380
Matthias Ernstberger,
Stefan Sagmeister
info@sagmeister.com
www.sagmeister.com

Salon Vektoria Germany
61, 98, 104, 161, 190, 195,
208, 260, 279, 292, 347,
370, 390, 408, 409, 425, 439
Benjamin Metz
hello@salonvektoria.com
www.salonvektoria.com

Emmi Salonen UK
31, 62, 80, 142, 192, 203,
286, 307, 326, 424
hello@emmi.co.uk
www.emmi.co.uk

Akira Sasaki Japan
66, 327
agrippa@pop21.odn.ne.jp

Sat One Germany
64, 100, 101, 129, 194, 236
grafx.design@gmx.de
www.satone.de

Loïc Sattler France
30, 51, 54, 61, 129, 427,
428
Loïc Sattler - Lysergid
contact@lysergid.com
www.lysergid.com

Joe A. Scerri Switzerland
41, 64, 67, 170, 189, 347,
353, 365, 395
limepin@runbox.com
www.joescerridesign.com

Georg Schatz Germany
24, 31, 33, 43, 60, 68, 144,
206, 327
g.schatz@swsp.de
www.swsp.de

Fons Schiedon Netherlands
109, 119, 149, 173, 302,
304, 305
office@fonztv.nl
www.fonztv.nl

seacreative Italy
240, 391
seacreative@tin.it
www.seacreative.net

Sektie Netherlands
102, 114, 124
Jeffrey Warlich
jeffreywarlich@yahoo.com
von-rudolf-art.livejour-
nal.com

selanra Germany
47, 73, 208
post@selanra.de
www.selanra.de

Sellout Industries Germany
141, 143, 146, 148, 149,
157, 172, 175, 188, 194,
225, 335, 352, 408, 409, 411
post@sellout-industries.org
www.sellout-industries.org

Semisans USA
48, 127, 187, 277, 328, 370,
391, 429
Aaron Tanner,
Matt Wagner
matt@semisans.com
www.semisans.com

Semitransparent Design Japan
64, 119, 126, 278
info@
semitransparentdesign.com
www.semitransparentdesign.
com

Sensus Design Factory
Croatia
27, 60, 70, 77, 95, 158
Nedjeljko Spoljar,
Kristina Spoljar
nedjeljko.spoljar@
zg.t-com.hr
www.sensusdesignfactory.com

Sesame Studio Australia
25, 26, 70, 76, 78, 95, 184,
207, 367, 457, 458
Anthony Rees
anthony@sesamestudio.com
www.sesamestudio.com

Matt Sewell UK
297
mattsewell@
jacuzzi.fsnet.co.uk
www.mattsewell.co.uk

seventysix Germany
33, 60, 446
Pascal Rohé
pascal@seventysix.de
www.seventysix.de

shivamat Germany
152, 153, 158, 201, 387,
388, 425, 442
Steffen Mackert
stfn@shivamat.com
www.shivamat.com

Shokl UK
409
info@shokl.com
www.shokl.com

Sidsel Stubbe Denmark
68, 90, 91
smile@sidselstubbe.dk
www.sidselstubbe.dk

SignalStrong
187, 188, 194, 197, 198,
199, 208, 361
Ahmed Sammy
signal@signalstrong.com
www.signalstrong.com

Simian Norway
37, 127, 138, 191, 206
Colin McMahon
simian@simian.no
www.simian.no

Simon & Goetz Germany
27, 38, 44, 48, 70, 73, 76,
226, 277, 422, 437, 446
info@simongoetz.de
www.brand-equity-group.de

Sito Austria
80, 120, 194, 306
Sito Schwarzenberger
ito@gmx.at
www.sito.ws

Skin Design
52, 116, 163, 438
post@skin.no
www@skin.no

Slang Germany
184, 349, 358
Nathanaël Hamon
nat@slanginternational.org
www.slanginternational.org

Mark Sloan USA
41, 194, 423, 447
mark@marksloan.net
www.marksloan.net

Hjärta Smärta Sweden
400
hjartasmarta@woo.se

Paul Snowden Germany
29, 371
ps@paul-snowden.com
www.paul-snowden.com

Iván Solbes Spain
102, 223
ivan@ivansolbes.com
www.ivansolbes.com

sopp collective Australia
277
Katja Hartung
contact@soppcollective.com
www.soppcollective.com

space3 Netherlands
328, 369, 405
Joost van der Heijden
info@space3.nl
www.space3.nl

Dan Sparkes UK
364, 366, 384, 385, 402,
407, 408, 411, 412, 455, 456
ECO
betty@kuildoosh.com
www.kuildoosh.com

Spild af Tid Denmark
29, 114
Jakob Thorbek,
Rasmus Meisler
info@spildaftid.dk
www.spildaftid.dk

spin UK
47, 411
Helen Dwyer, Joe Burrin,
Josh Young
patricia@spin.co.uk
www.spin.co.uk

ständige vertretung Germany
118, 127
nick kapica
office@svberlin.com
www.svberlin.com

Station Sweden
201, 369, 414
Rasmus Hägg
info@stationstation.com
www.stationstation.com

Sammy Stein France
357, 373, 389
sammyszx@gmail.com
sammy.stein.free.fr

Theres Steiner Switzerland
220, 279, 282
t.steiner@toi.ch

Stockbridge International
Italy
149, 150, 243, 251, 254,
264, 269, 335, 385, 393, 413
Alfredo Carlo
info@stockbridge.it
www.stockbridge.it

Stolen USA
26, 27, 114, 140, 279, 341
Thomas Brodahl
info@stolen.la
www.stolen.la

Strada Germany
32
Stefan Rueckerl
sr@studiostrada.de
www.studiostrada.de

strange//attraktor: Canada
23, 122, 280, 370, 389
Sködt D. McNalty
studio@strangeattraktor.com
strangeattraktor.com

Jakob Straub Germany
31, 91, 95
mail@jakobstraub.com
www.jakobstraub.com

struggle inc. USA
245, 275, 282, 311, 326,
352, 355, 365, 454
Struggle
info@struggleinc.com
www.struggleinc.com

Strukt Visual Network
Austria
28, 107, 405
iink
contact@strukt.at
www.strukt.at

Studio 3 Norway
33, 36, 39, 43, 52, 243, 245
Anja Sofie Haugen, Hedda
Haugen, Robert Arntsen,
Martine Eng Grønlund,
Gro Vik
kunde@studio3.no
www.studio3.no

Studio Dumbar Netherlands
28, 127, 277, 422
info@studiodumbar.nl
www.studiodumbar.nl

Studio Erosie Netherlands
407
Erosie
hello@erosie.net
www.erosie.net

Studio Five USA
32
Tatiana Arocha,
Melissa Gorman
hello@studiofiverocks.com
www.studiofiverocks.com

Studio Maverick Japan
308, 312, 407, 443
akira@picogram.jp
www.picogram.jp/maverick

Studio Oscar UK
144, 175, 200, 202, 224,
262, 263, 329
Oscar Wilson
info@studiooscar.com
www.studiooscar.com

Studio Output UK
43, 74, 243, 247, 266, 280,
299, 302, 307, 323, 329,
330, 337, 344, 361, 367,
370, 430
Dan Moore
info@studio-output.com
www.studio-output.com

Studio Sans Nom USA
186, 402
Dustin Hostetler
studio@withoutname.com
www.studiosansnom.com

Martha Stutteregger Austria
24, 78, 118
office@stutteregger
www.stutteregger.com

Stylepatrol.com Germany
44
Björn Hansen
studio@stylepatrol.com
www.stylepatrol.com

stylodesign UK
60, 67, 78, 277, 294, 437
Tom Lancaster
tom@stylodesign.co.uk
www.stylodesign.co.uk

stylorouge UK
357
Sharon Chai
info@stylorouge.co.uk
www.stylorouge.co.uk

substrat Germany
117, 232, 245, 252
contact@substratdesign.org
www.substratdesign.org

Sueellen Finland
56, 76
riku@sueellen.org
www.sueellen.org

Sunday-Vision Japan
191, 250
info@sunday-vision.com
www.sunday-vision.com

sunrise studios Germany
24, 35, 47, 140, 281, 296,
422, 425
Fabian Fischer
ff@sunrisestudios.de
www.sunrisestudios.de

superexpresso Italy
141, 328, 329
Michele Angelo
mike@superexpresso.com
www.superexpresso.com

Superfamous Netherlands
38, 43, 67, 74, 209
Folkert Gorter
folkert@superfamous.com
www.superfamous.com

Superlow Norway
70, 105, 120, 122, 123, 124,
126, 164, 177, 191, 423
Halvor Bodin
hal@superlow.com
www.superlow.com

Supermundane UK
95, 185, 188, 337, 455
i_love@supermundane.com
www.supermundane.com

Superpopstudio Belgium
390, 425, 426, 429
César Carrocera Giagnto
superpopstudio@
superpopstudio.com
www.superpopstudio.com

Supershapes Sweden
106, 250, 307, 330
Patrick Sundqvist
www.supershapes.com

surround USA
184
info@surround.ws
www@surround.ws

Syrup Helsinki Finland
90, 119, 139, 175, 237, 306,
362
office@syruphelsinki.com
www.syruphelsinki.com

Systm Iceland
24, 27, 62, 358, 441
Siggeir Hafsteinsson
digital@sys.is
www.sys.is/digital

T

Tabas France
196, 225, 360
cedric@tabas.fr
www.tabas.fr

Tado UK
46, 146, 148, 327
mikeandkatie@tado.co.uk
www.tado.co.uk

Takora Japan
96, 146, 147, 185, 199
Kimiyoshi Futori
(Cheap Pop)
info@graphictakora.com
www.graphictakora.com

Yoshi Tajima Japan
342, 349
tajima@radiographics.jp
www.radiographics.jp

Ken Tanabe USA
140, 295
ken@kentanabe.com
www.kentanabe.com

Ryohei Tanaka Japan
393, 395
ryonutsjp@yahoo.co.jp
www.utsubo.net/ryoheitanaka

tapetentiere Switzerland
42, 146, 148
syl
syl@tapetentiere.de
www.tapetentiere.de

Team Manila Philippines
96, 97, 102, 106, 107, 111,
115, 117, 125, 128, 155,
156, 203, 224, 238, 239,
246, 247, 371, 440
info@teammanila.com
www.teammanila.com

ten_do_ten Japan
125, 130, 244, 266, 362,
401, 407
ten@tententen.net
www.tententen.net

Tender USA
56, 128, 200
info@tendercreative.com
www.tendercreative.com

TGB design Japan
251, 292, 310, 346, 383, 451
Hideaki Komiyama
info@tgbdesign.com
www.tgbdesign.com

The KDU USA
115, 116, 190, 206, 246,
267, 427
Aerosyn-Lex
general@thekdu.com
www.thekdu.com

the Legalizer Denmark
105, 184, 195, 426
Laura Johanne G. Danielsen
info@legalizer.dk
www.legalizer.dk

the red is love Italy
32, 33, 38, 80, 237, 283,
312, 352, 356, 424, 447
Rosso aka Franzese Michele
Ciro
rosso@theredislove.com
www.theredislove.com

The Remingtons Switzerland
29, 64, 99, 128
Ludovic Balland
contact@theremingtons.ch
www.theremingtons.ch

The Skull Dezain Japan
145, 173, 222, 225, 231, 232,
236, 239, 240, 243, 244, 251,
252, 258, 261, 262, 266, 268,
269, 271, 272, 279, 280, 281,
284, 285, 331, 399, 407, 412
king@skull-dez.com
www.skull-dez.com

The Vacuum Design Canada
183, 402
Nate Smith
faceoff@vacuumsucks.com
www.vacuumsucks.com

the wilderness New Zealand
43, 75, 362
info@thewilderness.co.nz
www.thewilderness.co.nz

Amseldrossel Germany
140, 143, 175
Thomas Weyres
thomas@amseldrossel.com
www.pawone.de

Thonik Netherlands
68, 127
studio@thonik.nl
www.thonik.nl

Three Negative UK
60, 385, 388, 395
paddy@threenegative.com
www.threenegative.com

Tilt Germany
74, 75, 119, 149, 180, 360,
370
Dominic Bünning,
Marc Antosch,
Jan-Henrik Möller
info@tiltdesignstudio.com
www.tiltdesignstudio.com

Yorgo Tloupas UK
226, 280, 347, 439, 457, 458
yorgo@
intersectionmagazine.com
www.intersectionmagazine.com

Tnop™ & ΦbePOS|+|VE USA
209, 311, 413, 415, 456
Tnop Wangsillapakun
info@tnop.com
www.tnop.com

Toca Me Germany
139
info@toca-me.com
www.toca-me.com

Tohyto Venezuela
66, 102, 109, 123, 145, 160,
205, 209, 212, 225, 244,
254, 281, 303, 335, 351,
362, 397
Lopez
info@tohyto.net
www.tohyto.net

Tokidoki Italy
149, 231, 284
Simone Legno
www.tokidoki.it

Toko Australia
69, 100, 105, 118, 127, 196
Eva Dijkstra
info@toko.nu
www.toko.nu

Sophie Toporkoff France
122, 264
toporkoff@address.fr
www.rendezvousmagazine.fr

Fritz Torres Mexico
152
redoba501@yahoo.com

toxi UK
208
Karsten Schmidt
info@toxi.co.uk
www.toxi.co.uk

Toxic design Italy
27, 28, 52, 139
424, 439
Fabio Lattanzi Antinori
info@toxicdesignstudio.com
www.toxicdesignstudio.com

Trafik France
25, 67, 68, 438
trafik.lyon@wanadoo.fr
www.lavitrinedetrafik.com

Transittus
99, 189, 207, 442
Marianna Dutra
design@trasittus.com
www.transittus.com

Tsai-Fi USA
224
info@tsai-fi.com
www.tsai-fi.com

tstout inc. USA
225, 233, 337, 354, 355
Tyler Stout
tyler@tstout.com
www.tstout.com

Hiroki Tsukuda Japan
97, 365
voidvillage@snow.odn.ne.jp
www.tsukudahiroki.com

Tsutomu Umezawa Japan
165
Seishiro Rito Fujimoto
tsutomu.umezawa@gmail.com
www.umezawatsutomu.com

Jenni Tuominen, Jukka Pylväs
Finland
100, 387, 388, 414, 449, 452
Jenni Tuominen

Typeholics Germany
107, 261
contact@typeholics.de
www.typeholics.de

Typosition Germany
191, 208, 382
Jenna Limbach,
Peter Reichard
www.typosition.de

typotherapy+design Canada
114, 353, 361, 458
Noel Nanton
studio@typotherapy.com
www.typotherapy.com

U

ultrafris Netherlands
297
Anton Bensdorp,
Johannes Hogebrink
info@ultrafris.nl
www.ultrafris.nl

Umeric Australia
80, 353
inquire@umeric.com
www.umeric.com

underson Japan
102, 156, 159, 225, 236
Tsutomu Horiguchi
horiguchi@underson.com
www.underson.com

Underware Netherlands
116, 185
info@underware.nl
www.underware.nl

Unit c.m.a. Netherlands
182
Job Wouters
info@unit.nl
www.unit.nl

Upnorth USA
144, 228, 299, 303, 304,
308, 310
Justin Kay
studio@discover-upnorth.com
www.discover-upnorth.com

Urbanskiworkshop Germany
190
Denis März
contact@
urbanskiworkshop.com
www.urbanskiworkshop.com

urbn; Germany
229
Franka Futterlieb
reception@urbn.de
www.urbn.de

Catalina Estrada Uribe
Colombia
38, 47, 247, 336
catiestrada@gmail.com
www.katika.net

usugrow Japan
160, 247, 276, 357
usugrow@usugrow.com
www.usugrow.com

Povilas Utovka Lithuania
329, 389, 413
povilas@esu.lt
povilas.esu.lt

V

Vår Sweden
58, 266, 275, 366
Karl Grandin
grandin@woo.se

Laura Varsky Argentina
61
lv@lauravarsky.com.ar
www.lauravarsky.com.ar

Kjetil Vatne Norway
69, 97, 128, 222, 373
vatne@online.no
www.kvad.com

Vault49 USA
162
info@vault49.com
www.vault49.com

Velvet
23, 25, 30, 42, 58, 74, 77,
78, 82, 90, 92, 439
info@velvet.ee
www.velvet.ee

VIA01 Germany
429, 451
Chris Steurer
info@via01.de
www.via01.de

viagrafik Germany
59, 62, 65, 102, 116, 120,
126, 128, 153, 154, 175, 187,
188, 189, 193, 198, 219, 222,
226, 264, 269, 271, 272, 279,
285, 307, 308, 310, 311, 312,
331, 353, 358, 362, 368, 369,
389, 399, 402, 408, 409, 410,
412, 428, 439, 440, 441, 446,
450, 451, 455, 457, 458
André Nossek
mnwrks@viagrafik.com
www.viagrafik.com

Henrik Vibskov Denmark
226, 256, 282, 283, 285, 286
info@henrikvibskov.com
www.henrikvibskov.com

Vier5 France
117, 118
contact@vier5.de
www.vier5.de

David A. Ortiz Villegas
Mexico
297
davo.orz@gmail.com

visomat inc. Germany
117, 126, 127
Andrea Münch
info@visomat.com
www.visomat.com

Visual Mind Rockets Germany
31, 327, 383
Daniel Woessner
woessner@
visualmindrockets.com
www.visualmindrockets.com

Jonas Vögeli Switzerland
326
jonas@saalschutz.com

Vrontikis Design Office USA
151, 223
Ania Borysiewicz
pv@35k.com
www.35k.com

Leon Vymenets Canada
183, 390, 400
leon@stereo-eros.com
www.stereo-eros.com

W

Christian Walden Germany
185, 264, 352, 394
chris@dmyk.com
www.dmyk.com

Jun Watanabe Japan
57, 66, 153, 185, 200, 227,
243, 268, 269, 305, 369,
384, 409
info@harpoon.jp
www.junwatanabe.jp

M!ch Welfringer France
93, 96, 105, 125
Michel Welfringer
mich@designers-anonymes.com
www.designers-anonymes.com

weissraum.de(sign) Germany
44, 71, 78, 293, 324, 347,
360, 361, 368, 371, 382,
387, 443, 450
Lucas Buchholz, Bernd Brink
info@weissraum.de
www.weissraum.de

Lucias Westrup Denmark
110, 129, 142, 147, 152,
172, 197, 202, 210, 253
lucias291@gmail.com
www.lucias291.dk

Mikkel Grafixico Westrup
Denmark
38, 47, 124, 159, 173, 184,
188, 196, 309, 333, 369,
382, 385, 403, 408, 412
mikkel@grafixico.dk
www.grafixico.dk

WGD Norway
24, 32, 126, 182, 258, 259,
453
Erling Knudsen
wgd.grafisk@gmail.com

Klaus Wilhardt Denmark
52, 68, 414
klaus@wilhardt.com

Alexander Wise France
30, 73, 358, 455
info@alexanderwise.com
www.alexanderwise.com

Dennis Worden USA
336
dennis@dennisworden.com
www.dennisworden.com

X

Jun Xu USA
211
nuj716@gmail.com
www.junxu.com

XYZ.CH Switzerland
31, 61, 406
Alexander Meyer
schreib@xyz.ch
www.xyz.ch

Y

Masato Yamaguchi Japan
301
yamaguchi.m@gmail.com
www.works-m-yamaguchi.com

Shinpei Yamamori Japan
123, 455, 456, 457
Shinpei Yamamori [rtr]
snp@bysnp.com
www.bysnp.com

Shintaro Yarimizo Japan
151, 158, 205, 209, 210
yarimizoshintaro
info@yarimizo.com
www.yarimizo.com

YellowToothpick USA
55, 175, 282
Michelle Romo
michelle@
yellowtoothpick.com
www.yellowtoothpick.com

yippieyeah cooperative UK
79, 359, 373
Bauer, Borkowski
yy@yippieyeah.co.uk
www.yippieyeah.co.uk

Yo Freeman Finland
145, 152, 156, 175, 186,
226, 447, 457
Freeman
freeman@
controlskateboards.com
www.freeman.fi

Yok Australia
156, 390
Yok
yok@theyok.com
www.theyok.com

Yucca Studio Singapore
165, 200
Gerard & Agnes
hello@yuccastudio.com
www.yuccastudio.com

Russ Yusupov USA
70
workday@gmail.com
www.workdayprojects.com

Z

Judith Zaugg Switzerland
39, 424
contact@judithzaugg.ch
www.judithzaugg.ch

Zeek&Destroy Germany
116, 145, 173, 185, 189,
322, 323, 331, 341, 343, 373
Tim Kotmann
tim@zeekndestroy.com
www.zeekndestroy.com

Zetuei Fonts Japan
82, 188, 209, 264, 268
zetuei fonts
mail@zetuei.com
www.zetuei.com

zime SOL crew Netherlands
411
zime@solcrew.nl
www.solcrew.nl

Zinc Argentina
156
Cynthia Martinez
contact@zinc-design.com.ar
www.zinc-design.com.ar

zinestesia Spain
105, 304, 308, 310, 313
Diego Ramos
diego@zinestesia.net
www.zinestesia.net

Zion Graphics Sweden
21, 37, 56, 186, 223, 239,
245, 252, 275, 278, 280
Jonas Kjellberg
www.ziongraphics.com

ZIP Design UK
111, 263, 326, 335, 336,
342, 351, 406
Chrissie Abbott
www.zipdesign.co.uk

zookeeper France
37, 38, 90, 231, 233, 343,
423, 438, 439
dod
contact@zookeeper.fr
www.zookeeper.fr

zucker und pfeffer Germany
95, 205, 343
Denny Backhaus
denny@zuckerundpfeffer.com
www.zuckerundpfeffer.com

WORK INDEX

020.01 Atelier Télescopique
o: Tank architectes

021.01 Insect Design
o: The Old Truman
        Brewery
021.02 Discodoener
o: Efeu e.V.
021.03 Discodoener
o: Rudolf Architekten
021.04 Zion Graphics
o: Katamari

022.01 Fupete Studio
o: Onsee Srl
022.02 Rocholl Selected
        Designs
o: Volkswagen
022.03 David Maloney
o: Northland Connection
/:   Brain Magnet
022.04 Kontrapunkt
o: madeleines

023.01 Emil Hartvig
o: Bygteq
023.02 Flink
o: Antwerp Diamond Bank
023.03 strange//attraktor:
o: Questra Health
023.04 bleed
o: The Norwegian Church
023.05 Bionic Systems
o: Traksy.com / Yamaha
        Corporation
023.06 Futro
o: The Alliance
023.07 JDK
o: FMC
023.08 Borsellino & Co.
o: Plasse Projekt
023.09 Velvet
o: MolCode
023.10 Crush
o: wired sussex
023.11 KMS Team
o: Private Brauereien
        Deutschland
023.12 Alexander Fuchs
o: Kultusministerkonfe-
        renz der Länder
/:   Weißensee School of
        Art Berlin
023.13 Raredrop
o: crossing inc.
023.14 Rob Chiu
o: The Regional Forum
023.15 Rob Chiu
o: The Regional Forum

023.16 Annabelle Mehraein
o: Evalesc

024.01 Martha Stutteregger
o: Naturbad Amstetten
024.02 kw43
o: Audio Service
024.03 310k
o: dutchphone
024.04 Raredrop
o: coreworks
024.05 Axel Raidt
o: Berlin Stock Exchange
024.06 Jon Ari Helgason
o: Marel Food processing
        lines
024.07 WGD
024.08 Systm
o: Sound X
024.09 sunrise studios
o: Betha Service
024.10 makelike
o: Nikki Gersten
024.11 eduhirama
o: wide group
024.12 Georg Schatz
o: BrainagencyMedia
024.13 J6Studios
o: Chorus Technology
024.14 William Morrisey
o: International Marine
        Design
024.15 David Maloney
o: Red Energy
/:   Red Circle Agency
024.16 Jeffrey Kalmikoff
o: skinnyCorp

025.01 Pfadfinderei
025.02 Raredrop
o: Mitsubishi paper
        mills limited
025.03 KMS Team
o: Deutsche Rentenversi-
        cherung
025.04 Velvet
o: Stepford Finance
025.05 Sesame Studio
o: Air Refuel
025.06 Velvet
o: Tartu Kaubamaja
025.07 Mattisimo
o: Cingular Pocket
025.08 Rosendahl Grafikdesign
o: Homann Colormanagement
025.09 Insect Design
o: Blue Sky Films

025.10 Kimera
o: Bravado
/:   Bravado and Roberto
        Debayle
025.11 Velvet
o: Redman Real Estate
025.12 Trafik
o: LPtent
025.13 Balsi Grafik
o: agentur_01
/:   bern tourismus
025.14 nothing from outer
        space
o: cyon, switzerland
025.15 Velvet
o: Orangetime Event
        Marketing

026.01 archetype : interactive
o: Sun Win Logistics
        Limited
026.02 archetype : interactive
o: san woo group
026.03 Research Studios
        Berlin
o: Hankook
026.04 Stolen Inc.
o: MediaFlo
026.05 Borsellino & Co.
o: Digigroup
026.06 Research Studios
        Berlin
o: Video Network
        Research Studios
026.07 Norwegian Ink
o: Eccop
026.08 Futro
o: Studio Moderna
026.09 Sesame Studio
o: RDG
026.10 Sesame Studio
o: RDG
026.11 Sesame Studio
o: RDG
026.12 Sesame Studio
o: RDG
026.13 JDK
o: XBOX 360
026.14 Stolen Inc.
o: Adresse Immobilière
026.15 Axel Domke
o: Sartori und Berger
026.16 Carsten Raffel
o: buronord.ch

027.01 Flink
o: Federation of Belgian
        Diamond Bourses

027.02 Fluid Creativity
o: Timedon
027.03 Simon & Goetz
o: von Braun & Schreiber
027.04 nothing from outer
        space
027.05 Felix Braden
o: Herkules
/:   Cosmonaut Net.Work
027.06 GillespieFox
o: Madhima Gulgan Tours
027.07 Toxic design
o: Domina Hotels Group
/:   Leo Burnett Rome
027.08 Sensus Design Factory
o: Arakadabra, Zagreb
027.09 Systm
o: IGS
027.10 Toxic design
o: Clear Message
/:   Atomobravo
027.11 mateuniverse
o: Union Bank
027.12 Toxic design
o: Domina Hotels Group
/:   Leo Burnett Rome
027.13 Stolen Inc.
o: goFarm
027.14 Cape Arcona
        Typefoundry
o: Mart Shipping
027.15 Intégral Ruedi Baur
        et associés
o: Köln Bonn Airport
027.16 David Maloney
o: Red Circle Media
/:   Red Circle Agency

028.01 Chapter3
o: Idiogroup
028.02 Fluid Creativity
o: Fluid SMS
028.03 Attak
o: Gemeente 's-Hertogen-
        bosch
028.04 Emil Hartvig
o: Danmarks Radio
028.05 Strukt Visual Network
o: Birgit Kramer
028.06 Mutabor Design
o: Tallence
028.07 friederike preuschen
o: Paffrath
028.08 Mathilde Quartier
o: Novoptic
/:   Agence Polygone
028.09 Miha Artnak
o: ALU

028.10 Toxic design
o: 47THfloor
028.11 Studio Dumbar
028.12 nothing from outer
        space
028.13 Felix Braden
o: careforce-marketing &
        sales service
/:   Debüser+Bee Kommuni-
        kationsdesign
028.14 Labor für visuelles
        Wachstum
o: Kornberg im Taunus
028.15 blackjune
028.16 AmorfoDesignlab™
o: Chilorio™
/:   -1:0:1

029.01 Paul Snowden
o: Plateforme Bureau
029.02 Spild af Tid ApS
029.03 The Remingtons
o: Didier Pasquier
        Ludovic Balland
029.04 The Remingtons
o: Das Schiff

030.01 Crush
o: turnstyle consulting
030.02 Carsten Giese
o: Tischlerei Boege
030.03 2098
030.04 Christian Rothenhagen
o: beatnuts skateboards
030.05 Keep Left Studio
o: Transistor Studios
030.06 Double Standards
o: Bullet Events
030.07 I-Manifest
o: Potion Coffee Shop
030.08 Loïc Sattler
o: Iconed
030.09 Atomic Attack
030.10 Alexander Wise
o: Tirea
030.11 Velvet
o: Brilliant Marketing
        Communications
030.12 Velvet
o: Applause Music
        Management
030.13 Niels Shoe Meulman
o: FHV BBDO / Talpa
030.14 Emil Hartvig
o: Wind & Vanggaard
/:   Morten Windelev
030.15 310k
o: telefoontoataal

030.16 less rain
o: signal 7
031.01 Jakob Straub
o: Bar Roberto
    e Loredana
031.02 XYZ.CH
o: Coffeeshop
    Macchinetta
031.03 Georg Schatz
o: Caffè Tirreno
031.04 DigitalPlayground
    Studio
031.05 donat raetzo union
o: The Bean, London
/:   Assorted Images,
    London
031.06 morphor
031.07 Visual Mind Rockets
o: Suppe und Stulle
031.08 Attak
o: Martin van de
    Kimmenade
031.09 Nohemi Dicuru
o: Editora El Nacional
031.10 Emmi Salonen
o: Danny's Deli
031.11 La Superagencia
o: Cigarrera Bigott
031.12 Dimomedia Lab
o: Kebap da Demir
031.13 :phunk studio
o: Butter Factory
031.14 onrushdesign / front
o: Woo Restaurant
031.15 granit di Lioba
    Wackernell
o: Walthers' Restaurant

032.01 Studio Five
o: Expansion Team
032.02 AmorfoDesignlab™
o: Effiscience™
032.03 29 degres
o: Duru
/:   CB'a
032.04 Kanardo
o: Clusterphonic,
    creative cluster
    organisation
032.05 Kanardo
o: Buldo, restaurant
032.06 Martin Kvamme
o: Izza Nova
032.07 Moving Brands
o: Helicopter Film
    Services
032.08 Jon Ari Helgason
o: Esso

032.09 WGD
o: School project
032.10 Felix Braden
o: Kunz Handels
/:   Debüser + Bee
032.11 the red is love
o: Bitch Cafe
/:   Daniele Catapano
032.12 Rosendahl Grafikdesign
o: Jetfilm Verleih
032.13 Alexander Fuchs
o: Weißensee School of
    Art Berlin
032.14 Strada
o: Hofgut Hafnerleiten

033.01 asmallpercent
o: Gordon College
    Restore Creation
    Project
033.02 the red is love
033.03 Cuartopiso
o: Conciencia
033.04 Martin Kvamme
o: Naeringslivsdagene
033.05 Studio 3
o: Arkitekst
033.06 Lukatarina
o: PGD Ljubljana-Trnovo
    (fire brigade)
033.07 Grotesk aka Kimou
    Meyer
o: Grotesk
033.08 seventysix
o: Andrea Schwarz
033.09 feurer network ag
o: Deece Landscapes
033.10 Resin[sistem] design
o: Deece Landscapes
033.11 Sanjai Bhana
o: Ethnic Media
    Relations
033.12 onrushdesign / Front
o: LED
033.13 Georg Schatz
o: Eva Schatz,
    journalist
033.14 News
o: 100% Halal
033.15 Thomas Beyer Design
o: Staatsbibliothek zu
    Berlin, Preussischer
    Kulturbesitz

034.01 Guak
o: Bull
/:   Pau Misser
034.02 Muller
o: 7174 PTY

034.03 Thomas Nolfi
o: spinderiet
034.04 Marc Atlan
o: Emeco Industries
/:   Philippe Starck
034.05 Mattisimo
o: Gun It productions
034.06 morphor
034.07 Mattisimo
o: Phatburger
034.08 Mattisimo
o: Cold Cone
034.09 Mattisimo
o: Six Stitch
    alterations

035.01 Mattisimo
o: Saatchi LA
035.02 Katharina Leuzinger
o: Blinkink, London
035.03 Büro Destruct
o: Ping Pong Films
035.04 Felix Braden
o: Herkules
/:   Cosmonaut Net.Work
035.05 june
o: resonnances & cie /
    harraps
035.06 sunrise studios
o: Möbelwerft
035.07 Discodoener
o: Autohaus Labusch
/:   Sasa Zivkovic
035.08 Formikula
o: Heidemann
035.09 Carsten Raffel
o: 5special

036.01 NeoDG
o: MTV Networks
036.02 Naho Ogawa
o: brot zeit
036.03 bandage
o: Locals (commercial
    director team)
036.04 Atelier Télescopique
o: Azèle consultants
036.05 Atelier Télescopique
o: Bloc-A
036.06 Flexn
036.07 Miki Amano
o: Sophia Wallace
    Photography
036.08 Studio 3
036.09 Jeffrey Kalmikoff
o: Sports Alumni
    Nextwork
036.10 Axel Domke
o: Brand Central Station

037.01 zookeeper
o: Psycop coaching
037.02 fatbob
037.03 Paco Aguayo
o: Grupo Urrea
037.04 Paco Aguayo
o: Grupo Urrea
037.05 Simian
o: Wondertouch Llc.
037.06 Hayato Kamono
o: Polaris
037.07 Formikula
o: Affilinet
037.08 Raredrop
o: myself
037.09 Jeffrey Kalmikoff
o: A Life Once Lost
037.10 Zion Graphics
o: Hobby Film
037.11 44 flavours
o: Karlos
/:   Julio Rölle,
    Sebastian Bagge
037.12 Insect Design
o: www.picturesonwalls.
    com
037.13 Lorenzo Geiger
o: Tre Kokker

038.01 Labor fuer visuelles
    Wachstum
o: Da Enzo
038.02 Thomas Nolfi
o: hairdresser
038.03 Simon & Goetz
o: Brand Communication
    One
038.04 derek johnson
o: A3 Elements
038.05 Engine
o: Rembrandt Fusies &
    Overnames
/:   Locomotive B.V.
038.06 Superfamous
o: Selios
038.07 I Am Human
038.08 Balsi Grafik
o: headline hairstyling
038.09 Catalina Estrada
    Uribe
o: Jessica Bueno
038.10 zookeeper
o: Tribal touch
038.11 Mikkel Grafixico
    Westrup
o: The Voice

038.12 the red is love
o: Zig Zag
/:   Walter Luca
    Debartolomeis
038.13 Nathan Jobe
o: Soldier Unknown

039.01 Jon Burgerman
o: Creative
    Collaborations
039.02 Rinzen
o: Lychee Lounge
039.03 KesselsKramer
o: Wallie
/:   Wallie &
    KesselsKramer
039.04 Dr. Alderete
o: Madrid Comics
039.05 Studio 3
o: Fredrikstad Barne- og
    Ungdomsteater
039.06 FireGirl
o: Associação dos Comer-
    ciantes do Porto
039.07 Christian Rothenhagen
o: dailybuttons
/:   Mark Wiechert
039.08 Lousy Livincompany
o: Cleptomanicx
039.09 Lousy Livincompany
039.10 Judith Zaugg
o: Colmic, Michael
    Abplanalp
039.11 Jeremyville
o: Sydney Film Festival
039.12 Creative Pride
o: Ged Backland
039.13 austrianilllustra-
    tion.com
o: studio hollinger/wien
/:   tom mackinger
039.14 Alexander Fuchs
o: Protopark
039.15 Formikula
o: T-Online
039.16 IDolls
o: www.dasmiese.de
/:   Chima Okerenkwo

040.01 Yuu Imokawa
o: delotta
040.02 Lapin
040.03 eduhirama
o: restaurante nakombi
040.04 Attak
o: Achtung Gestaltung

041.01 red design
o: lansdowne place hotel

041.02 Joe A. Scerri
o: Woodpecker Holding
041.03 Amore Hirosuke
o: one note
041.04 Alphabetical Order®
o: Safrica
041.05 Mark Sloan
o: The Creo Vento
        Partnership
041.06 Jawa and Midwich
o: Baker PR
041.07 jl-prozess
o: black owl

042.01 Power Graphixx
042.02 Chapter3
o: Evoke
042.03 Axel Raidt
o: linuxhouse
042.04 Kontrapunkt
o: billund airport
042.05 Axel Domke
o: Fast Food
042.06 Maniackers Design
o: Little Luck Coffee &
        Maniackers Design
042.07 Velvet
o: Tallinn Children's
        Hospital Foundation
042.08 Bionic Systems
o: Mossbird Concept &
        Character, USA
042.09 Hayato Kamono
o: Brand New Peace
042.10 Cape Arcona
        Typefoundry
o: Grauraut Fotografie
042.11 tapetentiere
        consulting
042.12 344 Design, LLC
042.13 milchhof : atelier
o: Talk & Travel
042.14 Extraverage
        Productions
o: NetDragon
042.15 Labooo
042.16 Juju's Delivery
o: fuchs und gans
        catering

043.01 Superfamous
o: Clickstream Dynamics
043.02 Attak
o: Corazon
043.03 milchhof : atelier
o: Bigfish
043.04 GrafficTraffic
o: Moonfish Cafe
/:   FishMoon

043.05 Miha Artnak
o: ZEK advance
043.06 jum
o: form one
043.07 Oscar Salinas Losada
o: Tortas Hurakarrana
043.08 Maria Elena Velasco
        Rojas
o: Dental Care
043.09 the wilderness
o: Gorilla Technology
043.10 DED Associates
o: Animal Farm
043.11 Georg Schatz
o: katzito, art gallery
043.12 Studio Output
o: Fat Cat Group
043.13 Positron
o: heads
043.14 Studio 3
o: Norsk Filmforbund
043.15 Attak
o: Per Express
043.16 Mattisimo
o: Wow Wau Doggy
        Boutique

044.01 Seth Rementer
o: SC07 Conference
        Committee
044.02 fireondesign /
        herborize
o: Blue Lion, Restaurant
044.03 artless Inc
o: Doragon Concept
/:   illust: Tadashi Ura
044.04 Extraverage
        Productions
o: Horus Consulting
044.05 Rosendahl Grafikdesign
o: Löwe, Schwandt &
        Partner
044.06 raum mannheim
o: sable argent
044.07 Stylepatrol.com
o: Stephan Spindeler
044.08 weissraum.de(sign)
o: Marion's Country
        Kitchen, Woodstock,
        USA
044.09 chemicalbox
044.10 Felix Braden
o: Herkules
/:   Cosmonaut Net.Work
044.11 Simon & Goetz
o: Gebrüder Schaffrath
044.12 granit Di Lioba
        Wackernell
o: Hotel Greif, Bolzano

044.13 Extraverage
        Productions
o: NetDragon

045.01 bleed
o: Nutel
045.02 Kingsize
o: Woonderland
045.03 Felix Braden
o: Dr. Haas Management-
        beratung
/:   Debüser + Bee
045.04 Ottograph
o: bottomliners
        advertising
045.05 bleed
o: Lone
045.06 Miha Artnak
045.07 DigitalPlayground
        Studio
045.08 Labor für visuelles
        Wachstum
o: agrarion.com
/:   leo burnett
045.09 DTM_INC
o: De Beemsterboel
045.10 kong. funktion
        gestaltung
o: Swiss Red-Holstein
045.11 Oscar Salinas Losada
o: El Palomo
045.12 Keep Left Studio
o: Digital Pictures
045.13 Lunatiq
o: Concorde Meat and
        Poultry

046.01 Juli Gudehus
o: Interdisziplinäres
        Brustzentrum Kempten
046.02 Amen
o: Istria Tourist Board
046.03 Tado
o: MTV Greenhouse
/:   MTV Networks Interna-
        tional

047.01 Catalina Estrada
        Uribe
o: Flotarium
047.02 FireGirl
o: Associação dos Comer-
        ciantes do Porto
047.03 Annelia Armas
o: Bioparques
047.04 Gints Apsits
o: Latvian Forests /
        Mammadaba

047.05 Lukatarina
o: Dobrova elementary
        school
047.06 Catalina Estrada
        Uribe
o: Frankachela
047.07 Extraverage
        Productions
o: Air Workgroup
047.08 spin
o: Hilliard
047.09 AND
o: Messe Basel
047.10 Mikkel Grafixico
        Westrup
o: NewTaste
/:   Michael Oxvang
047.11 selanra grafikdesign
o: Geßler & Gotier
047.12 DTM_INC
o: Far West
047.13 sunrise studios
o: Green food
047.14 Cyklon
o: Mikkelsen Films
047.15 29 degres
o: Salatbar Azur

048.01 Discodoener
o: mash bier
048.02 Nohemi Dicuru
o: nefertum aromatherapy
048.03 29 degres
o: allegra | geschenk-
        werkstatt
/:   virus Ideenlabor
048.04 Extraverage
        Productions
o: EthnoBotanic
048.05 Jon Ari Helgason
o: Yndisauki Healthfood
048.06 büro uebele
o: Nestwerk gemein-
        nützige Stiftung
/:   Gerd Häußler
048.07 jl-prozess
o: eickelmann & deuschl
048.08 Mattisimo
o: Garden, gardening and
        landscaping
048.09 Designkitchen
o: Koprax Gartendesign
048.10 Simon & Goetz
o: Elenxis
048.11 Semisans
o: LA Flower Savers

048.12 austrianillustra-
        tion.com
o: 3dpool
/:   tom mackinger
048.13 Mattisimo
o: Treeline Studios,
        Broadcast production
048.14 David Maloney
o: St. Cloud Convention
        & Visitors Bureau
/:   Brain Magnet
048.15 A-Side Studio
o: Origin Coffee

049.01 Atelier Télescopique
o: Omnia. Restaurant et
        Bar

050.01 Doma
050.02 backyard 10
o: Royal Art Force
050.03 Colletivo Design
o: Mountain Dew
/:   Colletivo Design
        Studio
050.04 backyard 10

051.01 National Forest
o: Element Skateboards
051.02 Loic Sattler
o: Lysergid
051.03 Keep Left Studio
o: Mojo Publicis
        Advertising Agency

052.01 Discodoener
o: bootshaus club köln
052.02 Toxic design
o: Domina Hotels &
        Resorts
/:   Leo Burnett Rome
052.03 Skin Design AS
o: Borgestad Gård
052.04 Extraverage
        Productions
o: Családfa-kutató
        intézet
052.05 Klaus Wilhardt
o: Joachim Ulrik von
        Sperling
/:   Klaus Wilhardt
052.06 blackjune
o: Berlin Joker
052.07 Adhemas
o: Kedd London
052.08 Studio 3
o: Westerdals School of
        Communication

052.09 Extraverage
       Productions
o: Hofer
052.10 Le_Palmier Design
o: Die Familie
052.11 Skin Design
052.12 Alëxone
o: méthanol garage
052.13 Axel Domke
o: Seasons Magazine
052.14 raum mannheim
052.15 Designunion
o: Sepp Lehner

053.01 Katharina Leuzinger
o: 133 Productions,
       Paris
/:   unit9.creative.
       production

054.01 Accident Grotesk!
054.02 Loic Sattler
o: Red baron (bar)

055.01 Magma
055.02 Cassie Leedham
o: The PR Room
055.03 YellowToothpick
o: Crowded Teeth
055.04 Amen
o: Prisco Passage
055.05 Rosendahl Grafikdesign
o: Fräulein Schneider
055.06 anna-OM-line.com
o: Editorial Primeraper-
       sona
055.07 Caótica
o: Pândega Produções
       Culturais
055.08 Thomas Nolfi
055.09 Hydro74
o: E360 Magazine
055.10 Magma
o: bcubed
055.11 ROM studio
o: Origen y Comunicación
       /Spira/Invex/Visa
055.12 Power Graphixx

056.01 Catalogtree
056.02 Hula Hula
056.03 Sueellen
o: Valter Cafe
056.04 Thomas Beyer Design
o: Sabine Brand & Simona
       Fische
056.05 Tender
o: Debra Heft

056.06 William Morrisey
o: Annaliese Levaggi
       Luxurious Jewelry
056.07 Fósforo
o: Málaga D.O.
056.08 MvM
o: dende
056.09 Petr Babák, Laborator
o: DUM architekti
056.10 Jon Ari Helgason
o: Islenskir Blomabaendur
056.11 Norwegian Ink
o: Oilfield Tool
       Consultants
056.12 Miha Artnak
056.13 Holzschuherstrasse
o: Rokokon
056.14 Gazelle Communication
o: Sacla
056.15 Zion Graphics
o: Spendrups Bryggeri AB

057.01 Niels Shoe Meulman
       Christel Palace
057.02 Katharina Leuzinger
o: Moon Productions
/:   unit9.creative.
       production
057.03 Pietari Posti
o: Pigmentti, Art Supply
       Shop
057.04 BankerWessel
o: 802
057.05 Jun Watanabe
o: adbrain inc
057.06 Flexn
o: Smusie
057.07 Positron
o: heads
057.08 Nonstop
o: Studio Blick Oy
057.09 Resin[sistem] design
o: Koots-Modern French
       Cuisine
057.10 Dr. Alderete
o: Terraza bar

058.01 Laundry
o: Business 2.0 magazine
       about google
058.02 Vår
o: Riche Restaurant
058.03 AmorfoDesignlab™
o: Piñata Films™
058.04 Jeffrey Kalmikoff
o: skinnyCorp
058.05 44 flavours
o: clothesline
/:   fabian wolf

058.06 Miha Artnak
058.07 Velvet
o: Applause Music
       Management
058.08 KesselsKramer
o: Hans Brinker Budget
       Hotel
058.09 Escobas
058.10 Hula Hula
o: Condechi Restaurant
/:   Hula+Hula
058.11 Furi Furi Company
o: SkyPerfecTV!
/:   IMJ.
058.12 Freaklüb
o: Gabriel Urist

059.01 MWK - Zimmermann und
       Hähnel
o: Amira
059.02 Mattisimo
o: HBO, HBOX productions
059.03 Lorenzo Geiger
o: idées diverses
059.04 Martin Kvamme
o: Nordvik & Partners
059.05 Brighten the corners
       Studio for Design
       London & Stuttgart
o: Agency Arrangement
/:   bleed
059.06 viagrafik
o: You are here
059.07 büro uebele
o: Evangelische Stiftung
       Alsterdorf
/:   Alexandra Busse
059.08 viagrafik
o: at work werbeagentur
059.09 Designunion
o: Lydia Schulze
059.10 Tim Bjørn
o: Liguria Living
059.11 KMS Team
o: Ausstellungsgesell-
       schaft Zollverein
059.12 1508
o: Byggeriets Innovation
       / Building Lab_dk
059.13 Neeser & Müller
o: Druckerei Albdruck
059.14 44 flavours
o: corporate cool
/:   Sebastian Bagge
059.15 unfolded
o: huberlendorff /
       Fotografie

060.01 stylodesign
o: Eraser Computing

060.02 Läufer + Keichel
o: GASAG - Berliner
       Gaswerke AG
060.03 Nonstop
o: Anorak Agency
060.04 DTM_INC
o: Top Trends b.v.
060.05 Maik Brummundt
o: argon support
060.06 123buero
o: Maak Roberts Fotograf
060.07 seventysix
o: Carsten Demmerle
060.08 :phunk studio
o: Lau Photos
060.09 KesselsKramer
o: The City of Amsterdam
/:   Amsterdam Partners &
       KesselsKramer
060.10 Georg Schatz
o: bluefant.de
060.11 Muller
060.12 Sensus Design Factory
o: Dag Orsic
       Photography, Zagreb
060.13 radargraphics
o: Business Unusual
/:   Paulus Huitema
060.14 urbn;
o: Eight Studios
/:   Franka Futterlieb
060.15 Three Negative
o: Hillside Veneers
060.16 Ashi & office
       Greminger

061.01 Laura Varsky
o: Piojito
061.02 Accident Grotesk!
o: About Design Magazine
061.03 Etienne Heinrich
o: 7 GRAD
061.04 Glauco Diogenes
o: Sidney Tadeu Lopes
       - Ecóloga
061.05 Salon Vektoria
o: Fachhochschule
       Darmstadt
061.06 Rinzen
o: Chilli Padi
       Restaurant
061.07 actiondesigner
o: NSB
061.08 XYZ.CH
o: HGKZ/SVG
061.09 DTM_INC
o: Maido
061.10 Dimomedia Lab
o: Area 13

061.11 propella, konzept +
       design
o: Bamboo Massaasch
061.12 Loic Sattler
061.13 Emil Kozak
o: Inverse
061.14 Bringolf Irion Vögeli
o: Fokus Form
061.15 Hayato Kamono
o: refuel
061.16 Maniackers Design
o: Little Luck Coffee &
       Maniackers Design

062.01 Neubau.
o: NeubauLaden
062.02 Büro Destruct
o: Roberto Balmer
062.03 IDolls
/:   Josh Paul / Ruth
       Kutscheit
062.04 Carsten Giese
o: Elektra, technische
       produktionen
062.05 :phunk studio
o: 1)Be.Bike
       2)Whiteroom
       3)Stray
       4) Bulb
062.06 Neubau.
o: Atelier Mohr
       Mannequins
062.07 Neubau.
o: Optivo
062.08 Emmi Salonen
o: pod
062.09 Pfadfinderei
o: Get Physical Music
062.10 viagrafik
o: archos france
062.11 Jawa and Midwich
o: DNA Electronic
/:   James Oury DNA
       Electronic
062.12 Mattisimo
o: Rohr Shultze,
       Creative Recruitment
062.13 Extraverage
       Productions
o: 33 hz
062.14 Systm
o: M13
062.15 IDolls
o: www.dreiquellen.de
/:   Ulrich Lahn
062.16 44 flavours
/:   Sebastian Bagge

063.01 blackjune
o: Radio Skateboards
063.02 blackjune
o: ewerk berlin
063.03 Rinzen
o: Flaunt
063.04 red design
o: fringe bar cafe
063.05 Rob Meek
o: mondo23
        (Screenwriters)
063.06 Kallegraphics
o: Café Sør
063.07 Lukatarina
o: Livartis - art
        moulding
063.08 Norwegian Ink
o: Outland
063.09 Ottograph
o: kc films south africa
063.10 I&EYE
o: JetKontor Hamburg
063.11 Urs Lehni
o: Paranoia Skate- and
        Snowboarding
063.12 Keep Left Studio
o: Spring Time Upholstry
063.13 june
o: datem
063.14 Extraverage
        Productions
o: Alarm 365
063.15 Lunatiq

064.01 A-Side Studio
o: Liam Arthur
        Photography
064.02 Ashi & office
        Greminger
o: feld airlines
064.03 The Remingtons
o: Zoo Basel
064.04 A-Side Studio
o: Nick Baily
        Photography
064.05 A-Side Studio
o: Good Coffee Company
064.06 Joe A. Scerri
064.07 unfolded
o: taywa
064.08 Omochi
o: nuisance
064.09 Semitransparent
        Design
o: Geed
064.10 Sat One
064.11 Omochi
o: Momoiro

064.12 Carsten Raffel
o: buronord.ch
064.13 Borsellino & Co.
o: EDMW Gastronomie
064.14 Borsellino & Co.
o: Kofler & Company
064.15 Omochi
o: wividry
064.16 Omochi

065.01 Omochi
o: Chaqru
065.02 Omochi
o: thorn salad
065.03 Atomic Attack
065.04 AmorfoDesignlab™
o: Nusalt Laser™
/:   -1:0:1
065.05 44 flavours
o: dancerock157
/:   Lutz Lindemann
065.06 Cuartopiso
o: Giancarlo Mazzanti
        Arquitectos
065.07 Paco Aguayo
o: Vanguardia Europea
065.08 Jason Kochis
o: Eventfabrik, Altdorf
065.09 Büro Destruct
o: tintonic
065.10 viagrafik
065.11 Omochi
o: Raru
065.12 Koadzn
o: WDD
065.13 44 flavours
/:   patrick fuchs
065.14 bleed
o: Grønland Basar
065.15 44 flavours
o: Karlos
/:   Julio Rölle
065.16 44 flavours
o: SeSe
/:   Jackson Five

066.01 Freaklüb
o: Trust Nobody Gallery
066.02 Floor Wesseling Ix
        Opus Ada
o: ocean desert
        enterprises
066.03 Extraverage
        Productions
o: Bio Dynamix
066.04 Keep Left Studio
o: Redbull Australia

066.05 Airside
066.06 Akira Sasaki
o: ontonson
066.07 Jun Watanabe
066.08 red design
o: audio
066.09 AmorfoDesignlab™
o: Aloha™
066.10 raum mannheim
o: wilk
066.11 Omochi
o: Neo Under Gate
066.12 Extraverage
        Productions
o: Bio Dynamix
066.13 Crush
o: smirnoff
066.14 Kallegraphics
o: Data Roger
066.15 Tohyto
o: Caracas Arepa Bar

067.01 cabina
o: Aeropuertos Argentina
        2000
067.02 Mission Design Agency
o: Design Year 2005
067.03 Superfamous
o: Production Dept
067.04 Die Gestalten
/:   Sascha Minde
067.05 stylodesign
o: Quench Water Coolers
067.06 Axel Domke
o: Seasons Magazine
067.07 Paco Aguayo
o: Vértice Comunicación
067.08 Trafik
o: Le Voxx
067.09 Joe A. Scerri
o: Muttenz
        Wirtschaftsrat

068.01 Flink
o: Antwerp WaterWorks
068.02 A-Side Studio
o: Andrew Lewis
        Photography
068.03 martinaigner.com
o: andreas peter
        schaupensteiner
068.04 clandrei
o: Lopo Media
068.05 sidsel stubbe
o: antropologerne.com
068.06 Georg Schatz
o: Brand&Value, brand
        consulting

068.07 kw43
o: Bizzbase
068.08 Trafik
o: Bodypack
068.09 radargraphics
o: Business Unusual
/:   Paulus Huiteman
068.10 Emil Hartvig
o: Copenhagen Business
        Society
/:   Jørgen Andersen
068.11 Mwmcreative
o: Composite Mouldings
        Limited
/:   Warwick Buckley
068.12 Mattisimo
o: CTR Restaurant
068.13 Bo Lundberg
o: Dahl Agenturer
068.14 Klaus Wilhardt
o: das büro
068.15 Paco Aguayo
o: Elias Rizo Architects
068.16 Thonik
o: S.M.A.K., Jan Hoet,
        Jojanneke Gijsen
        Design: thonik

069.01 archetype : interactive
o: Eternal Power
069.02 makelike
o: Entermodal
069.03 Annabelle Mehraein
o: Ehrle Communications
069.04 chris bolton
o: Goodluck
069.05 Kjetil Vatne
o: Idefagskolen
069.06 Toko
o: great: ad agency
069.07 Moving Brands
o: GMP
069.08 Mutabor Design
o: germanwings
069.09 Velvet
o: Greentec
069.10 blackjune
o: GravyTrain
069.11 Out Of Order
o: Guerrilla Games
069.12 precursor
o: Harris McMillan
        Architecture and
        Design
069.13 Mathilde Quartier
o: Jacques Perritaz
069.14 Toko
o: Ke expeditie

069.15 And
o: Iutec, Lukas Berger,
        Basel, Switzerland
070.01 Simon & Goetz
o: Lessings
070.02 Superlow
o: Libris
070.03 martinaigner.com
o: rauscher michael
        architekt
070.04 Muller
070.05 Rocholl Selected
        Designs
o: Priony Timepieces
070.06 Sensus Design Factory
o: Plana papiri, Zagreb
070.07 MaMadesign AB
o: Printiva AB
070.08 Sesame Studio
o: inQbator
070.09 A-Side Studio
o: Refresh Images
070.10 Attak
o: Sapir
070.11 Le_Palmier Design
o: sprint
070.12 Tim Bjørn
o: Studio 45
070.13 Out Of Order
o: Salute gelato
070.14 Russ Yusupov
o: Association for
        Computing Machinery
070.15 Russ Yusupov
o: Association for
        Computing Machinery,
        IEEE

071.01 Moving Brands
o: Spacelab
        (Architects firm)
071.02 2Advanced Studios
o: Search Engine
        Optimization
071.03 weissraum.de(sign)
o: TV-Koch Tim Mälzer
071.04 Power Graphixx
071.05 Attak
o: Eindhoven Universitas
071.06 DTM_INC
o: Visual Touch
071.07 Sarah Grimaldi
o: veutro editore
071.08 Ketchup Arts
o: Warner Indies Network
071.09 GWG
o: yamaguchiya

071.10 Fiftyeight3d
071.11 iaah
o: Ad one to staff
/:   IAAH
071.12 :g / studio-gpop
o: Hemisphere One

072.01 Urs Lehni
o: Paranoia Skate- and
        Snowboarding

073.01 selonra grafikdesign
o: Geßler & Gotier
073.02 Mathilde Quartier
o: Osmose
073.03 Alexander Wise
o: Constellation Corp
073.04 Extraverage
        Productions
o: Bio Dynamix
073.05 Moniteurs
o: One Click Solutions
073.06 Simon & Goetz
o: Winning wheels /
        Urban solutions
073.07 DTM_INC
o: Zandee Communication
073.08 Extraverage
        Productions
o: apropo
073.09 Jeffrey Kalmikoff
o: Greg Fishman
073.10 a+morph
o: Enviro Pro
073.11 Pentagram
o: Corella Publishing
073.12 Extraverage
        Productions
o: sandstone
073.13 flat
o: Millennium hair-
        design
073.14 Mathilde Quartier

074.01 Tsuyoshi Hirooka
o: Newsic
074.02 Superfamous
o: Finley
074.03 Tilt
o: Silke C. Müller,
        Sports Eduction
074.04 Thomas Nolfi
o: cph business school
074.05 Katrin Acklin
o: cubeworxx

074.06 Extraverage
        Productions
o: AirCalc++
074.07 Velvet
o: Emajöe Waterworks
074.08 Muller
o: Mam Tor™ Publishing
074.09 Escobas
o: Teico
074.10 flat
o: SapTechnopole
074.11 Ottograph
o: go! gallery
074.12 kw43
o: Camcab
074.13 PMKFA
074.14 hijack graphics
o: jenswalterulrich.de
074.15 Studio Output
o: Pickled Egg
074.16 Neeser & Müller
o: Culm Office Link

075.01 Amen
o: Odeonsplatz München
075.02 Maniackers Design
o: East Japan Kiosk
075.03 austrianilllustra-
        tion.com
o: Wolfgang Hametner
075.04 A-Side Studio
o: Blas Burgerworks
075.05 Katrin Acklin
o: united mobile
075.06 jum
o: CK
075.07 29 degres
o: Merlini | Artigiano
        Pastaio
075.08 Büro Destruct
o: Kulturhallen Dampf-
        zentrale & Egger Bier
075.09 Doma
075.10 Maniackers Design
o: Ponkotsu
075.11 Resin[sistem] design
o: Nanotechnology
        Victoria
075.12 Tilt
o: Weltenbau (Diploma)
075.13 the wilderness
o: 420 Spring Water
075.14 GillespieFox
o: JDMyard
075.15 Mattisimo
o: Catherine Farah Hair
        Studio

076.01 unfolded
o: edit | bilder für
        architektur
076.02 GWG
o: tai on group co.
076.03 Simon & Goetz
o: Swarovski /Marangoni
076.04 Simon & Goetz
o: Grow
076.05 kw43
o: Wüstenrot Österreich
076.06 Sueellen
o: Aliya Geneva
/:   Pekka Koivikko
076.07 Accident Grotesk!
o: Walter Media
076.08 Engine
o: European Credit
        Control
/:   Locomotive
076.09 Ashi & office
        Greminger
o: 19 Mark Studio
076.10 Simon & Goetz
o: Billerbeck
076.11 Sesame Studio
o: Meta
076.12 Sesame Studio
o: Varsity
076.13 Jawa and Midwich
o: Stephen Lenthall
        Photography
076.14 Magma
076.15 GWG
o: T.B.S
076.16 Sesame Studio
o: Micronyx
/:   Sesame Studio

077.01 FoURPAcK ontwerpers
o: index technocen-
        trum midden- en
        westbrabant
077.02 112 Ocean Drive
o: Fryklund Wannfors
        Neuschütz
077.03 blackjune
o: Nadine Elfenbein
077.04 flat
o: Nugerol Holding SA
077.05 Velvet
o: Estonian Road Museum
077.06 Designunion
o: Illmer Unternehmens-
        gruppe
077.07 KesselsKramer
o: Stichting Wakker Dier

077.08 GillespieFox
o: Autopia
077.09 blackjune
o: Gebrüder Puschmann
077.10 evaq studio
o: RxR studio
077.11 Laborator
o: K4 architects and
        engineers
077.12 Niels Shoe Meulman
o: We Cut Heads
077.13 Resopal-Schallware
077.14 Intégral Ruedi Baur
        et associés
o: cité internationale
        universitaire de
        paris (CIUP)
077.15 Sensus Design Factory
o: Lakmus Paper, Zagreb

078.01 Martha Stutteregger
o: Institute of Visual
        Culture, Cambridge
078.02 Bringolf Irion Vögeli
o: Sky-Frame
/:   Bringolf Irion Vögeli
078.03 weissraum.de(sign)
o: Club and Restaurant
078.04 Velvet
o: Arhiruum Architecture
        Bureau
078.05 DTM_INC
o: DD Design
078.06 stylodesign
o: Escape Studios
078.07 Jeffrey Kalmikoff
o: skinnyCorp
078.08 Daniela Grundmann
o: Strich Architekten
078.09 Dimomedia Lab
o: Domus Immobiliare
078.10 Paco Aguayo
o: Office Now
078.11 Axel Peemöller
o: Pedanten
078.12 Sesame Studio
o: Metatron
078.13 red design
o: digital interactive
        telvision group
078.14 blackjune
o: Alexander Laljak
078.15 Crush
o: women in media

079.01 Labooo
079.02 raum mannheim
o: modul

079.03 La Superagencia
o: Grupo Garande
079.04 Extraverage
        Productions
o: Unio Pack
079.05 yippieyeah coopera-
        tive
o: ports united
079.06 310k
o: fko
079.07 morphor
079.08 Intégral Ruedi Baur
        et associés
o: La Cinémathèque
        française

080.01 Labor für visuelles
        Wachstum
o: Thewall
080.02 Paco Aguayo
o: Vanguardia Europea
080.03 Sarah Grimaldi
o: liah chesnokov
080.04 Umeric
080.05 martinaigner.com
080.06 fireondesign /
        herborize
o: personal identity
080.07 the red is love
o: Sandiego Srl
/:   Angelo Caldarelli
080.08 dextro.org
o: silverserver
080.09 Euro RSCG Fuel
        Worldwide
o: Volvo Car Corporation
080.10 Emmi Salonen
o: Mika Ohtsuki
080.11 Omochi
o: LAW
080.12 Sito
o: +43
080.13 Sito
o: ito
080.14 büro uebele
o: Viavai Winebar
/:   Beate Gerner
080.15 nothing from outer
        space
o: netmodule
/:   www.nothing.ch

081.01 raum mannheim
o: boxservice
081.02 Labor für visuelles
        Wachstum
o: Dachkonzept 25
/:   igelstudios

081.03 diamond
o: Arbeitsgemeinschaft
       industrieller Forsc-
       hungsvereinigungen
081.04 Pep Karsten
o: Carillion
/:   Gardette Associés
081.05 Katrin Acklin
o: Pathologie Praxis
081.06 makelike
o: Entermodal
081.07 Futro
o: Recyclarium
081.08 makelike
o: Entermodal
081.09 Jon Ari Helgason
o: Auglysingamidlun

082.01 Raredrop
o: Ryu corporation
082.02 Zetuei Fonts
o: teito archives
/:   (c)teito archives
082.03 Shinya Inamura
       (everyday icons)
o: 3B Scientific Japan,
       Inc.
/:   (C) 3B Scientific
       Japan, Inc.
082.04 Omochi
o: NICE CHOICES
082.05 Coldwater Graphiix
o: TOKYO GO!GO!
082.06 kame design
o: Mari's Catering
082.07 Omochi
o: Tangomango
082.08 Velvet
o: Tangomango
082.09 Maniackers Design
o: Challenger
082.10 Power Graphixx
o: Izumojuki
082.11 QuickHoney
082.12 Oscar Salinas Losada
o: Tortas Hurakarrana
082.13 Raredrop
o: abbot's choice
082.14 No-Domain
o: Donkey
082.15 Maniackers Design

083.01 Double Standards
o: Institut Fuer Musik
       Und Medien
083.02 Axel Peemöller
o: Marius Wolfram
083.03 IDolls
o: Pott Records
/:   Rüdiger Töpfer

088.01 Gianni Rossi
o: Officine Smeraldo
089.01 Form
o: Dazed & Confused /
       TopShop
089.02 Mai-Britt Amsler
o: The Danish Town
       Planning Institute
089.03 Pantiestudio
o: Asociación Amigos de
       la Catedral Metro-
       politana, A.C.
089.04 bleed
o: Gudbrandsdalen AL

090.01 GillespieFox
o: Building Sustain-
       ability Seminars
090.02 Syrup Helsinki
o: Design Forum Finland
090.03 Velvet
o: Estonian Windsurfing
       Association
090.04 FireGirl
o: Companhia Instável
090.05 asmallpercent
o: ecotone.com
090.06 jum
o: CK
090.07 fireondesign /
       herborize
o: University of Bari
090.08 fireondesign /
       herborize
o: City of Naples
090.09 Fósforo
o: Orquesta y Coro
       Nacionales de España
090.10 MaMadesign AB
o: Jewish Museum in
       Stockholm
090.11 zookeeper
o: High School 64
090.12 Miha Artnak
o: Egmont film
090.13 e-Types
o: The Royal Danish
       Theater
090.14 sidsel stubbe
o: Isfirsk Leikhus
090.15 fireondesign /
       herborize
o: città del libro
090.16 Perndl+Co
o: Volkstheater Wien

091.01 Pentagram
o: Europäische Mozart-
       Wege
091.02 Rosendahl Grafikdesign
o: Berlinale Talent
       Campus
091.03 Dimomedia Lab
o: Schering Plough
/:   Medical Communica-
       tions
091.04 Dimomedia Lab
o: Elisir
091.05 Laurent Fétis
o: Mudam (Musée
       d'Art moderne du
       Luxembourg)
091.06 44 flavours
o: heliumcowboy artspace
/:   jörg heikhaus
091.07 sidsel stubbe
o: Vraa Hojskole
091.08 Fósforo
o: Kitchen
091.09 urbn;
/:   Franka Futterlieb
091.10 3 deluxe
o: Cocoon Club Frankfurt
091.11 Thomas Beyer Design
o: Rafael Vostell,
       Berlin
091.12 Mathilde Quartier
o: Conservatoire Neuchâ-
       telois
091.13 Jakob Straub
o: Teatro Valle, Roma
/:   orecchio acerbo
091.14 Neeser & Müller
o: Gastspiel Exibition
091.15 3 deluxe
o: Cocoon Club
091.16 desres
o: Stefan Bressel

092.01 Magenta Creative
       Networks
o: Commune on North
       Galery
/:   Molly Gochman
092.02 Klauser Weibel Design
o: Aargauer Kuratorium
092.03 Velvet
o: Estonian Youth Work
       Centre
092.04 Velvet
o: Dancing Company Lee

093.01 M!ch Welfringer
o: Beauxarts magazine,
       France
/:   designers anonymes
093.02 KMS Team
o: Pinakothek der
       Moderne
093.03 Matthias Gephart
o: X.POSURE
093.04 raum mannheim
o: Stadt Mannheim
093.05 re-public
o: Royal Danish Art
       Academy
093.06 kummer & herrman
o: BAK, basis voor
       actuele kunst
093.07 Engine
o: Northampton County
       Council
093.08 Mai-Britt Amsler
o: Copenhagen X
093.09 kummer & herrman
o: Stichting Best
       Verzorgde Boeken
093.10 Alëxone
o: les inattendus art
       event
093.11 Fons Hickmann m23
o: roc berlin, Rundfunk
       Orchester und Chöre
       Berlin
093.12 Carsten Giese
o: exhibition Typotektur
093.13 Ariel Pintos
o: Editorialmente

094.01 milchhof : atelier
o: Maxim Gorki Theater

095.01 Sesame Studio
o: 88
095.02 unfolded
o: Schweizerischer
       Bühnenverband
095.03 unfolded
o: west95
095.04 Supermundane
o: Good For Nothing
095.05 Raredrop
o: Tokyo Metropolitan
       Museum of Photography
095.06 Cassie Leedham
o: SeaSwarm Arts Organi-
       sation
095.07 Cassie Leedham
o: SeaSwarm Arts Organi-
       sation

095.08 Sensus Design Factory
       Zagreb
o: Croatian Designers
       Society
095.09 310k
o: sugarfactory
095.10 Zucker und Pfeffer
095.11 eduhirama
o: mario cohen
095.12 cabina
o: Juana de Arco _
       Galeria de Arte
095.13 Grandpeople
o: BergArt
095.14 clandrei
o: Lolita Bar Kassel
095.15 Benwar Home Design
o: Radio Campus Orleans
o: Benoit Matrion
095.16 Jakob Straub
o: Gli Olimpici del
       Teatro

096.01 Dimomedia Lab
o: Kukua Happy Beach
       - Bordighera
096.02 Team Manila
096.03 Takora
o: Central East Tokyo
       Exhibition
/:   grAphic tAkorA +
       DontMind
096.04 La Superagencia®
o: The Brand Lab for
       Fundación Corp Group
096.05 M!ch Welfringer
o: Beauxarts magazine,
       France
/:   designers anonymes
096.06 M!ch Welfringer
o: Beauxarts magazine,
       France
/:   designers anonymes

097.01 Team Manila
o: Pambansang Tshirt
097.02 BEK03
097.03 Alexandre Orion
o: Metabiotica -
       Alexandre Orion
097.04 raum mannheim
o: k+ exhibition
097.05 Hiroki Tsukuda
o: SAL
097.06 Kjetil Vatne
o: FredFyltFugl /
       Bomuldsfabriken

097.07 Cassie Leedham
o: Non-descript Theatre
      Company
/:   Cassie Leedham
097.08 HandGun
o: Aesthetic Refuge
097.09 Kjetil Vatne
o: Anagadirri
      Productions
097.10 Rune Mortensen Design
      Studio
o: Oslo University
      College
097.11 Dimaquina
o: Cibele Pastre /
      Domenica Mantel
097.12 Kjetil Vatne
o: Glitterbird - art for
      the very young / Oslo
      Univeristy College

098.01 raum mannheim
o: k+ exhibition
098.02 raum mannheim
o: k+ exhibition
098.03 Keep Adding
o: Niko
098.04 Magnetofonica
o: cesar m inserny
098.05 Salon Vektoria
o: Dare Art
098.06 44 flavours
/:   Julio Rölle
098.07 Salon Vektoria
o: Fachhochschule
      Darmstadt

099.01 Escobas
o: Tecnologico de
      Monterrey
099.02 The Remingtons
o: Ueli Gerber
099.03 Transittus
o: Flavia Costa Dance
      Company
099.04 Judith Drews
o: berliner comicfesti-
      val
099.05 Attak
o: Achtung Gestaltung
099.06 Cyklon
o: Nollapan Stockholm
099.07 Benwar Home Design
o: CRAB
/:   Bernard Cadon
099.08 Miha Artnak
o: ZEK advance

099.09 QuickHoney
099.10 Amore Hirosuke
o: Lion Veterinary
099.11 DigitalPlayground
      Studio

100.01 Atelier Télescopique
o: ARA
100.02 Polygraph
100.03 News
o: Bitterzoet
100.04 Toko
o: ZT Hollandia
100.05 Sat One
100.06 310k
o: urban explorers
100.07 Attak
o: Achtung Gestaltung
100.08 J. Tuominen, Jukka
      Pylväs
o: Rikkaus
100.09 Fupete Studio
o: Tribu magazine
/:   StudentiMediaGroup
      Spa
100.10 Oscar Salinas Losada
o: Loompen
100.11 Grotesk
o: Refill Magazine
100.11 HardCase Design
o: Stare Foundation
100.12 Tohyto
o: Antizoo
100.13 Canefantasma Studio
o: Comune di Monterig-
      gioni
100.14 Jon Burgerman
o: Flying Cat / Jon
      Burgerman

101.01 FireGirl
o: Teatro Helena Sá e
      Costa
101.02 resistro®
o: Expresso Produções
      Artísticas
101.03 DTM_INC
o: Top Trends b.v.
101.04 Jürgen und ich
o: Grenzgang
101.05 karlssonwilker inc.
o: Art Directors Club
      global
101.06 ROM studio
o: O gallery
101.07 Sat One

101.08 Mariana de Vasconcel-
      los Lameiro da Costa
o: Brasilian week of
      tourism
101.09 HandGun
o: World Up

102.01 Team Manila
102.02 Norwegian Ink
o: Beat Magazine
/:   Jakob Kermit
102.03 Norwegian Ink
o: Lydia Laska
102.04 underson
102.05 Iván Solbes
o: ELR editorial
102.06 Emil Hartvig
o: Danish graphic arts
      institute
102.07 Jason Kochis
o: Senor Tees
102.08 bisdixit
o: Fundació Gala-
      Salvador Dalí
102.09 29 degres
o: MIA
102.10 viagrafik
o: Passage club
102.12 Koadzn
o: War Of Monstars /
      Lazy Dog
102.13 Resin[sistem] design
o: Elwood Civics
102.14 Sektie
o: Lucy Dee
102.15 Escobas
o: Tiypo Magazine
102.16 Miki Amano
o: Steve & Tom

103.01 Escobas
o: MetroSur Gallery
103.02 FireGirl
o: Teatro Helena Sá e
      Costa
103.03 Adam Cruickshank
o: Semi-Permanent
103.04 Pandarosa
103.05 Fupete Studio
o: Grab magazine
/:   Frenkie Snc

104.01 Salon Vektoria
o: Dare Art
104.02 Dimaquina
o: Dub Echoes
/:   Bruno Natal
104.03 Keep Left Studio
o: Refill Magazine

104.04 Mutabor Design
o: Kunsthalle Kiel

105.01 decoylab
o: Paragraph Gallery
105.02 the Legalizer ApS
o: Johan Knattrup Jensen
105.03 zinestesia
o: WYZ
105.04 Me, Me
o: Grafuck
105.05 A-Side Studio
o: Hall For Cornwall
105.06 Superlow
o: W139, Amsterdam
105.07 Superlow
o: Hundreårsmarkeringen
      Norge 2005
105.08 M!ch Welfringer
o: Beauxarts magazine,
      France
/:   designers anonymes
105.09 Molho
o: Virtuosi Interna-
      tional Music Festival
105.10 Toko
o: Stichting Bliksum
105.11 base
o: Ministère de la
      Culture, France

106.01 Team Manila
106.02 Supershapes
o: Embassy

107.01 Caótica
107.02 Team Manila
107.03 Typeholics
o: Golden Pudel Club
107.04 Strukt Visual Network
o: Mosquito Musikclub /
      Austria, Timelkam
/:   Staudinger Thomas
107.05 Caótica
o: Hermes Frederico
107.06 raum mannheim
o: k+ exhibition
107.07 Magma
o: Starshot
/:   Maurice Redmond

108.01 Floor Wesseling Ix
      Opus Ada
o: kultivator
108.02 raum mannheim
o: k+ exhibition
108.03 raum mannheim
o: k+ exhibition

109.01 Fons Schiedon
o: Museum Princessehof
      Leeuwarden
109.02 Tohyto
o: Caracas Arepa Bar
109.03 Ariel Pintos
o: Camelia Ediciones

110.01 Keep Left Studio
o: Refill Magazine
110.02 Extraverage
      Productions
o: swatchthis!
110.03 Keep Left Studio
o: Refill Magazine
110.04 Lucas Westrup
o: Rub A Dub

111.01 ZIP Design
o: Barbican
111.02 Laundry
o: Honda Joy
111.03 Masa
o: Simpl3 Productions
111.04 Team Manila

112.01 Lifelong Friendship
      Society
o: Cranbrook Video
      Festival

113.01 bleed
o: Going Underground
113.02 Molho
o: Interruptions Book
113.03 Canefantasma Studio
o: Visionaria

114.01 Meomi Design
o: Tokyo a la Mode
/:   ©Joypop & Meomi
      Design
114.02 Sektie
o: Pete Philly
114.03 Lukatarina
o: Fever show-dance
      group
114.04 Extraverage
      Productions
o: swatchthis!
114.05 typotherapy+design
      inc.
o: Design Exchange (DX)
114.06 BankerWessel
o: The Swedish Museum of
      Architecture
114.07 Stolen Inc.
o: Offline

114.08 Gastón Caba
o: Milk Magazine / Benetton
114.09 Bo Lundberg
o: SpotCo New York
114.10 Attaboy
o: Laughing Squid
114.11 Woo
o: BonnierCarlsen
114.12 Sektie
o: Club Risk
114.13 Spild af Tid
o: Nordic Centre For Performing Arts
114.14 Martin Kvamme
o: Soria Moria
114.15 Canefantasma Studio

115.01 Team Manila
115.02 milchhof : atelier
115.03 The KDU
o: The KDU + Triple 5 Soul _ OMERTA
115.04 HardCase Design Dmitri Lavrow
o: Scarlatti, Cavalli, Cesti & Compagnie, for: Innovative Communications
115.05 milchhof : atelier
o: garage Festival
115.06 Niels Shoe Meulman
o: Summum
115.07 MvM / Maarten van Maanen
o: Stedelijk Museum de Lakenhal
115.08 Michael Genovese
o: Public
115.09 a+morph
o: Salon Oriental
115.10 raum mannheim
o: k+ exhibition
115.11 Fupete Studio
o: Grab magazine
/:   Frenkie Snc
115.12 Parra
o: Niels Meulman
115.13 Catalogtree
o: MiA2005
115.14 Woo
o: Atlas Publishing House

116.01 Zeek&Destroy
o: Zakk e.V.
116.02 Underware
o: Typeradio

116.03 Skin Design AS
o: Grafill
116.04 The KDU
o: The KDU + LA FORET TOKYO
116.05 Skin Design AS
o: Colin Eik & Gaute Gjøl Dale
116.06 Luca Forlani
o: Amedeo Sheert
116.07 Zeek&Destroy
o: Metzgerei Schnitzel
116.08 Laurent Fétis
o: le plateau
116.09 viagrafik
o: DSL Fashion
116.10 viagrafik
o: passage club
116.11 Diqart Graphics
o: Arts Connect
116.12 Alëxone
116.13 Clrqa
o: The Royal Magazine
116.14 Luca Forlani
o: street art and T-shirt
/:   blast

117.01 Canefantasma Studio
o: Pro Helvetia
117.02 Alexander Fuchs
o: Neuer Berliner Kunstverein
/:   Weißensee School of Art Berlin
117.03 actiondesigner
117.04 Norwegian Ink
o: Artbeat magazine
/:   Frode Nordbø
117.05 Neeser & Müller
o: Stadtlicht Projekt
117.06 Vier5
o: CAC Brétigny
117.07 Lorenzo Geiger
o: Kunsthalle Bern
/:   HKB Hochschule der Künste Bern
117.08 A-Side Studio
o: Acorn Theatre
117.09 Lollek und Bollek
o: Total Recall - das Festival des nacherzählten Films
117.10 fireondesign / herborize
o: City of Ercolano, Italy

117.11 re-p
o: Fonds régional d'art contemporain de Lorraine, Metz
117.12 Team Manila
117.13 visomat inc.
o: M12 / visomat inc.
117.14 automatic
o: Everyday Art
117.15 substrat
o: Blindstadt - Labor für Reflexion

118.01 artless Inc
118.02 Julie Joliat
o: Baby! magazine
/:   Rene Eller
118.03 Fuenfwerken Design
o: atelier frankfurt, frankfurt am main
118.04 Magenta Creative Networks
o: Commune on North Galery
/:   Molly Gochman
118.05 Brighten the corners
o: Fake Theatre Production Company
118.06 archetype : interactive
o: manzportal.com
/:   Dicken Lee
118.07 Neeser & Müller
o: Portes Ouvertes Basel
118.08 Extraverage Productions
118.09 Flink
o: the Flink gallery
118.10 Martha Stutteregger
o: mumok - Museum moderner Kunst Stiftung Ludwig Wien
118.11 Toko
o: Het Zuidelijk Toneel
118.12 ständige vertretung
o: istanbul foundation for culture and arts
118.13 Fuenfwerken Design
118.14 Vier5
o: Museum für Angewandte Kunst Frankfurt
118.15 Double Standards
o: Reed Messe Wien
118.16 ADAPTER
o: Defstep
118.16 archetype : interactive
o: Hong Kong Creative Association
/:   joe cheng

119.01 Mutabor Design
o: Kunsthalle Kiel
119.02 Atelier Mühlberg
o: Aktive Archive
119.03 Formdusche
o: hans otto theater potsdam
119.04 Pentagram
o: Philharmonie Luxembourg
119.05 3 deluxe
o: Cocoon Club
119.06 Nish
o: TheBlowUp
119.07 Semitransparent Design
o: Beyes
119.08 Fons Schiedon
o: Io, Isabella International Film Week
119.09 Tilt
o: Muthesius Kunsthochschule, Kiel
119.10 Kontrapunkt
o: øksnehallen
119.11 Jonas Ganz
o: cinéart
119.12 Futro
o: Bumerang Music Awards
119.13 Syrup Helsinki
o: Kunsthalle Helsinki
119.14 Kontrapunkt
o: kunstindustrimuseet
119.15 310k
o: sugarfactory

120.01 propella, konzept + design
o: landesgartenschau NEU-ULM
120.02 viagrafik
o: passage club
120.03 Intercity
o: Creative Review
120.04 HelloBard.com
o: Tra
120.05 Sito
o: Cabeza
120.06 Axel Domke
120.07 backyard 10
o: Kafe Magazine
120.08 Extraverage Productions
o: streetsoul
120.09 DTM_INC
o: Urban Cult
120.10 Extraverage Productions
o: Fontos! Magazine

120.11 News
o: Stichting Postivisme
120.12 Superlow
o: NIFCA

121.01 granit di Lioba Wackernell
o: kuns Meran, Merano arte
121.02 Chris Bolton
o: University of Art & Design Helsinki
121.03 Lunatiq
o: Derush

122.01 Floor Wesseling Ix Opus Ada
o: kalmar konst museum
122.02 Paco Aguayo
o: Centro Cultural Universitario
122.03 red design
o: University of Brighton
122.04 29 degres
o: TAF - Transit Artwork Foundation
122.05 strange//attraktor:
o: The Pause Festival
122.06 Superlow
o: Nifca
122.07 artless Inc
122.08 Caótica
o: Companhia de Dança Deborah Colker
122.09 hirschindustries
o: Musee d'Art Moderne Grand-Duc Jean Luxembourg
122.10 Sophie Toporkoff
o: Rendez-Vous magazine
/:   Sophie Toporkoff / Rendez-Vous magazine
122.11 unfolded
o: west95
122.12 Niels Shoe Meulman
o: Suburbia
122.13 Laurent Fétis
o: Caisse des dépots et consignations / Palais de Tokyo
122.14 No-Domain
o: Intro
122.15 Jürgen und ich
o: Sandra Stein
122.16 jewboy Corporation™
o: Sitra-Ahra Book Publishing

123.01 Niels Shoe Meulman
o: Annejes van Liempd
123.02 Superlow
o: Aschehoug
123.03 Superlow
o: Aschehoug
123.04 Tohyto
o: Suborn
123.05 rtr
o: NWBA
123.06 Nish
o: n/a
123.07 Plastic Kid
o: Expo Kong
123.08 No-Domain
o: Ambulante
123.09 Atomic Attack
o: Chalk Magazine
123.10 Raredrop
o: Kunekuneshi
123.11 Martin Kvamme
o: Soria Moria
123.12 archetype : interactive
o: RTHK
123.13 Power Graphixx

124.01 GrafficTraffic
o: Snafu Magazine
/:   High 5 Entertainment
124.02 3 deluxe
o: Peko Peko
124.03 3 deluxe
124.04 jewboy Corporation™
o: Reign' art project
       events
124.05 La Superagencia®
o: The Brand Lab for
       Fundación Corp Group
124.06 Superlow
o: Nifca
124.07 Superlow
o: Nifca
124.08 Caótica
o: Companhia de Dança
       Deborah Colker
124.09 ruse76
o: ink tank magazine
124.10 Extraverage
       Productions
o: nasty
124.11 Mikkel Grafixico
       Westrup
o: Pestol.dk
124.12 JAKe
o: Badjuju
124.13 paulroberts.tv
o: Anrick Bregman

124.14 44 flavours
o: spanish fly
/:   Patrick Fuchs
124.15 44 flavours
/:   Patrick Fuchs
124.16 Sektie
o: Daan

125.01 Hausgrafik
o: Salzhaus Winterthur
125.02 hirschindustries
o: Musee d'Art Moderne
       Grand-Duc Jean
       Luxembourg
125.03 Extraverage
       Productions
/:   www.drezign.hu
125.04 Formgeber
o: exhibition project
       (Kunstverein
       Heidelberg)
125.05 ten_do_ten
o: visualogue
125.06 env-design
o: zephyr / raum fuer
       forografie / mannheim
125.07 Molho
o: DES - Design Gráfico
       Brasileiro
125.08 123Buero
125.09 Formgeber
o: exhibition project
       (Kunstverein
       Heidelberg)
125.10 Laurent Fétis
o: Caisse des Dépots et
       consignations / Parc
       de La Villette
125.11 Out Of Order
o: CJP
125.12 Team Manila
125.13 Dimomedia Lab
o: Sidemast 2006
/:   Medical Com
125.14 M!ch Welfringer
o: Beauxarts magazine,
       France
/:   designers anonymes
125.15 büro uebele
o: UIA 2005 Istanbul
       Congress
/:   Frank Geiger

126.01 Razauno
o: Complex Magazine
126.02 Konstantinos
       Gargaletsos
o: Prenelle Gallery

126.03 viagrafik
o: co pop köln
126.04 WGD
o: School project.
       furniture exhibition
126.05 Semitransparent
       Design
o: Bit Things (YCAM)
126.06 bleed
o: Norwegian Design
       Council
126.07 Superlow
o: Danse og teatersen-
       trum (DTS)
126.08 William Morrisey
o: Espaço Documenta
126.09 Brighten the corners
       Studio for Design
       London & Stuttgart
o: Architektur Stadt
       Münster
126.10 Fons Hickmann m23
o: Diakonie in
       Düsseldorf
126.11 visomat inc.
o: M12 / visomat inc.
126.12 Le_Palmier Design
o: Bönig & Company /
       Camel
126.13 Otherways 5th Floor
       Studio
o: het Bureel
/:   Otherways
126.14 granit di Lioba
       Wackernell
o: kuns Meran, Merano
       arte
126.15 Floor Wesseling
o: 16-2.org

127.01 Attak
o: Uitpunt ,s-Hertogen-
       bosch
127.02 FireGirl
o: Associação dos Comer-
       ciantes do Porto
127.03 Thonik
o: Centraal Museum
       Utrecht
127.04 visomat inc.
o: M12 / visomat inc.
127.05 Simian
o: Oslo International
       Film Festival
127.06 29 degres
o: GT29
127.07 Studio Dumbar
o: H+F Collection

127.08 Semisans
o: Juvenile Guidaance
       Foundation
127.09 dainippon
o: Brutus, Magazine
       House
127.10 ständige vertretung
o: werkstatt der
       kulturen
127.11 raum mannheim
o: k+ exhibition
127.12 Jonas Ganz
o: Musiktheater Laut
/:   Jonas Ganz
127.13 Keep Left Studio
o: Refill Magazine
127.14 Toko
o: TeDoen Artprojects
127.15 derek johnson
o: V Gallery, Basel
127.16 Pentagram
o: Mozarthaus Vienna

128.01 News
o: Hiscox
128.02 The Remingtons
o: Der Anker
128.03 Accident Grotesk!
128.04 Team Manila
128.05 Flexn / Bank
o: Lodown
128.06 Catalogtree
o: MiA2005
128.07 Kjetil Vatne
o: Finn Eirik Modahl /
       Råstølen Sculpture
       Complex
128.08 Tender
o: Two Bravo
128.09 fireondesign /
       herborize
o: unione industriali
128.10 Annabelle Mehraein
o: Lothringer 13
128.11 makelike
o: Portland Institute
       for Contemporary Art
       (PICA)
128.12 3volt Design
128.13 3volt Design
128.14 3volt Design
128.15 viagrafik
o: Via Electronic
       Department

129.01 Atelier Télescopique
129.02 Balsi Grafik
o: tripleeight club
       lounge

129.03 Annella Armas
o: Instituto del
       Patrimonio Cultural.
       Venezuela
129.04 Annella Armas
o: Museo Histórico
       Clarines. Venezuela
129.05 Matthias Gephart
o: X.POSURE
129.06 Annella Armas
o: Ministerio de la
       Cultura. Venezuela
129.07 Pantiestudio
o: Eje 7
129.08 FireGirl
o: Teatro Helena Sá e
       Costa
129.09 Laundry
o: Yaris
129.10 Loïc Sattler
o: Museum für Form
129.11 Lucias Westrup
o: Toiletpapir
129.12 Axel Raidt
o: Schlie & Werner,
       landscape architects
129.13 Laundry
o: Yaris
129.14 Sat One

130.01 ten_do_ten
o: yasu gallery
130.02 chris bolton
o: University of Art &
       Design Helsinki
130.03 Fons Hickmann m23
o: ifa Gallery

131.01 karlssonwilker
o: The Goldman Warehouse
131.03 Creative Review
/:   Design: The Projects
       (Daniel Mair and
       Gareth Holt). Pho-
       tographer: Dan Tobin
       Smith. Assistant:
       Alistair Strong.
       Compositor: Martin
       Pryor
131.03 Tsuyoshi Kusano
       Design
o: Japan Science and
       Technology Agency

131.04 Creative Review
/:   Design: The Projects
     (Daniel Mair,
     Gareth Holt). Photo:
     Dan Tobin Smith.
     Assistant: Alistair
     Strong. Compositor:
     Martin Pryor

136.01 Keep Left Studio
o: Refill Magazine

137.01 newoslo

138.01 Labor für visuelles
     Wachstum™
o: designsatelite
138.02 Pantiestudio
138.03 Fupete Studio
138.04 Kosta Lazarevski
o: O communication
     - advertising agency
138.05 Futro
o: Brumen Design
     Biennale
/:   Fundacija Brumen
138.06 Insect
o: Red Represents
/:   insect.co.uk
138.07 Borsellino & Co.
o: M-109 Network
138.08 Intercity
o: Fusion
138.09 Simian
o: superstar

139.01 Intercity
139.02 brandigloo
139.03 Toca Me
139.04 donat raetzo union
o: Pixelprinz, screen/
     prepress, Bern
139.05 FireGirl
o: O Baú da Maria
139.06 Toxic design
o: Atomobravo
139.07 resistro®
o: Gibson Hinds / Hinds
     Design
139.08 Emil Hartvig
o: Danish Development
/:   Jakob Brahe Pedersen
139.09 moxi
o: Spax Architekten
139.10 moxi
o: Fabian Blaser, oro
     verde

139.11 David Maloney
o: EyeSpeak
/:   Airhart & Co.
139.12 lindedesign
o: Wissenswerft
139.13 Dimomedia Lab
o: Lorenzo Mascherpa
139.14 Dimomedia Lab
o: Marco Cornagli
139.15 Syrup Helsinki
o: Huippu Design
     Management

140.01 Amseldrossel
o: www.pawone.de
140.02 Cruz Creative
140.03 Keloide.net
o: 7 espinas produc-
     ciones
140.04 Resin[sistem] design
o: Studio ON
140.05 Resin[sistem] design
140.06 Ken Tanabe
140.07 Rob Chiu
140.08 Stolen Inc.
140.09 Extraverage
     Productions
140.10 Colletivo Design
140.11 sunrise studios
140.12 DigitalPlayground
     Studio
140.13 123Buero
o: Sayimsorry
/:   Silke Krieg

141.01 Michele Angelo
141.02 cubegrafik - 100%
     Digital
o: Sixlab - Research,
     Design & Development
141.03 Alexandre Orion
o: Tela.tv
/:   Alexandre Orion
141.04 Norwegian Ink
o: Nordisk Film as
141.05 Dr. Alderete
141.05 Sellout Industries
141.06 Lapin
141.07 Ninjacruise
o: The BrandingFarm
141.09 Chris Hutchinson
141.10 Mattisimo
141.11 Jeremyville
o: Mokem, Australia
141.13 Frederique Daubal
o: Matthias Koslik
141.14 Frederique Daubal
o: Matthias Koslik

141.16 Masa
o: DGV - Die Gestalten
     Verlag

142.01 Extraverage
     Productions
142.02 Extraverage
     Productions
142.03 BEKO3
142.04 BEKO3
142.05 Keep Left Studio
o: Refill Magazine
142.06 Carsten Raffel
o: United States of the
     Art
142.07 Emmi Salonen
142.08 Lunatiq
o: Eagle Star Petroleum
     Corp.
142.09 jum
o: USotA
142.10 Felix Braden
o: Debüser+Bee Kommuni-
     kationsdesign
142.11 Lucias Westrup
o: Lucias

143.01 Sellout Industries
143.02 Thomas Weyres
o: CEH PLUS PLUS
143.03 Blu Design
o: tiypo
143.04 QuickHoney
o: Future Music Magazine
143.05 Heiko Hoos
143.06 actiondesigner
143.07 Matthias Gephart
o: Own Business
143.08 Nish
o: Obelisk
143.09 Extraverage
     Productions
143.10 Draplin
o: camworld.com
/:   BlogCorp
143.11 Extraverage
     Productions
143.12 Emil Kozak
o: Evolver
/:   Tobias Munk Åkesson
143.13 less rain

144.01 Extraverage
     Productions
144.02 DesignChapel
144.03 BEKO3
144.04 2Advanced Studios
o: Grafika66

144.05 BEKO3
144.06 interspectacular
144.07 DesignChapel
o: North Kingdom
144.08 Canefantasma Studio
o: Itaca
144.09 Cupco!
o: FEWMANY
144.10 BEKO3
144.11 apishAngel
144.12 apishAngel
144.13 Georg Schatz
144.14 Nish
o: WDDG
144.15 Studio Oscar
o: Levi's
144.16 Upnorth

145.01 The Skull Dezain
o: Vicious Flavor from
     bishop.inc
145.02 Microbot
145.03 hijack graphics
145.04 hijack graphics
145.05 No-Domain
145.06 ROM studio
o: Pachteca
145.07 Yo Freeman
o: CTRL Crushers
145.08 44 flavours
/:   Julio Rölle
145.09 Zeek&Destroy
145.10 Glauco Diogenes
145.11 Tohyto
o: Coachella

146.01 Rolitoland
146.02 Tado
o: Flying Cat
146.03 Tado
o: Freshnessmag
146.04 Tado
o: Freshnessmag
146.05 Tado
o: Freshnessmag
146.06 Cupco!
146.07 Tado
o: Flying Cat
146.08 Tado
o: Tado
146.09 Tado
o: Freshnessmag
146.10 Takora
o: Metro Minute
146.11 Takora
o: Sony Stiyle Store
146.12 Sellout Industries
146.13 tapetentiere

146.14 redaktion »echtzeit«
o: international dust
146.15 Alexander Fuchs
o: Fux

147.01 44 flavours
/:   Julio Rölle
147.02 Attak
o: Attak und Arillo
147.03 Cuartopiso
147.04 A-Side Studio
147.05 Lapin
o: Cadaver Exquisito
147.06 Lucias Westrup
o: Tom Box
147.07 Takora
147.08 Lunatiq
147.09 Jeremyville
o: I Love You Baby book
147.10 Rolitoland
147.11 La Superagencia
o: Studio T

148.01 lindedesign
o: MilkMyMusic.com
148.02 Tado
o: Flying Cat
148.03 Sellout Industries
148.04 Lukatarina
148.05 Norwegian Ink
o: Creatoy
148.06 Attak
148.07 Attak
148.08 Extraverage
     Productions
148.09 DigitalPlayground
     Studio
148.10 lindedesign
o: MilkMyMusic.com
148.11 leBeat
o: leBeat //
     graphic&animation
148.12 Attak
148.13 Extraverage
     Productions
148.14 lindedesign
148.15 tapetentiere
148.16 Regina

149.01 Axel Peemöller
o: Soliloqueen
149.02 AmorfoDesignlab™
o: Pastilla Digital™
149.03 Stockbridge Interna-
     tional
o: Parco Corno alle
     Scale

149.04 Designbolaget
o: taburet
/:   Henrik Schleisner
149.05 Tokidoki LLC
149.06 Fons Schiedon
o: Submarinechannel
149.07 Fons Schiedon
o: Submarinechannel
149.08 Fons Schiedon
o: Submarinechannel
149.09 Tilt
149.10 Chris Hutchinson
149.11 Sellout Industries
149.12 Tokidoki LLC
149.13 mateuniverse
o: typografschaft
149.14 BEK03
149.15 :g / studio-gpop
o: The Happy Pill
149.16 Chris Rubino
o: Deep Focus

150.01 Cupco!
o: Fewmany
150.02 Lapin
o: Antifanzine
/:   Jorge Navarro
        Herradon(lapin) Pedro
        Mogrovejo Lucitron
150.03 Stockbridge Interna-
        tional
o: Hang Ten
150.04 Designkitchen
150.05 Felix Braden
o: Timetwist
150.06 Labor für visuelles
        Wachstum™
o: grellschwarz
150.07 Kimera
150.08 Pandarosa
150.09 44 flavours
/:   Sebastian Bagge
150.10 hijack graphics
o: clubmilk

151.01 Vrontikis Design
        Office
o: Via Motif, San
        Raphel, USA
151.02 Extraverage
        Productions
151.03 Dr. Alderete
151.04 Cuartopiso
o: Ovum
151.05 Extraverage
        Productions
151.06 Cuban Council
o: Beetle Farm

151.07 redaktion »echtzeit«
151.08 DigitalPlayground
        Studio
151.09 Cassie Leedham
o: Pixel Bettie
151.10 Kanardo
151.11 Bianca Strauch
151.12 Nando Costa
o: Modernista!
/:   Gary Koepke & Lance
        Jensen
151.13 Norwegian Ink
o: Lydia Laska
151.14 Fase
o: TEC
151.15 Extraverage
        Productions
151.16 Shintaro Yarimizo

152.01 Lucias Westrup
o: Lucian
152.02 Furi Furi Company
o: Girls Power Manifesto
152.03 Jon Burgerman
152.04 Attak
152.05 Escobas
152.06 Raffaele Primitivo
152.07 Gastón Caba
152.08 Attak
152.09 Jeremyville
o: Fused magazine, UK
152.10 Gianni Rossi
o: wp lavori in corso
152.11 Yo Freeman
o: CTRL Clothing
152.12 Shivamat
152.13 Fritz Torres
o: nortec
152.14 Dr. Morbito &
        1000Changos
o: 1000changos
/:   Omar Mijangos
152.15 Carsten Raffel
152.16 Fellow Designers

153.01 viagrafik
153.02 Jun Watanabe
o: Devilock
153.03 Cherrybox Studios
o: Jakdup
/:   Jessica Knapp
153.04 mateuniverse
o: tonk
153.05 Ashi & office
        Greminger
o: stirato
153.06 Atomic Attack
153.07 Norwegian Ink
o: Nordisk Film as

153.08 Lapin
153.09 Jun Watanabe
o: ZYGORD
153.10 No-Domain
153.11 Dr. Morbito &
        1000Changos
o: Revista Tiypo
/:   Omar Mijangos/
        1000changos
153.12 DigitalPlayground
        Studio
153.13 Shivamat

154.01 iaah
o: Threadless
154.02 Attak
154.03 viagrafik
o: Volkswagen AG

155.01 Roya Hamburger
155.02 Team Manila
o: United Tinikling
/:   Inksurge, Electroly-
        chee, Teammanila,
        Everywhereweshoot
155.03 Nathan Jobe
o: Soldier Unknown
155.04 No-Domain
155.05 No-Domain

156.01 YOK
o: GRASP Great ape
        survival project
/:   Yok
156.02 Team Manila
156.03 Yo Freeman
o: CTRL Clothing
156.04 Nathan Jobe
o: Soldier Unknown
156.05 Attak
o: The Hunter
156.06 HKI - Hellohikimori
o: Overage4design
156.07 Zinc
o: Cynthia Martinez
156.08 Masa
o: VW - FOX Hotel
156.09 Clrqa
156.10 Yo Freeman
o: CTRL Clothing
156.11 Caótica
156.12 QuickHoney
156.13 underson
156.14 Emil Hartvig
o: Adpassion
/:   Rene P
156.15 DigitalPlayground
        Studio
o: Popcorn Club

157.01 Norwegian Ink
o: Nordisk Film as
157.02 2Advanced Studios
o: Grafika66
157.03 Formgeber
157.04 Attak
o: Boomerang
157.05 iaah
o: Bass Center
/:   IAAH
157.06 Kosta Lazarevski
157.07 Cupco!
o: Fewmany
157.08 BEK03
o: movie twins
157.09 hijack graphics
157.10 Magma
157.11 Sellout Industries
157.12 Plastic Kid

158.01 Sensus Design Factory
        Zagreb
o: Ulupuh Zagreb
158.02 Sensus Design Factory
        Zagreb
o: Ulupuh Zagreb
158.03 Shintaro Yarimizo
158.04 Flavio Bagioli
o: desorg
158.05 kw43
o: Charles Green
158.06 44 flavours
o: kingdrips.de
/:   Lutz Lindemann
158.07 Shivamat
/:   mutabor
158.08 iaah
o: Incines / Cammami
        Design
/:   Cammami Design
158.09 Crush
o: union Square
158.10 Nathan Jobe
o: Soldier Unknown
158.11 Matthias Gephart
o: German Writers Crew
        »463«
158.12 Calliope Studios
158.13 Dennis Eriksson
o: Stop-ill Publishing
158.14 actiondesigner
158.15 Shivamat
158.16 Insect
o: sixlegsarebetter.com
/:   insect.co.uk

159.01 Nathan Jobe
o: adidas
159.02 Flexn / Bank

159.03 Dr. Alderete
159.04 Masa
159.05 Mikkel Grafixico
        Westrup
159.06 underson
159.07 Hula Hula
159.08 Furi Furi Company
159.09 Hydro74
159.10 Lapin
159.11 Dr. Alderete
o: Spatium magazine
159.12 Braveland Design
o: Kick Media
159.13 I&Eye
o: FH Dortmund
159.14 kw43
o: Sieger Design
159.15 Felix Braden
o: Langmeiers Marketing
        Kommunikation
/:   debüser + bee kom-
        munikationsdesign

160.01 Tohyto
160.02 Extraverage
        Productions
160.03 usugrow
o: organic contrast (own
        office)
160.04 Nuuro
o: n/a
160.05 Keloide.net
o: Ruben Coca Produccio-
        nes Cinematograficas
160.06 Christian Rothenhagen
o: dlxsf
160.07 Fupete Studio
160.08 onrushdesign / Front
o: Umemi design

161.01 Tatiana Arocha
161.02 Deanne Cheuk
o: Tokion Magazine
161.03 Deanne Cheuk
o: Tokion Magazine
161.04 Razauno
161.05 Extraverage
        Productions
161.06 Coutworks
o: MdN Magazine
161.07 Salon Vektoria
161.08 Felix Braden
o: Floodfonts
161.09 Norwegian Ink
o: Jon Sindre
161.10 Blink Blink
161.11 Blu Design
o: tiypo

161.12 Resin[sistem] design
o: Superbia design
161.13 Keloide.net
o: Babylon Motorhome

162.01 Vault49
162.02 redaktion »echtzeit«
o: echtzeit magazin
162.03 Formgeber
o: Jotopia | Visual
    Noise
162.04 ROM studio

163.01 Skin Design
o: Grafill
163.02 AmorfoDesignlab™
o: Cedim™ & Design Week
    Monterrey™
/:   A+Positivo™
163.03 DigitalPlayground
    Studio
163.04 Hydro74
o: Manifest Worldwide
163.05 radargraphics
o: Boomerang Media
163.06 Hydro74
o: Steelo
163.07 Labor für visuelles
    Wachstum™
o: grellschwarz
163.08 FL@33
/:   Aerial Photography by
    Fenwick Helicopters,
    Paris
163.09 Out Of Order
163.10 Cape Arcona
    Typefoundry
o: [ths] Design
163.11 Niels Shoe Meulman
o: Badboek

164.01 Superlow
164.02 Sarah Grimaldi
o: bambistar™
164.03 BEK03
o: iea

165.01 Sarah Grimaldi
o: bambistar™
165.02 Designkitchen
o: HomeCare
/:   Richard Balstedt
165.03 Dimomedia Lab
o: Dimomedia Lab -
    Massimo Sirelli
165.04 Yucca Studio
o: GreenDonkey

165.05 Extraverage
    Productions
o: fortrock clo-thing
165.06 Tsutomu Umezawa
o: kirin
165.07 Flexn / Bank
165.08 Otherways 5th Floor
    Studio
o: Ninaber van Eyben
/:   Gerrit-Jan Ninaber
    van Eyben
165.09 Labor für visuelles
    Wachstum™
o: grellschwarz
165.10 Microbot

166.01 redaktion »echtzeit«
o: echtzeit magazin
166.02 Creative Pride
/:   Matt Kenyon

167.01 DigitalPlayground
    Studio
167.02 DigitalPlayground
    Studio
167.03 DigitalPlayground
    Studio
167.04 Cuartopiso

168.01 Peter Anderson
o: cafe paul rankin
/:   The Rankin Group
168.02 Extraverage
    Productions

169.01 Inocuodesign
169.02 Nando Costa
o: Modernista!
/:   Gary Koepke & Lance
    Jensen
169.03 Inocuodesign
169.04 Instant

170.01 Petra Börner
170.02 Roya Hamburger
170.03 Miki Amano
170.04 Joe A. Scerri
o: Ten Studio

171.01 Molho
171.02 Formgeber
o: Jotopia
171.03 Ashi & office
    Greminger
o: Design Embassy
171.04 Masa
o: KONG - Tienda /
    Galeria

172.01 Kallegraphics
172.02 PMKFA
172.03 PMKFA
172.04 Oscar Salinas Losada
172.05 JDK
o: sanctuary
172.06 3 deluxe
172.07 3 deluxe
172.08 Sellout Industries
172.09 44 flavours
/:   Patrick Fuchs
172.10 Carsten Raffel
o: United States of the
    Art
172.11 Muller
o: Mam Tor™ Publishing
172.12 Jawa and Midwich
o: Uncommunicative
/:   Nils Davey Uncom-
    municative
172.13 Extraverage
    Productions
172.14 Lucias Westrup
o: Lucias 291
172.15 Lousy Livincompany
172.16 Adam Cruickshank
o: Regular Product

173.01 Fons Schiedon
o: I love dust
173.02 The Skull Dezain
o: Vicious Flavor from
    bishop.inc
173.03 Fons Schiedon
o: I Love Dust
/:   Fons Schiedon
173.04 Oc/Om/Oy/Ok
173.05 Zeek&Destroy
173.06 Magnetofonica
/:   Laura Sofia González
    R.
173.07 Parra
o: Cathal McKee
173.08 Furi Furi Company
173.09 Parra
173.10 I-Manifest
173.11 BEK03
173.12 Mikkel Grafixico
    Westrup
o: Pestol.dk

174.01 Insect Design
o: Quiksilver Europe
174.02 Flexn / Bank
174.03 Nohemi Dicuru-fash-
    iongraphic

175.01 :g / studio-gpop
o: Fat Statement

175.02 Extraverage
    Productions
175.03 Koadzn
o: Koa
175.04 Cupco!
175.05 Syrup Helsinki
175.06 Thomas Weyres
o: Vresno
175.07 viagrafik
o: pyramid editions
175.08 Studio Oscar
o: Ben Wilson Design
/:   Oscar Wilson
175.09 Norwegian Ink
o: Peter Opsvik
175.10 Sellout Industries
175.11 Yo Freeman
o: CTRL Clothing
175.12 Yo Freeman
o: CTRL Clothing
175.13 YellowToothpick
o: Go Outside
175.14 Akinori Oishi
175.15 Yo Freeman
o: CTRL Clothing

176.01 Fakir
o: Fakir
176.02 Raphazen
176.03 Kallegraphics
176.04 Deanne Cheuk
o: Tokion Magazine

177.01 Superlow
177.02 Cybu Richli
177.03 Mone Maurer
177.04 Frederique Daubal

178.01 Deanne Cheuk
o: Tokion Magazine
178.02 Deanne Cheuk
o: Tokion Magazine
178.03 Deanne Cheuk
o: Tokion Magazine
178.04 Deanne Cheuk
o: Tokion Magazine

179.01 Lifelong Friendship
    Society
179.02 Deanne Cheuk
o: Tokion Magazine
179.03 Miha Artnak
o: ZEK advance
179.04 Miha Artnak
o: ZEK advance
179.05 Miha Artnak
o: ZEK advance

180.01 Inocuodesign

180.02 Laundry
180.03 Tilt
o: Stylefetish
    Designlabs
180.04 BEK03
o: POW

181.01 Hydro74
o: Devoid of Yesterday
181.02 Carsten Raffel
181.03 dzgnbio
o: spootnick.com
181.04 I-Manifest
181.05 dzgnbio
181.06 Extraverage
    Productions
181.07 3 deluxe
o: Rockamora
181.08 Hydro74
o: ReeCall

182.01 Unit c.m.a.
o: Disco Exota
/:   i.c.w. Xelor
182.02 Keloide.net
182.03 WGD
o: Norwegian Ink

183.01 Peter Anderson
o: rain city
/:   The Rankin Group
183.02 The Vacuum Design
o: Snickers
183.03 William Morrisey
183.04 Leon Vymenets
o: Lamar
183.05 I-Manifest
183.06 Kimera

184.01 Instant
o: Brau Union Österreich
184.02 Sesame Studio
o: Soap Creative
184.03 the Legalizer
184.04 Mikkel Grafixico
    Westrup
o: Pestol.dk
184.05 the Legalizer
o: General G
184.06 Slang
184.07 Matthias Gephart
o: Kore, Writers »463«
184.08 Keloide.net
o: RCPC
184.09 Keep Left Studio
o: Vietnamese Student
    Association
184.10 Resin[sistem] design
184.11 Resin[sistem] design

184.12 ehquestionmark
o: minipips
184.13 Raphazen
182.14 Lapin
184.15 surround
o: MTV Networks

185.01 Laundry
185.02 Norwegian Ink
o: Oslo-TV
185.03 Takora
o: Readymade Magazine
/:   Cheap Pop
185.04 Underware
o: Susannah Huntington,
     Paddington
185.05 Underware
185.06 Jun Watanabe
185.07 Analog.Systm
o: Systm
185.08 Fupete Studio
185.09 Zeek&Destroy
o: NUI Graffngraph
185.10 Mattisimo
o: Matthew Richard
     Schneider
185.11 lindedesign
o: zoofuku
185.12 Plastic Kid
185.13 Kosta Lazarevski
o: rad fabrik
185.14 Christian Walden
o: dmyk
185.15 Supermundane

186.01 Felix Braden
o: 7p5
/:   debüser + bee
     kommunikationsdesign
186.02 Nando Costa
o: Violet
/:   Gary Koepke & Lance
     Jensen
186.03 Studio Sans Nom
186.04 onrushdesign / front
o: Friday Fans
186.05 inkgraphix
o: Skank Clothing
/:   Mattias Lundin
186.06 Crush
o: William Grant & sons
186.07 Büro Brendel
186.08 Koadzn
o: Koa
186.09 Dennis Eriksson
o: Stop-ill Publishing
186.10 Neasden Control
     Centre
o: MTV UK

186.11 Nuuro
o: DGeral
186.12 Resin[sistem] design
186.13 Kallegraphics
186.14 Digart Graphics
186.15 Zion Graphics
o: J.Lindeberg
186.16 Yo Freeman
o: CTRL Clothing

187.01 viagrafik
o: Volkswagen AG
187.02 Ninjacruise
o: Imagefed
187.03 Keep Left Studio
o: Jenny Lloyd
     Copywriter
187.04 Adapter
o: NWBA
187.05 SignalStrong
o: None
187.06 dzgnbio
o: 5K
187.07 Boris Dworschak
o: Vektoria Magazine
187.08 Semisans
187.09 Abraka design
o: rue de la clé
187.10 29 degres
o: rekap
187.11 Hydro74
o: E360 Magazine
187.12 Hydro74
o: Conform Consume
187.13 Attaboy
o: Hi Fructose Magazine
187.14 cubemen studio
187.15 Axel Peemöller

188.01 Hayato Kamono
188.02 Mikkel Grafixico
     Westrup
o: Jukas Design
/:   Jesse Jakob Jensen
188.03 Flink
188.04 projekttriangle
o: Plasmic
188.05 Raffaele Primitivo
188.06 Oc/Om/Oy/Ok
o: Telos Origin
188.08 modo
188.09 Bodara, Büro für
     Gebrauchsgrafik
o: Brandwatcher
188.10 viagrafik
o: booth & cliborn
     Publishing
188.11 Supermundane
o: faesthetic
188.12 Norwegian Ink

188.13 SignalStrong
o: None
188.14 Sellout Industries
188.15 Zetuei Fonts
o: azb
188.16 june

189.01 Magnetofonica
189.02 Magnetofonica
189.03 Muller
o: Ashley Wood
189.04 paulroberts.tv
189.05 Bionyc Industries
o: Crush Licensing
189.06 Clrqa
o: Oruga Films
189.07 Clrqa
o: Mono Magazine
189.08 Clrqa
o: Oruga Films
189.09 Mode
o: Dalton Maag
/:   Mode
189.10 Joe A. Scerri
189.11 Zeek&Destroy
189.12 AmorfoDesignlab™
o: Brand™
189.13 Transittus
189.14 AmorfoDesignlab™
189.15 AmorfoDesignlab™
o: -1:0:1™
189.16 viagrafik
o: Volkswagen AG

190.01 310k
o: drukkerij kahle
190.02 Made
o: Made™
190.03 Hydro74
o: Relevant
190.04 The KDU
o: The KDU + nonTYPE
190.05 Tatiana Arocha
o: Camila Arocha
190.06 Salon Vektoria
190.07 Fósforo
190.08 Kontrapunkt
190.09 actiondesigner
190.10 Accident Grotesk!
o: Vectorjockey VJ
     Software
190.11 Rocholl Selected
     Designs
o: Brandwatcher
190.12 Attak
190.13 Urbanskiworkshop

191.01 Julie Joliat
o: Schöningh & Wulffrat

191.02 Typosition
o: spatium magazine
191.03 Superlow
o: Oslo Collective
191.04 Amen
o: Formstelle
191.05 Krv Kurva
191.06 Rocholl Selected
     Designs
o: KearneyRocholl
191.07 Simian
191.08 june
191.09 Sunday-Vision
o: AGARI design
191.10 derek johnson
o: INDE design studio
/:   Ina Johnson
192.11 Raffaele Primitivo
192.13 Insect
o: Red Represents
192.15 Emmi Salonen
192.16 Designanorak / DSNRK

193.01 Raffaele Primitivo
193.02 A-Side Studio
193.03 Attak
193.04 Raffaele Primitivo
193.05 Mitch Paone
o: Almost Minimal
193.06 Neubau.
o: Neubau Laden
193.07 Ketchup Arts
193.08 viagrafik
o: Pyramid editions
193.09 viagrafik
193.10 viagrafik
o: pyramid editions
193.11 viagrafik
o: NPY editions
193.12 viagrafik
o: pyramid editions

194.01 Sito
o: Ichiban
194.02 Sito
194.03 SignalStrong
194.04 MvM / Maarten van
     Maanen
194.05 hijack graphics
194.06 Raffaele Primitivo
194.07 Emil Hartvig
194.08 Extraverage
     Productions
194.09 Plasticbag
o: United Situation
194.10 mateuniverse
o: pirat
194.11 Sat One

194.12 Mark Sloan
o: sloan
194.13 Sellout Industries
194.14 projekttriangle
o: RED Research Eingi-
     neering and Design
194.15 dzgnbio

195.01 Clrqa
o: Simpl3 Crew
195.02 PMKFA
195.03 Mode
o: Dalton Maag
195.04 Keep Left Studio
o: Keep Left Magazine
195.05 fireondesign /
     herborize
o: iblog, chubbz
195.06 2Advanced Studios
o: 2Advanced Studios
195.07 Out Of Order
o: Technation
195.08 NYK
195.09 Salon Vektoria
195.10 HandGun
195.11 the Legalizer
o: GoPingPong

196.01 Nuuro
o: n/a
196.02 Dimomedia Lab
o: Unbit.it
196.03 Miha Artnak
o: ZEK advance
196.04 Ash
/:   Victor Ash
196.05 Dimomedia Lab
o: Unbit
196.06 NYK
196.07 La Superagencia
o: Suspicious Design
     Group
196.08 Tabas
o: La société Modern
196.09 Mikkel Grafixico
     Westrup
o: Golden9
196.10 NYK
196.11 moxi
o: Fabian Blaser, od
196.12 Toko

197.01 Keep Left Studio
o: Refill Magazine
197.02 SignalStrong
197.03 Miha Artnak
o: ZEK advance
197.04 Keloide.net
o: Divididos

197.05 Lucias Westrup
o: Lucias 291
197.06 Furi Furi Company
197.07 Ketchup Arts
197.08 Keloide.net
197.09 Mule Industry
o: Neubau / Stefan Gandl
197.10 Mattisimo
197.11 Axel Peemöller
o: Kontainer
197.12 Keloide.net
o: morphotypo
197.13 Extraverage
       Productions
197.14 Extraverage
       Productions

198.01 NYK
198.02 Hayato Kamono
198.03 viagrafik
o: essentials
198.04 DigitalPlayground
       Studio
198.05 Extraverage
       Productions
198.06 Extraverage
       Productions
198.07 Labor für visuelles
       Wachstum™
o: Fruit Berlin
198.08 HKI - Hellohikimori
198.09 I&EYE
o: Artack
198.10 I&EYE
o: DKOR8
198.11 3volt Design
198.12 Microbot
198.13 Floor Wesseling Ix
       Opus Ada
o: upperclasz
198.14 jum
198.15 SignalStrong
o: None
198.16 Jan-Kristof Lipp
o: NewLocalShit
199.01 Faith
199.02 hijack graphics
199.03 La Superagencia
o: Suspicious Design
       Group
199.04 Flexn / Bank
o: Backjumps
199.05 Furi Furi Company
199.06 BEKO3
199.07 Takora
o: Bandai
/:   Kirakirajapan Project

199.08 hijack graphics
199.09 Microbot
199.10 Microbot
199.11 hijack graphics
199.12 SignalStrong
o: None
199.13 Caótica
199.14 Coutworks
o: New Collective
199.15 cubemen studio
o: avatag
199.16 cubemen studio

200.01 asmallpercent
200.02 Tender
o: Rhode Island School
       of Design
200.03 HKI - Hellohikimori
o: Overage4design
200.04 Kosta Lazarevski o:
       rushersdieyoung
200.05 Intercity
o: Karpinski Design
200.06 Jawa and Midwich
o: Jawa and Midwich
200.07 Yucca Studio
o: Junkflea
200.08 Keloide.net
200.09 Grandpeople
o: Dans For Voksne
200.10 Extraverage
       Productions
o: Logikwear
200.11 Jun Watanabe
o: Contrast inc
200.12 Neubau.
200.13 Raredrop
200.14 Maak
o: HandGraphicDesign™
200.15 Miha Artnak
o: ZEK advance
200.16 Studio Oscar

201.01 HKI - Hellohikimori
o: Overage4design
201.02 viagrafik
o: pyramid editions
201.03 Keloide.net
201.04 Station
201.05 Miha Artnak
o: ZEK advance
201.06 Designanorak / DSNRK
201.07 Extraverage
       Productions
201.08 Axel Peemöller
o: Kontainer
201.09 Resin[sistem] design
201.10 cisma
201.11 Escobas

201.12 Shivamat
201.13 Extraverage
       Productions
/:   www.logikwear.com

202.01 Furi Furi Company
202.02 FL@33
202.03 Erik Jarlsson
o: Syrup
202.04 Studio Oscar
o: Stussy
/:   Oscar Wilson
202.05 Lucias Westrup
o: Lucias

203.01 Team Manila
203.02 Emmi Salonen
203.03 cisma
203.04 Extraverage
       Productions

204.01 Mitch Paone
o: Dreamers Ink
       Aesthetics
204.02 Ketchup Arts
204.03 Kallegraphics
204.04 MH grafik
/:   Max Henschel
204.05 Yuu Imokawa
o: brownsuger
204.06 Attak
o: Corazon
204.07 Retron / Richard
       øiestad
o: Eurodata computer
       club
204.08 Attak
204.09 Resin[sistem] design
204.10 Lindedesign
o: Alive
204.11 Jawa and Midwich
o: Simple Shape
/:   Simon Dovar Simple
       Shape
204.12 Formgeber
o: Jotopia | Visual
       Noise
204.13 David Clavadetscher
o: design network
       switzerland
204.14 Dimomedia Lab
204.15 Ashi & office
       Greminger
204.16 44 flavours
/:   patrick fuchs

205.01 Shintaro Yarimizo
o: yamatodamashii
205.02 Shintaro Yarimizo

205.03 Shintaro Yarimizo
205.04 Shintaro Yarimizo
205.05 Fase
205.06 Shintaro Yarimizo
205.07 Amen
205.08 :phunk studio
205.09 FireGirl
o: Casa dos Noivos
205.10 resistro®
205.11 Positron
o: ROHTO
205.12 David Maloney
o: Brain Magnet
205.13 Tohyto
205.14 Matthias Gephart
o: Own Writing/Design
       Project
205.15 Laborator
o: Magnum design
205.16 zucker und pfeffer

206.01 e-Types A/S
o: OeO Design
       Consultancy
206.02 44 flavours
/:   Lutz Lindemann
206.03 Mattisimo
o: 65 Media
206.04 Attak
206.05 Jawa and Midwich
o: Beauty Links LLP
206.06 Accident Groteska!
206.07 The KDU
o: The KDU _ ALMS llc
206.08 Extraverage
       Productions
o: Ark Design
206.09 Georg Schatz
206.10 Borsellino & Co.
206.11 Chris Rubino
o: Badger & Partners Inc
206.12 Braveland Design
o: Carbon 14
206.13 Mwmcreative
o: Cass-Creative Design
       Studio
/:   Cassandra St Louis
206.14 Chris Rubino
206.15 Draplin
206.16 Simian
o: egz

207.01 Hyl Design
o: FormFollows
/:   c2006 Hyl Design
207.02 Chris Rubino
o: ige
207.03 Hyl Design
207.04 Hyl Design

207.05 jl-prozess
207.06 Pep Karsten
o: Alkaa
207.07 fatbob
207.08 Ketchup Arts
207.09 Coldwater Graphiix
o: Beach HousE corp.
207.10 Maniackers Design
o: Mami Kobayashi
207.11 june
o: thomson
207.12 june
o: thomson
207.13 2098
o: ralphheinsohn.com
207.14 Sesame Studio
o: Halfnine Media
207.15 Sesame Studio
207.16 Transittus

208.01 Fellow Designers
o: Hybrid
208.02 Salon Vektoria
o: Klub Kamikaze
208.03 Salon Vektoria
o: la famille
208.04 Salon Vektoria
o: la famille
208.05 44 flavours
o: SeSe
/:   Jackson Five
208.06 Attak
208.07 archetype : interactive
o: Hong Kong Design
       Community
208.08 SignalStrong
208.09 Mattisimo
o: Mattisimo, mmo
208.10 Attak
208.11 selanra grafikdesign
208.12 Typosition
o: spatium magazine
208.13 Chris Rubino
o: aol
/:   Deep Focus
208.14 La Superagencia
o: Suspicious Design
       Group
208.15 toxi
o: toxi.co.uk
208.16 Mattisimo
o: Forma Industrial
       Design Studio

209.01 Nando Costa
o: Lard & Joy
209.02 :g / studio-gpop
o: Gpop

209.03 Axel Peemöller
o: Kontainer
209.04 NYK
209.05 2Advanced Studios
o: 2Advanced.Net Hosting
209.06 Tnop™ & ®bePOS|+|VE
o: CHM®systems, Bangkok
209.07 Furi Furi Company
/:   (C)Furi Furi Company
      & Chinjyu expedition
      team
209.08 2Advanced Studios
209.09 Superfamous
o: Deluxe
209.10 Shintaro Yarimizo
209.11 decoylab
209.12 Zetuei Fonts
o: teito re-construction
      plan
/:   hitoyo karino
209.13 Tohyto
209.14 Tohyto
209.15 Engine
209.16 Maak
o: Oak Creative

210.01 Raphazen
o: die gestalten
210.02 dextro.org
o: turux.org
210.03 Shintaro Yarimizo
210.04 Shintaro Yarimizo
210.05 Polygraph
210.06 Cybu Richli
210.07 Lucias Westrup
210.08 cisma
o: Resfest
211.01 eP_ design in progress
211.02 Ketchup Arts
211.03 dzgnbio
211.04 Blu Design
211.05 Jun Xu
211.06 Mwmcreative
/:   Maria da Gandra
211.07 Muller
211.08 Plasticbag
211.09 No-Domain
211.10 decoylab
211.11 Chris Hutchinson
211.12 Danny Franzreb
o: Tanbot

212.01 Tohyto
o: Latino
212.02 Nando Costa
212.03 Nuuro

213.01 red design
213.02 red design

213.03 red design
213.04 BEKO3
o: avila delux

218.01 blackjune
o: Radio Skateboards
219.01 viagrafik
o: Triplus clothing
219.02 blackjune
o: Radio Skateboards
219.03 A-Side Studio
o: FSC
219.04 blackjune
o: Converse

220.01 Theres Steiner
o: sog. dinge und
      kleider

221.01 News
o: Bbuild
221.02 La Mirona

222.01 blackjune
o: Premium Exhibitions
222.02 Kjetil Vatne
o: Grand lovestory
222.03 Extraverage
      Productions
o: Mayo Chix
222.04 Abraka Design
o: la fabrique
222.05 viagrafik
o: sykum footwear
222.06 viagrafik
o: ETF
222.07 flat
o: Tsuru
222.08 The Skull Dezain
o: R8Spide from
      Routeburn
222.09 blackjune
o: Radio Skateboards
222.10 GWG
o: Air To Ground A-
      seven(Descente)
222.11 Visual Mind Rockets
o: Ruffer
222.12 Borsellino & Co.
o: Vektoriat

223.01 Yuu Imokawa
o: Collcooration
223.02 Amore Hirosake
o: Lulu
223.03 asmallpercent
o: nest - modern baby
      products

223.04 Vrontikis Design
      Office
o: Overbreak, Los
      Angeles, USA
223.05 Axel Domke
o: Christiane Prien
223.06 Futro
o: Fabrika
223.07 Zion Graphics
o: Peak Performance
223.08 KesselsKramer
o: 55DSL
223.09 blackjune
o: Radio Skateboards
223.10 Iván Solbes
o: Casiopea
223.11 artless Inc
o: Stylife
223.12 Inksurge

224.01 blackjune
o: Radio Skateboards
224.02 Team Manila
224.03 Jeremyville
o: Adio Footwear
224.04 Studio Oscar
o: Levi's
224.05 FL@33
o: toi com moi, Paris
224.06 Tsai-Fi
224.07 Raffaele Primitivo
224.08 Studio Oscar
o: Levi's
224.09 Fase
o: CHEMIRE
224.10 Neeser & Müller
o: Tarzan
224.11 Miki Amano
o: Scottex
/:   Bradley Flickstein

225.01 chemicalbox
o: chemicalbox shirt
225.02 tstout inc.
o: Concepts
225.03 Christian Rothenhagen
o: record
225.04 Raffaele Primitivo
o: Flat Store
225.05 The Skull Dezain
o: R8Spide from
      Routeburn
225.06 backyard 10
o: Levi's
225.07 Sellout Industries
o: play
225.08 Tabas
o: Cam a yeux

225.09 underson
o: miranda co.
/:   cozy corporation
225.10 Grotesk
/:   Upper Playground
225.11 Tohyto
o: Coachella

226.01 bleed
o: Arkaden
226.02 Die Seiner
o: SEIN
226.03 Yorgo Tloupas
o: 33-1 R-lax fashion
      store
226.04 Intercity
o: Millc
226.05 Canefantasma Studio
o: Aloe&Wolf
226.06 dopepope
o: Ca$hmere
226.07 Simon & Goetz
o: Casué
226.08 june
o: juundso
226.09 Parra
o: Ben G skatestore
226.10 projekttriangle
o: Full Artist Control
226.11 Henrik Vibskov
226.12 Raffaele Primitivo
o: Hvana Brand
226.13 DTM_INC
o: Frogbite
226.14 viagrafik
o: Red Moose Clothing
226.15 Yo Freeman
o: CTRL Clothing

227.01 Jun Watanabe
o: CONTRAST inc
227.02 GWG
o: LOTUSPOND
227.03 Hammarnäs
o: Björn Borg
227.04 Magma
o: Kult Industries
227.05 Jason Kochis
o: Fashion Victim
227.06 Calliope Studios
227.07 Furi Furi Company
o: Girls Power Manifesto
227.08 DED Associates
o: Graniph
227.09 austrianillustra-
      tion.com
o: Ponytale
/:   Fabienne Feltus

228.01 Nish
o: Infamous
228.02 K-Berg Projects
/:   Ultranajs
/:   D.Kjellberg
228.03 cabina
o: Juana de Arco
228.04 No-Domain
o: Intro
228.05 decoylab
o: Early Jewelry
228.06 austrianillustra-
      tion.com
o: Ponytale
/:   Fabienne Feltus
228.07 HandGun
o: Alone
228.08 Lloyd & Associates
o: Strenesse
228.09 Yuu Imokawa
228.10 Upnorth
o: 2k by gingham
228.11 Christian Rothenhagen
/:   berlinNATIVE
228.12 Carsten Raffel
o: station zwei - bfd

229.01 Graeme McMillan
o: adidas Y-3
/:   adidas
229.02 urbn;
o: Earlybirds-Shop
/:   Jörn Alraun
229.03 Christian Rothenhagen
o: deerBLN
229.04 Matthias Ernstberger
o: AKDMKS Ladies
/:   Kemistre 8 LLC
229.05 Carsten Raffel
o: station zwei - bfd

230.01 Keep Left Studio
o: 2k Tshirts
230.02 Hydro74
o: Vans
230.03 Jules
o: Furesshu Clothing
230.04 Masa
230.05 123klan
o: Stussy
230.06 Jason Kochis
o: Sony Signatures
/:   Dirtbag Clothing Inc.
230.07 Polygraph
o: One-Eyed Willy
230.08 AmorfoDesignlab™
o: Pastilla Digital™

230.09 Tsuyoshi Hirooka
o: Beams T

231.01 Extraverage Productions
o: fortrock clo-thing
231.02 zookeeper
o: Spootnick
231.03 Positron
o: Sweep Zweep
231.04 zookeeper
o: Spootnick
231.04 Keep Left Studio
o: O'Neill Surf
231.06 Masa
231.07 Masa
231.08 zookeeper
o: Spootnick
231.09 Formgeber
o: Sabotage
231.10 Ninjacruise
o: Threadless
231.11 Tokidoki
231.12 The Skull Dezain
o: R8Spide from Routeburn

232.01 Tsuyoshi Hirooka
o: 2K
232.02 Tsuyoshi Hirooka
o: Unnon
232.03 The Skull Dezain
o: Routeburn
232.04 Formgeber
o: Suspect
232.05 substrat
o: Florinda Schnitzel
232.06 raum mannheim
o: kaufhalle
232.07 Plastic Kid
o: Pestol
232.08 austrianillustra-
       tion.com
o: Fabienne Feltus

233.01 Masa
233.02 human empire
o: human empire shop
233.03 tstout inc.
o: QWST Clothing
233.04 Meomi
o: Trendy Tadpole
233.05 zookeeper
o: Spootnick
233.06 blackjune
o: Radio Skateboards
233.07 zookeeper
o: Spootnick
233.08 Furi Furi Company
o: Girls Power Manifesto

234.01 Grotesk
o: uniqlo / staple
234.02 Jon Burgerman
o: Love Rabby / Crown
       Creative
234.03 Jeremyville
234.04 jum
o: superyou
234.05 jewboy Corporation™
o: Gusta
234.06 Maniackers Design
o: Inner life corp.
234.07 Calliope Studios
o: Yoya Inc.
234.08 derek johnson
o: special clothing
/:   derek johnson
234.09 human empire
o: human empire shop
234.10 Jon Burgerman
o: Love Rabby / Crown
       Creative
234.11 Flying Förtress
o: Rockaway Bear
234.12 Flying Förtress
o: Stüssy Inc.
234.13 Gianni Rossi
o: Wp lavori in corso
234.14 Naho Ogawa
o: Anna Sui
234.15 Fiftyeight3d
o: Burg&Schild
234.16 automatic
o: Burton Snowboards

235.01 Formgeber
o: Jotopia | Urban Wear
235.02 DesignChapel
235.03 automatic
o: Analog
235.04 Kingsize
o: 5th Avenue Shoerepair
       / Resteröds

236.01 The Skull Dezain
o: Sacrifice from
       Routeburn
236.02 Sat One
o: Mogul
236.03 Sat One
o: Mogul
236.04 William Morrisey
o: Concealed.
236.05 A-Side Studio
o: FSC
236.06 Positron
o: Destroyder

236.07 underson
o: miranda co.
/:   cozy corporation
236.08 Sat One
236.09 Dimomedia Lab
o: BinbiSi

237.01 Amore Hirosuke
o: Comoesta Yaegashi
237.02 Syrup Helsinki
o: Le Shop Stockholm
237.03 the red is love
o: Isd
/:   Isd Napoli
237.04 Out Of Order
o: Supernatural
237.05 Lynn Hatzius
o: Kate Harwood
237.06 Grotesk
237.07 Polygraph
237.08 Furi Furi Company
o: Girls Power Manifesto
237.09 Fellow Designers
o: Lindex
237.10 the red is love
o: Baco moda
/:   Gaetano Giamundo
237.11 Grotesk
o: Spike Lee
/:   Spike Lee + Marc Ecko
237.12 Tsuyoshi Hirooka
o: Unnon

238.01 blackjune
o: Radio Skateboards
238.02 Jason Kochis
o: Fashion Victim
/:   copyright Fashion
       Victim, Inc.
238.03 Jason Kochis
o: Senor Tees
238.04 Insect Design
o: Infected T-shirts /
       London
238.05 Jason Kochis
o: Senor Tees
238.06 Jason Kochis
o: Senor Tees
238.07 Jason Kochis
o: Senor Tees
238.08 Ashi & office
       Greminger
o: Pavilion Hotel London
238.09 Miki Amano
238.10 Team Manila
238.11 dragon

239.01 Out Of Order
o: Supernatural

239.02 The Skull Dezain
o: R8Spide from
       Routeburn
239.03 Zion Graphics
o: J.Lindeberg
239.04 Masa
239.05 Team Manila
239.06 Amore Hirosuke
o: blue dress

240.01 Masa
240.02 Christian Rothenhagen
o: r. castelli art
       projects
240.03 Keren Richter
o: blood is the new
       black
240.04 Keren Richter
o: blood is the new
       black
240.05 NeoDG
o: rulo fightwear
/:   neodg
240.06 seacreative
o: zoojunkie
240.07 Lunatiq
o: Lunatiq
240.08 The Skull Dezain
o: R8Spide from
       Routeburn
240.09 Hula Hula
o: Cartoon Network
/:   Hula+Hula / CN
240.10 Magma
o: Starshot
/:   Denise Kaufmann
240.11 Akiza
240.12 KesselsKramer
o: Diesel
/:   Diesel & KesselsK-
       ramer

241.01 dzgnbio
o: spootnick.com
241.02 Akiza
241.03 Akiza

242.01 bleed
o: djuice
242.02 Keep Left Studio
o: Nylon Sound Studios
242.03 Deanne Cheuk
o: Tokion Magazine
242.04 Faith
o: Lush Magazine

243.01 red design
243.02 Mikko Rantanen
o: Lailatay

243.03 Deanne Cheuk
o: Tokion Magazine
243.04 Stockbridge Interna-
       tional
o: Hang Ten
243.05 Studio Output
o: Walé Adeyemi
243.06 Studio 3
o: Bik Bok
243.08 Jun Watanabe
o: Devilock
243.17 The Skull Dezain
o: Vicious Flavor from
       bishop.inc

244.01 ten_do_ten
o: parco
244.02 Extraverage
       Productions
o: Logikwear
244.03 chemicalbox
o: chemicalbox shirt
244.04 Tohyto
o: Intro Store BCN
244.05 The Skull Dezain
o: Vicious Flavor from
       bishop.inc
244.06 ten_do_ten
o: little more

245.01 cabina
o: Juana de Arco
245.02 Zion Graphics
o: Peak Performance
245.03 struggle inc.
o: Nikao Youth Projects
245.04 Studio 3
o: Bik Bok
245.05 Studio 3
o: Bik Bok
245.06 substrat
o: Florinda Schnitzel
245.07 Razauno
o: Ecko Unlimited
245.08 A-Side Studio
o: FSC

246.01 derfaber
246.02 Team Manila
o: Re/public
246.03 Faith
o: Lush Magazine
246.04 The KDU
o: The KDU + SVSV
246.05 Furi Furi Company
o: GPM
246.06 Furi Furi Company
o: GPM

247.01 derfaber
247.02 Team Manila
o: Tru Youth
/:   Rosario Herera
247.03 Catalina Estrada
       Uribe
o: Juliana Gonzales
247.04 Jason Kochis
o: Project E Clothing
247.05 usugrow
o: slap
247.06 Nohemi Dicuru
o: Le boudoir store
247.07 blackjune
o: Radio Skateboards
247.08 Studio Output
o: Acorn Conceptual
       Textiles

248.01 Lloyd & Associates
o: Apparel Label
       Capitalism™

249.01 Magma
o: Starshot

250.01 HandGun
o: Alone
250.02 K-Berg Projects
o: Ultranajs
/:   D.Kjellberg
250.03 Supershapes
o: Rizzo
250.04 Furi Furi Company
o: GPM
250.05 Yuu Imokawa
o: Collaboration
250.06 Maak
250.07 Furi Furi Company
o: GPM
250.08 Furi Furi Company
o: GPM
250.09 Sunday-Vision
o: John Lawrence Sullivan

251.01 The Skull Dezain
o: R8Spide from
       Routeburn
251.02 Stockbridge Interna-
       tional
o: Law&Order
251.03 TGB design
o: UCS
251.04 Yuu Imokawa
o: Collaboration
251.05 Palle Bruun Rasmussen
o: Revolution and
       Redrabbit WS Engros
       Aps

251.06 Palle Bruun Rasmussen
o: Revolution and
       Redrabbit WS Engros
251.07 Extraverage
       Productions
o: fortrock clo-thing
251.08 AmorfoDesignlab™
o: Deftones™
/:   BIchikori™
251.09 Hydro74
o: Split

252.01 jum
252.02 Fiftyeight3d
o: burg&schild
252.03 I-Manifest
252.04 Lloyd & Associates
o: Apparel Label
       Capitalism™
252.05 Binatural
o: Anni Futuri
252.06 Nohemi Dicuru
o: Neutroni clothing
252.07 Sarah Grimaldi
o: bambistar™
252.08 Extraverage Productions
o: fortrock clo-thing
252.09 The Skull Dezain
o: Vicious Flavor from
       bishop.inc
252.10 Tsuyoshi Hirooka
o: Unnon
252.11 ehquestionmark
o: adidas
252.12 substrat
o: Florinda Schnitzel
252.13 Zion Graphics
o: Peak Performance
252.14 dzgnbio
o: spootnick.com
252.15 A-Side Studio
o: FSC
252.16 Resin[sistem] design
o: 2 For the Show

253.01 Flexn / Bank
o: In Juli
253.02 AmorfoDesignlab™
o: Fresco Gear™
253.03 AmorfoDesignlab™
o: Deftones™
/:   Bichikori™
253.04 Lucias Westrup
o: Lion Kings With
       Golden Wings
/:   LKWGW
253.05 Koadzn
o: Level Art
/:   Koa

253.06 Hydro74
o: SVRN
253.07 Power Graphixx
o: BQE
253.08 backyard 10
o: UsualSuspect
253.09 NeoDG
o: Rulo Fightwear
/:   neodg

254.01 Julie Joliat
o: Christien Meindertsma
254.02 Stockbridge Interna-
       tional
o: Law&Order
254.03 Inocuodesign
o: EAST ERIK
254.04 Tohyto
o: Coachella

255.01 Keep Left Studio
o: O'Neill Surf
255.02 Hydro74
o: SVRN
255.03 Keep Left Studio
o: O'Neill Surf
255.04 Keep Left Studio
o: O'Neill Surf

256.01 Keep Left Studio
o: ShadyKids.com
256.02 Henrik Vibskov
256.03 Niels Shoe Meulman
o: Umbro girls
256.04 Michael Genovese
o: STUSSY

257.01 Ninjacruise
o: Android8
/:   Glen Lieberman

258.01 Masa
258.02 Lousy Livincompany
o: Cleptomanicx
258.03 Niels Shoe Meulman
o: Unruly
256.04 Keep Left Studio
o: ShadyKids.com
256.05 Keep Left Studio
256.06 Keep Left Studio
258.07 The Skull Dezain
o: Hurley International
258.08 WGD
o: Bik Bok
258.09 Faith
o: Lush Magazine

259.01 WGD
o: Bik Bok

259.02 Hydro74
o: Exo Skate Shop
259.03 Nohemi Dicuru
o: Simulacro E fashion
       designers
259.04 Mitch Paone
o: Old Navy
/:   Logan, Alexei Tylevich
259.06 Hydro74
o: Burton Snowboards

260.01 Koadzn
o: Science Skateboards
260.02 Out Of Order
o: Supernatural
260.03 inkgraphix
o: Skank Clothing
/:   Mattias Lundin
260.04 A-Side Studio
o: Stilo Clothing
260.05 Keep Left Studio
o: Soul Clothing
260.06 blackjune
o: Radio Skateboards
260.07 Parra
o: Ben G skatestore
260.08 Razauno
o: Chevere
260.09 Salon Vektoria

261.01 Keep Left Studio
o: O'Neill Surf
261.02 Koadzn
o: Mood
261.03 backyard 10
o: UsualSuspect
261.04 Axel Peemöller
o: DEWAR
261.05 JB CLASSICS
261.06 123klan
261.07 The Skull Dezain
o: Games From Senri
       Boeki Corporation
261.08 Extraverage Productions
261.09 Masa
o: The LIFT
261.10 Furi Furi Company
o: GPM
261.11 Typeholics.
o: Illmatic/Typeholics
261.12 123klan
o: Stussy

262.01 Koadzn
o: Triiad
262.02 bandage
o: BlackBoxMagazine

262.03 Raphazen
262.04 Studio Oscar
262.05 The Skull Dezain
o: Sacrifice from Routeburn
262.06 310k
o: hemp hoodlamb

263.01 Magma
o: Starshot
263.02 Adhemas
o: FoxyLady
263.03 Dimomedia Lab
o: NatiMatti
263.04 Keep Left Studio
o: General Pants Group
263.05 Studio Oscar
o: Levi's
263.06 ZIP Design
o: Harvey Nichols
       Department Store
263.07 Raffaele Primitivo
263.08 Raffaele Primitivo
263.09 Matthias Gephart
o: HipHop/Sportswear
       Company Kickz
263.10 Formgeber
o: Steffi

264.01 Carlos Bêla
o: Maruxia handcraft
264.02 Stockbridge
       International
o: Woolrich
264.03 FL@33
o: Stereohype.com
264.04 Christian Walden
o: Riot Ape Foundation
264.05 Sophie Toporkoff
o: PSP Fashion / colette
264.06 Retron
o: Caesars Casual Wardrobe
264.07 Binatural
o: Ano 21
264.08 Lousy Livincompany
264.09 Labor für visuelles
       Wachstum™
o: gigi.lin Berlin
264.10 Zetuei Fonts
o: azb
264.11 newoslo
o: Swims A/S
264.12 viagrafik
o: women's secret

265.01 Oc/Om/Oy/Ok
o: Royal Gráfico
265.02 Caótica
o: Sandpiper

265.03 evaq studio
o: Mioko Miochizuko /
      Senritsu
265.04 Marc Atlan
o: Comme des Garçons
      Parfums

266.01 milchhof : atelier
o: Fuzzi
266.02 The Skull Dezain
o: Vicious Flavor from
      bishop.inc
266.03 ten_do_ten
o: chico
266.04 Tsuyoshi Hirooka
266.05 Niels Shoe Meulman
      MAG Boots
266.06 Studio Output
o: Walé Adeyemi
266.07 I-Manifest
266.08 Vår
o: Sunday Sun

267.01 Keep Left Studio
o: O'Neill Surf
267.02 Keep Left Studio
o: Nike USA
267.03 Keep Left Studio
o: O'Neill Surf
267.04 evaq studio
267.05 The KDU
o: The KDU + SVSV
267.06 Emil Kozak
o: Norris

268.01 Zetuei Fonts
o: azb
268.02 Carsten Raffel
268.03 The Skull Dezain
o: Sacrifice from
      Routeburn
268.04 Oc/Om/Oy/Ok
o: LDN
268.05 Jun Watanabe
o: Flavor
268.06 Lunatiq

269.01 Keep Left Studio
o: Nike USA
269.02 Keep Left Studio
o: Soul Clothing
269.03 Keep Left Studio
o: Nike USA
269.04 Jun Watanabe
o: Contrast
269.05 Coldwater Graphiix
o: ENGINE
269.06 viagrafik
o: Glizmo Streetwear

269.07 Neubau.
o: Atelier Mohr Mannequins
269.08 Hydro74
o: Burton Snowboards
269.09 The Skull Dezain
o: R8Spide from Routeburn
269.10 Tsuyoshi Hirooka
o: Unnon
269.11 Jun Watanabe
o: Devilock
269.12 Hydro74
o: Westbeach Apparel
269.13 Atelier télescopique
o: Wassingue
269.14 Stockbridge Interna-
      tional
o: Law&Order
269.15 The Skull Dezain
o: R8Spide from Routeburn
269.16 Jun Watanabe
o: Devilock

270.01 Parra
o: Rockwell Clothing
270.02 cabina
o: Juana de Arco
270.03 44 flavours
/:   patrick fuchs
270.04 Raffaele Primitivo
270.05 Raffaele Primitivo
270.06 44 flavours
o: dancerock157
/:   Lutz Lindemann
270.07 A-Side Studio
270.08 fatbob
o: huffer
270.09 fatbob
o: huffer

271.01 No-Domain
o: Intro
271.02 Paco Aguayo
o: Galeria del Calzado
271.03 The Skull Dezain
o: Sacrifice from Routeburn
271.04 Tsuyoshi Hirooka
o: Beams T
271.05 Kallegraphics
o: Selena
271.06 Axel Peemöller
o: Dewar
271.07 Karen Jane
o: ultrafinebrand.com
271.08 Karen Jane
o: ultrafinebrand.com
271.09 blackjune
o: Radio Skateboards
271.10 Clrqa
o: Hidrophoniq.com

271.11 viagrafik
o: airbag craftworks
271.12 Emil Kozak
o: Roots
271.13 :phunk studio
o: 1)Holy Grail
      2)White Room
      3)Staple
271.14 Attak
o: Corazon
271.15 automatic
o: Analog
271.16 cisma
o: Zoomp

272.01 Hammarnäs
o: D&G/Dolce & Gabbana
272.02 viagrafik
o: Kauzwear
272.03 44 flavours
o: 24-7unique
/:   Julio Rölle
272.04 backyard 10
o: Levi's
272.05 The Skull Dezain
o: Vicious Flavor from
      bishop.inc
272.06 Axel Peemöller
o: Dewar
272.07 DTM_INC
272.08 Raffaele Primitivo
272.09 Flying Förtress
o: Stüssy Inc.

273.01 PMKFA
o: Wood Wood
273.02 Tsuyoshi Hirooka
o: Beams T
273.03 Power Graphixx
o: Refer

274.01 bandage
o: Döner Magazine
274.02 Inocuodesign
o: Belio Magazine
274.03 Büro Otto Sauhaus
o: hamansutra

275.01 Niels Shoe Meulman
o: Hype Type
275.02 blackjune
o: Converse
275.03 Zion Graphics
o: J.Lindeberg
275.04 Raffaele Primitivo
275.05 Vår
o: Sunday Sun
275.06 struggle inc.
o: 2K

275.07 Axel Peemöller
275.08 A-Side Studio
o: FSC
275.09 :q / studio-qpop
o: OkiDoki
275.10 Deanne Cheuk
o: Beams T
/:   Gas
276.01 Karen Jane
o: ultrafinebrand.com
276.02 Hydro74
o: Burton Snowboards
276.03 Laborator
o: Monidee
276.04 usugrow
o: slap
276.05 Marc Atlan
o: 2K T-Shirts
276.06 blackjune
o: Radio Skateboards
276.07 Formikula
o: Freeman T. Porter
276.08 Raffaele Primitivo
276.09 Pandarosa
276.10 Designbolaget
o: B.Young
/:   Claus Due
276.11 Thomas Nolfi
o: missya underwear

277.01 stylodesign
o: Lulu & Red
277.02 re-public
o: Kopenhagen Fur
277.03 Hydro74
o: Split
277.04 Carsten Raffel
277.05 AmorfoDesignlab™
o: BIchikori™
/:   -1:0:1™
277.06 Codeluxe
o: siebenschoen
277.07 Semisans
o: Kip Farmer Design
277.08 Studio Dumbar
o: Marlies Dekkers
277.09 Simon & Goetz
o: René Lezard
277.10 sopp collective
o: Bianca Spender
277.11 MH grafik
o: Cream S.A
277.12 Büro Destruct
o: Luzi de Beaufort

278.01 Lloyd & Associates
o: Apparel Label
      Capitalism
/:   Kimberly Lloyd

278.02 blackjune
o: Radio Skateboards
278.03-04 Zion Graphics
o: Peak Performance
278.05 Laborator
o: Monidee
278.06-08 Zion Graphics
o: Peak Performance
278.09 344 Design, LLC
o: iwasateenage.com
278.10 Semitransparent
      Design
o: Laug(h) tab Floor
278.11 Yuu Imokawa
o: Collaboration
278.12 Neeser & Müller
o: Tarzan

279.01 Stolen Inc.
o: StolenShirts
279.02 Koadzn
o: Owl Movement
279.03 Theres Steiner
o: sog. dinge und kleider
279.04 Salon Vektoria
o: Rodriguez&Rodriguez
279.05 Flavio Bagioli
o: Magdalena Perez
279.06 Tsuyoshi Hirooka
o: Beams T
279.07 viagrafik
o: women's secret
279.08 Formgeber
o: sabotage
279.09 Formgeber
o: Sabotage
279.10 The Skull Dezain
o: Sacrifice from
      Routeburn

280.01 Resin[sistem] design
o: Angela Winterbottom
      Jewellery
280.02 Ketchup Arts
280.03 3 deluxe
o: Rockamora
280.04 Resin[sistem] design
280.05 Tsuyoshi Hirooka
280.06 Koadzn
o: Mood
280.07 Polygraph
o: Dune
280.08 The Skull Dezain
o: R8Spide from Routeburn
280.09 Extraverage
      Productions
o: fortrock clo-thing
280.10 Zion Graphics
o: Peak Performance

280.11 Yorgo Tloupas
o: AndA
280.12 strange//attraktor:
o: Black Market Clothing
280.13 Studio Output
o: Montane
280.14 Zion Graphics
o: Peak Performance
280.15 Extraverage
       Productions
o: The Lab
280.16 Atomic Attack
o: Ming Ming

281.01 Tohyto
o: Intro Store BCN
281.02 Mattisimo
o: 25 Temple Clothing
281.03 310k
o: hemp hoodlamb
281.04 backyard 10
o: UsualSuspect
281.05 Microbot
o: Rebelkid
281.06 310k
o: razk
281.07 The Skull Dezain
o: Vicious Flavor from
       bishop.inc
281.08 Form
o: UniForm
/:   UniForm
281.09 Fase
o: Lindo Killer
281.10 Tsuyoshi Hirooka
o: Beams T
281.11 :g / studio-gpop
o: Designer Clobber
281.12 Balsi Grafik
o: wolfsmilch
281.13 sunrise studios
o: C-Arrow Magazines
281.14 Tsuyoshi Hirooka
o: Unnon

282.01 44 flavours
o: 24-7unique
/:   Julio Rölle
282.02 Christian Albriktsen
o: Village Apparel
282.03 Theres Steiner
o: sog. dinge und
       kleider
282.04 DigitalPlayground
       Studio
282.05 struggle inc.
o: 2K
282.06 Tsuyoshi Hirooka
o: Unnon

282.07 Masa
282.08 Tsuyoshi Hirooka
o: Beams T
282.09 Kosta Lazarevski
o: flexy
282.10 Keren Richter
o: blood is the new
       black
282.11 YellowToothpick
o: Crowded Teeth
282.12 Henrik Vibskov
282.14 Marc Atlan
o: Comme des Garçons
       Parfums

283.01 Henrik Vibskov
283.02 Oc/Om/Oy/Ok
283.03 Henrik Vibskov
283.04 Henrik Vibskov
283.05 the red is love
o: Opengate
/:   Pasquale Pagano
283.06 Power Graphixx
o: Tab

284.01 The Skull Dezain
o: R8Spide from
       Routeburn
284.02 The Skull Dezain
o: Vicious Flavor from
       bishop.inc
284.03 Fluid Creativity
o: Brand Neusense
284.04 Tsuyoshi Hirooka
o: Unnon
284.05 Gastón Caba
o: Muy Mono
284.06 Tokidoki LLC
284.07 Ottograph
o: drippie clothing
284.08 Ohio Girl Design
o: The Quiet Life
284.09 Attak
o: Corazon

285.01 Magma
o: Starshot
285.02 Mattisimo
o: Savvy Samurai
285.03 Lousy Livincompany
285.04 Tsuyoshi Kusano
       Design
o: Beams
285.05 The Skull Dezain
o: R8Spide from
       Routeburn
285.06 Laborator
o: Monidee

285.07 Henrik Vibskov
285.08 viagrafik
o: kauzwear
285.09 Keren Richter
o: holy terror

286.01 Henrik Vibskov
286.02 Emmi Salonen
o: Candy & Gertrud
286.03 Lousy Livincompany
286.04 Tsuyoshi Hirooka
o: Unnon
286.05 Keep Left Studio
o: 2k Tshirts

287.01 Petra Börner
o: Louis Vuitton
       (Accessories)
/:   LVH

292.01 Rocholl Selected
       Designs
o: The Europe Group
/:   CTVN
292.02 Salon Vektoria
292.04 Tsuyoshi Kusano
       Design
o: NAMCO BANDAI Holdings
       Inc.
293.05 weissraum.de(sign)
o: Flare Film
293.07 Rocholl Selected
       Designs
o: Area Magazine
293.13 weissraum.de(sign)
o: Überland
       Internetagentur

294.01 stylodesign
o: Double Knot
294.02 Adam Cruickshank
o: Mess+Noise
294.03 Power Graphixx
o: MTV JAPAN
294.04 310k
o: beamlab
/:   310k
294.05 Mutabor Design
o: Lenqit
294.06 Mutabor Design
294.07 Calliope Studios
o: Adobe
294.08 Mutabor Design
294.09 29 degres
o: Invaders (FR) CH
294.10 Futro
o: Interseek
294.11 Futro
o: Sekvenca

294.12 Mutabor Design
o: voyo.tv
294.13 Raredrop
o: MOVIDA Holdings
294.14 Bionic Systems
o: VIVA Fernsehen
294.15 Borsellino & Co.
o: Vektoriat Magazine
294.16 Borsellino & Co.
o: Emdash Magazine

295.01 David Maloney
o: Front Porch
       Productions
/:   Airhart & Co.
295.02 jum
o: CK
295.03 Ken Tanabe
o: Switch
/:   Switch 646 894 0809
       a@iheartswitch.com
295.04 Bionic Systems
o: Viva Fernsehen
295.05 Masa
o: Sony Entertainment
       Television Latin
       America
295.06 Anónimo Studio
o: ABC News
/:   Anónimo Studio
295.07 Power Graphixx
295.08 JDK
o: MTV
295.09 Ketchup Arts
o: thrasher japan
       magazine
295.10 Polygraph
o: Sony Computer Enter-
       tainment Inc.
295.11 Emil Hartvig
o: Rhinosaurus
295.12 JDK
o: XBOX 360
295.13 cabina
o: Sergio Resumil + El
       Oso Producciones
295.14 Kontrapunkt
o: nordisk film
295.15 Luca Marchettoni
295.16 Sanjai Bhana
o: Matthew Lima Web
       Media Design &
       Development

296.01 Emil Hartvig
o: Fotokompagniet
/:   Flemming Gottfredsen
296.02 Futro
o: MTV Adria

296.03 FilmGraphik
o: Hanno Olderdissen /
       ifs Köln
296.04 june
296.05 Gints Apsits
o: Apsits motion
       division
296.06 Gints Apsits
o: Apsits motion
       division
296.07 Masa
o: 3 Malandros Films
296.08 Magnetofonica
o: Carlos Malavé
296.09 FilmGraphik
o: dffb
296.10 Tsuyoshi Kusano
       Design
296.11 sunrise studios
o: Game Convention
       Worldwide
296.12 A-Side Studio
o: MTV Networks
/:   Buter Design

297.01 La Fusée
o: La Fusée Games
/:   Clément Perrotte
297.02 jl-prozess
o: mathilda
297.03 Matt Sewell
o: Candela Films
297.04 JDK
o: Cartoon Network
297.05 ultrafris
o: Eliace
297.06 Kosta Lazarevski
o: SK clan - Ravenshield
       (game) Macedonian-
       Holland clan
297.07 29 degres
o: The Pirate
297.08 Hula Hula
o: Instituto Mexicano de
       la Radio
297.09 Hula Hula
o: Taller Público
297.10 Hula Hula
o: Chinelo Entertainment
/:   Hula+Hula / Joaquin
       Fernández
297.11 David Ortiz Villegas
o: Hell's Cuisine
       Productions
297.12 Polygraph
o: Sony Computer
       Entertainment Inc.

297.13 Ketchup Arts
o: thrasher japan
      magazine
297.14 Ketchup Arts
o: ollie magazine
297.15 Ketchup Arts
o: Famitsu 64+
/:   enterbrain

298.01 Peter Anderson
o: David Barrie Talkback
      Channel Four
/:   David Barrie Talkback
      Channel Four
298.02 Fakir
o: Revista Complot

299.01 Rob Chiu
o: Beyond™
299.02 bleed
o: Fantefilm
299.03 Konstantinos
      Gargaletsos
o: Pulse
/:   Point Blank Inc
299.04 Upnorth
o: complex magazine
299.05 Colourmovie
o: Music Video
      Production
      Association
299.06 Studio Output
o: BBC Radio 1
299.07 Upnorth
o: complex magazine
299.08 Upnorth
o: complex magazine
299.09 Chris Rubino
o: Cinefile Anthology

300.01 HandGun
o: Nike

301.01 No-Domain
o: Heineken
/:   snowfort06
301.02 No-Domain
o: Heineken
301.04 Lukatarina
o: L#5
301.05 FilmGraphik
o: Clemens Pichler /
      hff muc
301.06 Hugh Morse
o: Warner Music Group
/:   Hugh Morse
301.07 No-Domain
o: Heineken

302.01 Fons Schiedon
o: MTV ASIA
/:   MTV ASIA
302.02 Sarah Grimaldi
o: greenmedia srl
302.03 Glauco Diogenes
o: MTV BRASIL
302.04 FilmGraphik
o: Freitstil Medien
302.05 Studio Output
o: BBC Radio 1
302.06 Engine
o: MTV UK
302.07 Bionyc Industries
o: NICKELODEON
302.08 Colletivo Design
o: Battle Lab Motion
      Studio
302.09 Engine
o: Redline Magazine

303.01 No-Domain
o: Levi's
303.02 Upnorth
o: complex magazine
303.03 Tohyto
o: Platanoverde
303.04 interspectacular
o: Stash DVD Magazine
303.05 Engine
o: Redline Magazine

304.01 Tsuyoshi Hirooka
o: MTV Japan
304.02 Fase
o: GZ
304.03 Fons Schiedon
o: MTV ASIA
304.04 Bionic Systems
o: VIVA Fernsehen
304.05 Masa
o: Sony Entertainment
      Television Latin
      America
304.06 NeoDG
o: Proyect for mtv
/:   neodg
304.07 Insect
o: Sony Playstation
/:   insect.co.uk
304.08 cisma
o: AXN
304.09 Upnorth
o: complex magazine
304.10 zinestesia
o: MTV Latin America

305.01 Tsuyoshi Hirooka
o: D.D.Wave

305.02 Kingsize
o: Kanal 5
305.03 JAKe
o: The Mighty Boosh
305.04 Dimomedia Lab
o: Pixel M
305.05 Bionyc Industries
o: Nickelodeon/Bermuda
      Shorts
305.06 A-Side Studio
o: MTV Networks
/:   Buster Design
305.07 Jun Watanabe
o: Levorg
305.08 cisma
o: AXN
305.09 Faith
o: EP Magazine
305.10 A-Side Studio
o: Buster Design
305.11 JAKe
o: The Mighty Boosh
305.12 A-Side Studio
o: MTV Networks
/:   Buster Design
305.13 No-Domain
305.14 Etienne Heinrich
o: viva media ag
305.15 Fons Schiedon
o: MTV ASIA
305.16 Kingsize
o: SVT

306.01 Polygraph
o: KP
306.02 Sito
o: Cabeza
306.03 A-Side Studio
o: Buster Design
306.04 A-Side Studio
o: Shopping Channel
/:   Buster Design
306.05 Rinzen
306.06 Alphabetical Order®
o: Johan Palmgren & Åsa
      Blanck
306.07 FilmGraphik
o: Philipp Ruch /
      Textwerft
306.08 Martin Kvamme
o: Sub Productions
306.09 FilmGraphik
o: Philipp Ruch /
      Textwerft
306.10 Peter Anderson
o: Eroica BBC 1
      Television
/:   BBC Broadcasting

306.11 loyalkaspar
o: Vh1
/:   Viacom
306.12 Syrup Helsinki
o: Aula Design
306.13 Hula Hula
o: Instituto Mexicano de
      la Radio

307.01 Engine
o: Synopsis Film
307.02 Emmi Salonen
o: Eatock
307.03 viagrafik
o: NPY editions
307.04 loyalkaspar
o: Rainbow Media
/:   Voom
307.05 Studio Output
o: Ambience Media
307.06 viagrafik
o: brett magazine
307.07 viagrafik
o: candyspace england
307.08 Emil Hartvig
o: Ultralyd
/:   Danmarks Radio
307.09 Timo Novotny
/:   Timo Novotny /
      inLoops Ulrich
      Gehmacher / Orbrock
      Masahito Hanzawa /
      power-graphixx
307.10 Kallegraphics
o: Hyperion
307.11 viagrafik
o: via motion
307.13 Supershapes
307.14 Adhemas
o: Sensorama
307.15 viagrafik
o: brain damage magazine

308.01 Carlos Bêla
o: MTV Brazil
308.02 Plastic Kid
o: in2media
308.03 Plastic Kid
o: In2media
308.04 Carsten Raffel
o: Virtual Fight Club
      (vfc)
308.05 viagrafik
o: brain damage magazine
308.06 zinestesia
o: MTV Latin America
308.07 Microbot
o: Lowend Deluxe

308.08 Power Graphixx
o: Timo Novotny
308.09 viagrafik
o: juice magazine
308.10 Dimaquina
o: Nako
308.11 viagrafik
o: toca me magazine
308.12 Studio Maverick
o: brights
308.13 Anónimo Studio
o: Puma TV
/:   Anónimo Studio
308.14 Polygraph
o: Atari Japan
308.15 Upnorth
o: complex magazine
308.16 Norwegian Ink
o: Lydia Laska

309.01 Raredrop
o: Shueisha
309.02 Laundry
o: G4 Networks, USA
309.03 Mitch Paone
o: Non-Static
309.04 Ketchup Arts
o: Music Machine
309.05 Maniackers Design
o: Sony Magazines
309.06 Maniackers Design
o: Ai-LAND
309.07 Ketchup Arts
o: enterbrain
309.08 Ketchup Arts
o: Famitsu 64+
/:   enterbrain
309.09 Raredrop
o: Dogma Publishing
309.10 Ketchup Arts
o: tattoo trival
309.11 Maniackers Design
o: Bic Funning
309.12 344 Design, LLC
o: Googly Films
309.13 Tsuyoshi Hirooka
o: enterbrain
309.14 Rinzen
o: DC Comics
309.15 Mikkel Grafixico
      Westrup
o: Mad Comix

310.01 Catalogtree
o: Close Encounters
      Ypenburg
/:   artoteek den haag
310.02 viagrafik
o: batterie mag

310.03 Creative Pride
o: Weargame
/:   ©Weargame
310.04 viagrafik
o: batterie mag
310.05 Upnorth
o: complex magazine
310.06 zinestesia
310.07 TGB design
o: MXTV
310.08 Gints Apsits
o: Fabrica Comics
        Department
310.09 Matthias Gephart
o: Nicki Hebestreit

311.01 Tsuyoshi Kusano
       Design
o: Shiseido Company,
        Limited
311.02 anna-OM-line.com
311.04 struggle inc.
o: Atari
311.05 Büro Destruct
o: Roland Müller, The
        Shanghai Story Book
311.06 blackjune
o: klm games
311.07 Tnop™ & ®bePOS|+|VE
o: G4 Video Game
        Television
311.08 Tsuyoshi Kusano
       Design
311.09 Faith
o: Canadian Broadcasting
        Corporation
311.10 asmallpercent
o: Technology Task Force
        - Gordon College
311.11 viagrafik
o: wag magazine
311.13 Maniackers Design
o: Clubking
311.12 Colourmovie
o: Warner Brothers
        Records/Reprise
/:   Alpha Visual Intel-
        ligence

312.01 Sarah Grimaldi
o: sony pictures home
        entertainment
/:   Sphe
312.02 Kosta Lazarevski
o: ZBRC fanzine
312.03 Carsten Raffel
o: Carlo Krüger

312.04 Chris Rubino
o: CourtTV
/:   Amalgamated
312.05 William Morrisey
o: 3FM Amsterdam Radio
312.06 viagrafik
o: blond magazine
312.07 the red is love
o: Peetza Magazine
312.08 Fase
o: gravedad zero
312.09 automatic
o: Sell Your Sins
312.10 Jürgen und ich
o: Feedmee Design/Viva
        Fernsehen
312.11 dainippon
o: M.Co.
312.12 2098
o: alien-action.com
312.13 Studio Maverick
o: Ambivalence
312.14 Chris Rubino
o: aol
/:   Deep Focus
312.15 Chico Jofilsan
/:   gp2
312.16 Katrin Acklin
o: time to print
        publishing

313.01 Fakir
313.02 zinestesia
o: Fuel Italy
/:   Fox Internationa
        Channels Italy
313.03 Adapter
o: Pics

314.01 Laundry
o: MTV networks, USA

315.01 Laundry
o: G4 Networks
/:   National Television

320.01 human empire
o: morr music

321.01 Sagmeister Inc.
o: Sister Ray Enterprises,
        Lou Reed

322.01 Bionic Systems
o: Open Source Festival,
        Germany
/:   Bionic Systems
322.02 Zeek&Destroy
o: Combination Records

322.03 blackjune
o: Hidden Industries
322.04 multifresh
o: outward sound

323.01 Engine
o: Effenaar / Red Zone
323.02 Engine
o: Subtitles Music
323.03 Dirk Rudolph
o: Motor Music
323.04 Jason Kochis
o: Daniel Miller
323.05 Pfadfinderei
o: Native Instruments
323.06 Labooo
323.07 Studio Output
o: Supreme Audio Pro
323.08 AmorfoDesignlab™
o: PastillaDigital™
/:   -1:0:1
323.09 johnjayart.com
323.10 DTM_INC
o: Homebrew Recordings
323.11 Zeek&Destroy
o: Andreas Schiko
323.12 Ketchup Arts
o: schneider

324.01 Pfadfinderei
o: Partysan Media &
        Verlag
324.02 Attak
o: Caspion
324.03 Pfadfinderei
o: Dalbin
324.04 Braveland Design
o: Aztec Records
324.05 onrushdesign / front
o: Ni Tónlistarskólinn -
        The New Music School
324.06 Attak
o: Liberty Valance
324.07 weissraum.de(sign)
o: Audiomatique
        Recordings
324.08 310k
o: djbroadcast
324.09 johnjayart.com
o: ebbergreene
324.10 jl-prozess
o: dj miss shapes
324.11 Borsellino & Co.
o: FFM Dance Dept.
324.12 Axel Domke
o: Diynamic Music HH
325.01 Niels Shoe Meulman
o: Bitter Zoet

325.02 Gastón Caba
o: Flavia & the Motonets
325.03 Dirk Rudolph
325.04 Blindresearch
o: Die Gestalten
        Designstudio/Naidoo
        Herberger Produktion
325.05 re-public
o: Danish Jazz
        Federation
325.06 Ashi & office
        Greminger
o: Hifi Usagi

326.01 Pfadfinderei
o: MDR Sputnik
326.02 struggle inc.
o: Sonotheque
326.03 Attak
o: Jazzwerkplaats Den
        Bosch
326.04 Ottograph
o: eufprods / jazzmeterors
326.05 Ketchup Arts
o: Music Machine
326.06 Kosta Lazarevski
o: Sure Shotz Entertain-
        ment
326.07 Ottograph
o: club hopping radio
326.08 Keren Richter
o: hartley goldstein
326.09 Emmi Salonen
326.10 Die Seiner
o: DJ Razor Cut
326.11 ZIP Design
o: Shyboy Productions
326.12 Designbolaget
o: Rar Lyd
/:   Claus Due
326.13 Plastic Kid
o: Cassette Jam Records
326.14 Jonas Vögeli
o: Holzpop Records
326.15 struggle inc.
o: Sonotheque
326.16 Instant

327.01 112 Ocean Drive
o: Monza
327.02 Tado
o: Holiphonic Records
327.03 Jussi Jääskeläinen
o: Senator Records
327.04 Mattisimo
o: Sandwich Records
327.05 frans carlquist
o: Flora & Fauna Records

327.06 Annabelle Mehraein
o: Homing Sound
        production, CI-Design
        (not realized)
327.07 National Forest
o: Ubiquity Records
327.08 jum
o: Radio Infiniverse
327.09 Out Of Order
o: Asucar Records
327.10 DTM_INC
327.11 Luca Marchettoni
o: Muzzle
327.12 Kosta Lazarevski
o: Nema Labavo Records
327.13 Visual Mind Rockets
o: PP Sales Forces
327.14 Georg Schatz
o: homing,
        musicproduction
327.15 Akira Sasaki
o: weather
327.16 Jawa and Midwich
o: Buttercuts Records
/:   Andy Oury Buttercuts
        Records

328.01 Michele Angelo
o: Super Elastic Bubble
        Plastic
328.02 Kingsize
o: Autohorse
328.03 Laurent Fétis
o: Miao! (Music
        Consultant Company)
328.04 artless Inc
o: Soundgraphics Inc
/:   Tadashi Ura
328.05 raum mannheim
o: wildnis
328.06 backyard 10
o: Universal Music
328.07 Floor Wesseling Ix
       Opus Ada
o: dub pirates
328.08 jl-prozess
o: dj brigitte
328.09 space3
o: Effenaar
328.10 Cabine
o: Stereo Total/Disko B
328.11 clandrei
o: Danger League
328.12 Semisans
o: First Flight Record
        Label
328.13 backyard 10
o: Music Express
        Magazine

328.14 Ottograph
o: spicy goat
328.15 Woo
o: Luger/Mondo,
       Stockholm

329.01 inkgraphix
o: Perola Productions
/:   Mattias Lundin
329.02 Studio Oscar
o: Base Planning Tokyo
329.03 Povilas Utovka
o: Lama rec.
329.04 Maya Hayuk
o: Dearly Beloved
       Records
329.05 desres design group
o: guilty76
329.06 radargraphics
o: Earforce records
329.07 Ninjacruise
o: nest
329.08 Studio Output
o: Mantis Recordings
329.09 boris dworschak
o: At Home Records
329.10 Michele Angelo
o: dj mouse up / mouse
       down

330.01 Labooo
330.02 Labooo
330.03 Fluid Creativity
330.04 Discodoener
o: Bond Bar - Club
330.05 Gianni Rossi
o: Dejavu Records
330.06 Michaël Pinto
330.07 La Fusée
o: Virgo Music
/:   Clément Perrotte
330.08 Supershapes
o: DC3
330.09 Kallegraphics
o: Stereo Rodeo Studio
330.10 Airside
o: People in Planes
       (Wind-Up Records NY)
330.11 Studio Output
o: Ministry of Sound
330.12 Labor für visuelles
       Wachstum™
o: Monopol Mannheim

331.01 MH grafik
o: Disidente
/:   Pedro Mendoza

331.02 Atelier Télescopique
o: La BIC. Brigade
       d'interventions
       culturelles
331.03 Ashi & office
       Greminger
o: Kick the Balls
331.04 Attak
o: Dynamo Eindhoven
331.05 Zeek&Destroy
o: LaCosaMia Records
331.06 viagrafik
o: expo club köln
331.07 andrew rae
o: Orson Records
331.08 The Skull Dezain
o: T-skrabble DJ'S
331.09 Positron
o: Ace Killer Union

332.01 iaah
o: City Stages
/:   IAAH
332.02 Finsta
o: King of Kings records

333.01 Mikkel Grafixico
       Westrup
o: Organiseret
       Riminalitet
/:   Organiseret
       Riminalitet - Khalern
       - LarsEFX - Slogan
       - KoolJep - DJ Jett
333.02 Resin[sistem] design
o: Rail Records Store
333.03 Maya Hayuk
o: wooster collective/
       vinnie ray
333.04 Masa
o: Los Amigos Invisibles
       - Gozadera Records

334.01 Masa
o: Los Amigos Invisibles
       - Gozadera Records
334.02 Le_Palmier Design
o: poolside records
334.03 Emil Hartvig
o: Sinatra Recordings
/:   Nancy Sinatra
334.04 Roya Hamburger
o: Foolmoon Band
/:   Jasper den Dulk
334.05 Konstantinos
       Gargaletsos
o: Clever Brains Fryin'
/:   Point Blank Inc

334.06 Le_Palmier Design
o: die poolfamilie
334.07 human empire
o: morr music
334.08 kame design
o: Ann Oyama
/:   (c) 2005 Ann Oyama
       and kame design
334.09 Ottograph
o: supperclub
334.10 Raffaele Primitivo

335.01 ZIP Design
o: Club Rock
335.02 Stockbridge Interna-
       tional
o: Baseshot/Law&Order
335.03 Attak
o: Liberty Valance
335.04 Norwegian Ink
o: Lydia Laska
335.05 Parra
o: Carl Craig & Gamall
335.06 Alëxone
o: the heatshkok
       project band
335.07 Sellout Industries
o: The Good People
335.08 Tohyto
o: Nosordo & Aa Records
335.09 jewboy Corporation™
o: Teder Music

336.01 Parra
o: Bitterzoet
336.02 DTM_INC
o: Homebrew Recordings
336.03 Dimaquina
o: Lontra Music
/:   João Rodrigues João
       Filho
336.04 Alëxone
o: SAKO
336.05 Naho Ogawa
o: Bamboo Stream
336.06 112 Ocean Drive
o: Ove med skägget
336.07 Dennis Worden
o: Feuled By Ramen Inc.
336.08 ZIP Design
o: 6 Feet Records
336.09 human empire
o: morr music
336.10 Crush
o: Union
336.11 nem
o: lina
336.12 Ottograph
o: MAW

336.13 Catalina Estrada
       Uribe
o: All Stars DJ's
       Festival
336.14 dynamo-ville
o: Sea Otter (band)
336.15 Formdusche
o: rio bravo

337.01 tstout inc.
o: The Standard
337.02 Form
o: Polydor Records
/:   Form
337.03 Fase
o: PANDA LAB
337.04 Raffaele Primitivo
o: Hydra DJ Set
337.05 Raffaele Primitivo
o: Brigand recordings
337.06 Studio Output
o: Brass Monkey
337.07 Supermundane
o: Hassle Records
337.08 Chris Bolton
o: Escalator Records
337.09 Engine
o: DnBXXL™
337.10 Raffaele Primitivo
o: Hydra DJ Set
337.11 Dr. Alderete
o: The Mutants - Ranch
       Records
337.12 Jason Kochis
o: Lowlife Superhero
/:   copyright Lowlife
       Superhero
337.13 Positron
o: Victor Entertainment
337.14 nem
o: susie
337.15 Attak
o: Black Rebel
       Motorcycle Club
337.16 dzgnbio
o: peace off

338.01 Hypnoteis
o: Skip The Rush
338.02 Discodoener
o: emi music
338.03 newoslo
o: MIX
338.04 red design
o: rise robots rise

339.01 Dirk Rudolph

339.02 evaq studio
o: Beck / Interscope
       Records
339.03 AmorfoDesignlab™
o: PastillaDigital™
339.04 3 deluxe
o: The Dalles

340.01 Lifelong Friendship
       Society
o: Favourite Sons
340.02 Jussi Jääskeläinen
o: Players Paradise
       Recordings
340.03 Chris Bolton
o: Bikini Wax

341.01 Zeek&Destroy
o: Buddy Records / Edel
       Records
341.02 Le_Palmier Design
o: Universal Music
341.03 Stolen Inc.
o: Vespertine
341.04 Dirk Rudolph
342.01 Adapter
o: Yamaha Corporation
342.02 ZIP Design
o: Nebula Music
342.03 Maya Hayuk
o: Jackie-O Mother-
       fucker/ ATP Records
342.04 Martin Kvamme
o: Sony/BMG
342.05 Büro Destruct
o: Lovebugs
342.06 Out Of Order
o: Hot-kitchen
342.07 Yoshi Tajima
o: Fate Records
/:   Yoshi Tajima

343.01 Cape Arcona
       Typefoundry
o: The Sound Of Animals
       Fighting
343.02 Engine
o: Ministry Of Sound
343.03 AmorfoDesignlab™
o: Buddy Akai
343.04 Ohio Girl Design
o: Ambulete / Capitol
       Records
/:   Andy Mueller
343.05 Miha Artnak
o: DaIIra
343.06 Zeek&Destroy
o: Combination Records

343.07 Martin Kvamme
o: Karin Park
343.08 Grandpeople
o: Hot Hot Hot!
343.09 ROM studio
o: Black Cherry Band
343.10 zookeeper
o: Small is beautiful
343.11 ROM studio
o: Black Cherry Band
343.12 Atelier télescopique
o: Natacha Tertone
343.13 zucker und pfeffer
o: Remute
343.14 Carlos Bêla
o: Inker + Squat

344.01 Power Graphixx
o: Womb
344.02 Tsuyoshi Hirooka
o: shop33
344.03 Studio Output
o: Brass Monkey
344.04 Hydro74
o: Flicker Records

345.01 Herbert Baglione
o: Gigolo Records
345.02 Moving Brands
o: Keane
345.03 No-Domain
o: LAE
345.04 Jared Connor
o: The Mars Volta
/:   Jared Connor and
        Jermaine Rogers

346.01 No-Domain
o: Sonar
346.02 Anónimo Studio
o: Subcultura
/:   Anónimo Studio
346.03 DTM_INC
o: Homebrew Recordings
346.04 Extraverage
        Productions
o: mamarecords
346.05 Braveland Design
o: Grand Royal
346.06 Braveland Design
o: Spirite & Grand Royal
346.07 Rinzen
o: The Brides of Frank
346.08 Le_Palmier Design
o: Universal Music
346.09 C100
o: zerwirk
346.10 Hula Hula

346.11 TGB design
o: Form
346.12 Plastic Kid
o: Atreyu

347.01 weissraum.de(sign)
o: DJ DaBrink
347.02 Yorgo Tloupas
o: Set Grand Prix
347.03 Dimomedia Lab
o: Big Martino
347.04 Salon Vektoria
o: Colourful Grey
347.05 Keep Adding
o: Finish The Fight
/:   Finish the Fight
347.06 Rinzen
o: Ponyloaf
347.07 ehquestionmark
o: awakenings
/:   awakenings
347.08 Joe A. Scerri
347.09 Barbara Lippe
o: Club Cerberus Vienna
        (Oliver Riebenbauer)
347.10 Inocuodesign
o: Urban Funke
347.11 Raffaele Primitivo
o: hydra DJ Set
347.12 Jason Kochis
o: One Way Letter

348.01 red design
o: tru thoughts
348.02 Insect Design
o: IE Music/London

349.01 Yoshi Tajima
o: International Deejay
        Gigolo Records
349.02 Lifelong Friendship
        Society
o: The Favourite Sons
349.03 Slang
o: Proptronix

350.01 Parra
o: Bitterzoet
350.02 Inocuodesign
/:   Ninja Tunes
350.03 ehquestionmark
o: lex records
350.04 ehquestionmark
o: lex records
/:   lex records   Alexis
        Griszka
351.02 Tohyto
o: Simple Parties

351.03 ZIP Design
o: The Sanderson Pitch

352.01 Laundry
o: mtv networks, USA
/:   for Stardust Studios
352.02 Nish
o: Thugfucker
352.03 struggle inc.
o: Sonotheque
352.04 Jeremyville
o: Jamm 4 Genes
352.05 Sellout Industries
o: the saint
352.06 Sellout Industries
o: momentan music
352.07 human empire
o: morr music
352.08 human empire
o: morr music
352.09 Christian Walden
o: Köllifornia
352.10 Hugh Morse
o: Warner Music Group
/:   Hugh Morse
352.11 inkgraphix
o: DJ Flax
/:   Mattias Lundin
352.12 Lifelong Friendship
        Society
o: The Favourite Sons
352.13 human empire
o: morr music
352.14 Lousy Livincompany
o: Smallville
352.15 the red is love
o: Paura
/:   Francesco Curci
352.16 Grandpeople
o: Platebutikken Tiger

353.01 Hyl Design
o: Ai Records
/:   c2006 Hyl Design
353.02 red design
o: skint records
353.03 Joe A. Scerri
353.04 Crush
o: palm pictures
353.05 viagrafik
o: surogat
353.06 Neubau.
o: Mamasweed Music
        353.07 viagrafik
o: fatcat sounds
353.08 Grandpeople
o: Melektronikk

353.09 Umeric
o: MTV Networks
        Australia
/:   Umeric /
MTV Networks Australia.
353.10 Engine
o: About a Kid
353.11 typotherapy+design
        inc.
o: PITB music
353.12 typotherapy+design
        inc.
o: ptr music
353.13 Laundry
o: mtv networks, USA
/:   for Stardust Studios
353.14 viagrafik
o: kanister records
353.15 Miha Artnak
o: Kosta
353.16 Ketchup Arts
o: DJ Die

354.01 DTM_INC
o: Homebrew Recordings
354.02 ehquestionmark
o: lex records
354.03 tstout inc.
o: WRUV Radio
354.04 Jussi Jääskeläinen
o: Moodmusic Records

355.01 Out Of Order
o: Supernatural
355.02 Pietari Posti
o: Wolmar Viski &
        Haaveet, The Band
/:   Pietari Posti
355.03 Parra
o: Paradiso & Mr. Wix
355.04 Parra
o: Paradiso & Mr. Wix
355.05 Parra
o: waxwell record store
355.06 Out Of Order
o: Supernatural
355.07 Rinzen
o: Heavy Trash
355.08 JDK
o: Higher Ground
355.09 Parra
o: Jimmy Woo
355.10 Parra
o: Jimmy Woo
355.11 Parra
o: rushhour
355.12 Nonstop
o: Poko Rekords Oy

355.13 tstout inc.
o: Dolorean
355.14 Oliver Kartak
o: Uptight Recordings
355.15 Raffaele Primitivo
o: Hydra DJ Set
355.16 struggle inc.
o: Dooka Records Bootleg

356.01 Hula Hula
o: Fobia /Sony BMG
356.02 A-Side Studio
o: Fishaman Records
356.03 the red is love
o: Paura
/:   Francesco Curci
356.04 clandrei
o: Danger League
356.05 Form
o: Mercury Records
/:   Form
356.06 nem
o: purejam
356.07 Kallegraphics
o: Dupassdegdudentomp
356.08 the red is love
o: Paura
/:   Francesco Curci
356.09 PMKFA
o: Rickard Jäverling
356.10 No-Domain
o: Dead Beat
356.11 Hausgrafik
o: Tamedia AG
356.12 Masa

357.01 usugrow
o: SMD
357.02 Nando Costa
o: Plastiq Phantom
357.03 stylorouge
o: 679 Recordings
/:   Stylorouge / 679
        Recordings
357.04 Akiza
o: Prikosnovénie
357.05 Martin Kvamme
o: Universal Music
357.06 Akiza
o: Prikosnovénie
357.07 Cape Arcona
        Typefoundry
o: Festland
357.08 derfaber
357.09 Nohemi Dicuru
o: Kremadelik
        onlineradio
357.10 Sammy Stein
o: renardo crew

358.01 Flavio Bagioli
o: Super 45 music e-
       magazine
358.02 C100
o: Bohannon
358.03 Keloide.net
o: Famas loop
358.04 Codeluxe
358.05 red design
o: tru thoughts
358.06 Systm
o: Funk Harmony Park
358.07 Slang
o: Kid606
358.08 Pfadfinderei
o: kommerz.ch - online
       music magazin
358.09 Magenta Creative
       Networks
o: AFC Music
/:   Francisco Allendes
358.10 :phunk studio
o: MTV ASIA
358.11 Axel Domke
o: Nanda ZIP
358.12 Bionic Systems
o: Jenna G, UK
/:   Bionic Systems
358.13 viagrafik
o: 0611 club
358.14 Alexander Wise
o: Elias
358.15 viagrafik
o: zorn records
358.16 Positron
o: Muture Communications

359.01 Grandpeople
o: Paraplay
359.02 evoq studio
o: Kudu
359.03 Laundry
o: mtv networks, USA
/:   for Stardust Studios
359.04 Creative Pride
o: Gatecrasher
359.05 QuickHoney
359.06 Flavio Bagioli
o: Umho Negro
359.07 dzgnbio
o: L.T.R Records
359.08 Engine
359.09 Hyl Design
o: Concrete Plastic
/:   c2006 Hyl Design
359.10 Mattisimo
o: Heroine, band

359.11 AmorfoDesignlab™
o: The Grocery™
/:   -1:0:1
359.12 Yuu Imokawa
o: R and C
/:   Yuu Imokawa
359.13 yippieyeah coopera-
       tive
o: ny sushi

360.01 Tilt
o: Luna Club, Kiel
360.02 Pep Karsten
o: N-Rec
360.03 Oliver Kartak
o: G-stone Recordings
360.04 Out Of Order
o: Nieuwe Revu
360.05 Maniackers Design
o: Yoshimoto Kogyo
360.06 archetype : interactive
o: wave music company
360.07 Tabas
o: Cannes pantiero music
       festival
360.08 Hyl Design
o: Concrete Plastic
/:   c2006 Hyl Design
360.09 archetype : interactive
o: Musicad
360.10 Out Of Order
o: Supernatural
360.11 desres design group
o: Pooledmusic /
       Ian Pooley
360.12 radargraphics
o: Koninklijk Concertge-
       bouw Amsterdam
360.13 DesignChapel
o: Station Åtta
360.14 weissraum.de(sign)
o: Dualism Music
360.15 Attak
o: Primal Grunt
360.16 Pep Karsten
o: Segment Records
/:   Pep Karsten

361.01 Magenta Creative
       Networks
o: Unabombaz
361.02 CityDeep Music
361.03 weissraum.de(sign)
o: EastWest Records
361.04 red design
o: tru thoughts
361.05 Hyl Design
o: Ai Records
/:   c2006 Hyl Design

361.06 Form
o: For Life Records
       (Japan)
/:   Form
361.07 Raffaele Primitivo
o: Hydra DJ Set
361.08 Studio Output
o: Ministry of Sound
361.09 No-Domain
361.10 dzgnbio
o: peace off
361.11 weissraum.de(sign)
o: Danced Records
361.12 Ketchup Arts
o: meltarea
361.13 SignalStrong
o: ChemicalLens
361.14 red design
o: tru thoughts
361.15 typotherapy+design
       inc.
o: Green Nicks Records

362.01 ten_do_ten
o: fiji rock festival
       2004
/:   cool sound
362.02 ten_do_ten
o: cybird
/:   plug.inc
362.03 dzgnbio
o: duumvirat
362.04 the wilderness
o: Concord Dawn
362.05 Floor Wesseling Ix
       Opus Ada
o: beatcase productions
362.06 resistro®
o: DJ Nado Leal
362.07 Syrup Helsinki
o: Design Forum Finland
362.08 Resin[sistem] design
o: Simian Army
362.09 Tohyto
o: Simple Parties
362.10 viagrafik
o: ballerstatus usa
362.11 JDK
       Higher Ground
362.12 Raffaele Primitivo

363.01 Jason Kochis
o: Sony Signatures
/:   copyright Sony Signa-
       tures, Inc.
363.02 Floor Wesseling Ix
       Opus Ada
o: minstrel productions

363.03 Inocuodesign
o: Dj vadim / Ninja
       Tunes
/:   Ninja Tunes
363.04 Hydro74
o: Flicker Records
363.05 Yuu Imokawa
o: R and C
363.06 dainippon
363.07 archetype : interactive
o: Alpha Visual
       Intelligence
363.08 apishAngel
o: Dope Dragon records
363.09 Ketchup Arts
o: kitchen
363.10 Raredrop
o: Wavemaster
363.11 Raredrop
o: MTV Japan
363.12 Raredrop
o: Risk System Recorded
       Things

364.01 Raffaele Primitivo
o: The Dreamers
364.02 Dan Sparkes
o: Nathan Daniel
/:   Graham Dews
364.03 Insect
o: Ministry of sound
/:   insect.co.uk
364.04 Atelier télescopique
o: Dazed
/:   Dazed
364.05 Raffaele Primitivo
364.06 Raffaele Primitivo
o: Hydra DJ Set
364.07 Raffaele Primitivo
o: Hydra DJ Set
364.08 Raffaele Primitivo
o: Hydra DJ Set
364.09 Dan Sparkes
o: Warp Records
/:   Graham Dews

365.01 struggle inc.
o: Sonotheque
365.02 Hiroki Tsukuda
o: simone
365.03 Raffaele Primitivo
o: Serious Seriez
365.04 News
o: Cinnaman
365.05 C100
o: Cafe am Hochhaus
365.06 No-Domain
o: Sleep Debt

365.07 PMKFA
o: Junior Senior
365.08 Joe A. Scerri
365.09 PMKFA
o: La Vida Locash
       records

366.01 Nish
o: Thugfucker
366.02 Vår
o: Celebrity Lifestyle
366.03 resistro®
o: Titàs + Sony/Bmg
366.04 Dan Sparkes
o: Warp Records
/:   Graham Dews

367.01 ehquestionmark
o: skam recordings
367.02 ehquestionmark
o: skam recordings
367.03 Laurent Fétis
o: Atmosphériques
367.04 Laurent Fétis
o: Escalator Records
367.05 frans carlquist
o: Von Records
367.06 DTM_INC
o: Headrush
367.07 PMKFA
o: Lo-Fi-Fnk/La Vida
       Locash records
367.08 eduhirama
o: collected_beats
367.09 Studio Output
o: Renaissance
367.10 Nish
o: MTV: Mhd
367.11 Sesame Studio
o: Cleave

368.01 Attak
o: The Sympathizers
368.02 Cape Arcona
       Typefoundry
o: Quartermania Record
       Label
/:   Andrew Quarterman
368.03 multifresh
o: holocene music
368.04 Ottograph
o: martinez move
368.05 Hellebek + Lemvig
o: Copenhagen Jazz
       Festival (not used)
368.06 viagrafik
o: coldcur rec.
368.07 raum mannheim
o: ambrose

368.08 Carsten Giese
o: Indiebase.org
368.09 backyard 10
o: Coolibah Music Bank
368.10 Engine
o: Darkestra Media
      Initiatives
368.11 GrafficTraffic
o: We Yo Nee
368.12 Maniackers Design
:   Yoshimoto Kogyo
368.13 weissraum.de(sign)
o: In Focus
368.14 Kasia Korczak / Slavs
o: Exclaim / Jad Wio
368.15 Masa
o: Gozadera Records
368.16 resistro®
o: O Roda
/:   Creative Director -
      Billy Bacon Developed
      at Nú-Dës

369.01 Engine
o: Asylum
369.02 viagrafik
o: skoladdin
369.03 Station
o: Ideal Recordings
369.04 DigitalPlayground
      Studio
o: Stephanie Döring
369.05 Axel Domke
o: Diynamic Music HH
369.06 Tsuyoshi Kusano
      Design
o: Victor Entertainment,
      Inc.
/:   Victor Entertainment,
      Inc.
369.07 Rune Mortensen
o: Trailerpark
      Recordings
369.08 red design
o: estereo
369.09 resistro®
o: DJ Nado Leal
369.10 Station
o: Ideal Recordings
369.11 Grandpeople
o: Grandpeople
369.12 space3
o: Fair Deal Records
369.13 Jun Watanabe
o: Shin Murohime
369.14 Mikkel Grafixico
      Westrup
o: Locals Gang
/:   Mick Murder

369.15 Sagmeister Inc.
o: Lou Reed Music, Lou
      Reed
369.16 Engine
o: Asylum

370.01 strange//attraktor:
o: Organik Rekords
370.02 Danny Franzreb
o: Fourknox
370.03 Engine
o: i.T
370.04 Studio Output
o: Metropolis Music
370.05 Semisans
o: Higher Step Records
370.06 onrushdesign / front
o: Breakbeat.is
370.07 precursor
o: G Groove
370.08 News
o: Last Night On Earth 2
370.09 Salon Vektoria
o: Roxyrainbow
370.10 Crush
o: Union
370.11 Tilt
o: Frank Stallone & The
      Astronauts (Band)
370.12 onrushdesign / front
o: Breakbeat.is
370.13 Attak
o: Pieter Humo
370.14 310k
o: satamile records
370.15 No-Domain
o: Sonar
370.16 ehquestionmark
o: lex records

371.01 Accept & Proceed
o: Doseldorf
371.02 Team Manila
o: Iced Out Records
/:   Richard Gutierrez
371.03 Paul Snowden
o: Modus Operandi
371.04 weissraum.de(sign)
o: Tripple Hill Movement
371.05 News
o: Last Night On Earth 3
371.06 Formgeber
o: Benea
371.07 Labor für visuelles
      Wachstum™
o: grellschwarz
371.08 Le_Palmier Design
o: die poolfamilie

371.09 hintzegruppen
o: club of molecules
371.10 Nando Costa
o: Plastiq Phantom
/:   Plastiq Phantom
371.11 GillespieFox
o: FBi 94.5FM
371.12 Labor für visuelles
      Wachstum™
o: FreeForm Records HH
371.13 Lorenzo Geiger
o: The Clients Funk
      Society

372.01 Michaël Pinto
372.02 Floor Wesseling Ix
      Opus Ada
o: Jeffrey Croese
372.03 Luca Marchettoni
372.04 Attak
o: Achtung Gestaltung
372.05 Gianni Rossi
o: Tam Tam Studio
      Recordings
372.06 Raffaele Primitivo
o: dj primitivo
372.07 News
o: Travelling
372.08 Tsuyoshi Hirooka
o: Victor Entertainment,
      Japan

373.01 Miha Artnak
o: Oru
373.02 raum mannheim
o: ann eleven
373.03 Sammy Stein
o: renardo crew
373.04 yippieyeah coopera-
      tive
o: ny sushi
373.05 clandrei
o: Flowkati
373.06 Miha Artnak
o: Slon in Sadez
373.07 Kjetil Vatne
o: Mongrel Records
373.08 Le_Palmier Design
o: Die Plattenkiste
      Hamburg
373.09 Zeek&Destroy
o: Buddy Records / Edel
      Records
373.10 Raffaele Primitivo
o: hydra DJ Set
373.11 frans carlquist
o: Flora & Fauna Records
373.12 AmorfoDesignlab™
o: Pastilla Digital™

374.01 Grandpeople
o: Safe as Milk
374.02 red design
o: tru thoughts
374.03 Pfadfinderei
o: Bpitchcontrol
374.04 human empire
o: morr music

375.01 Cuartopiso
o: Mélodie Lounge
/:   Photography:
      Diana Montoya
375.02 PMKFA
o: King
375.03 Tsuyoshi Hirooka
o: Soviet

380.01 Sagmeister Inc.
o: The Antler,
      Restaurant
381.02 Carlos Bêla

382.01 JDK
o: Meadow Ceres
382.02 Manuel Musilli
382.03 Muller
o: Tom Muller
382.04 Manuel Musilli
382.05 Formgeber
o: Mechamythology /
      Jochen Eeuwyk
382.06 Typosition
o: free project for
      local city
382.07 iaah
o: Soundworks
/:   IAAH
382.08 HardCase Design
      Dmitri Lavrow
o: K&P Kuzmenkov &
      Partners
382.09 Mikkel Grafixico
      Westrup
o: Galleriga
382.09 weissraum.de(sign)
o: Global
382.10 Analog.Systm
o: Helgafell

383.01 Carlos Bêla
383.02 TGB design
o: Technick
383.03 Resin[sistem] design
o: Monash Jewellery and
      Metalsmith club
383.04 Visual Mind Rockets
o: Rudolf Virchow
      Zentrum Würzburg

383.05 Dimaquina
o: Box4 Art Gallery
/:   Juliana Cintra
383.06 Engine
o: Audio+Visual
383.07 Carsten Raffel
o: Familie Wüstefeld
383.08 Flavio Bagioli
o: Michelle Letelier
383.09 Coldwater Graphiix
o: Beams
383.10 Canefantasma Studio

384.01 Coutworks
o: IKI,inc
384.02 AKA
o: Cloudy
384.03 backyard 10
384.04 Jun Watanabe
384.05 human empire
384.06 Hula Hula
o: Domestica Magazine
      México
384.07 Nanospore
384.08 Dan Sparkes
o: Wet Shame
/:   Mat Moran

385.01 chemicalbox
385.02 Three Negative
385.03 backyard 10
385.04 Stockbridge
      International
o: Rustage
385.05 Mikkel Grafixico
      Westrup
o: South Habour
      Copenhagen
/:   Grafixico
385.06 Dan Sparkes
o: Wet Shame
/:   Mat Moran
385.07 actiondesigner

386.01 decoylab
386.02 Gints Apsits
o: AA
386.03 Gints Apsits
o: AA deer
386.04 cubemen studio
o: tilemag

387.01 weissraum.de(sign)
o: ON Kiteboards
387.02 A-Side Studio
387.03 boris dworschak
o: Prickie

387.04 J. Tuominen, Jukka
       Pylväs
o: Jenni&Jukka
387.05 Magnetofonica
o: Isabella Henriquez
387.06 Makak Factory
387.07 Makak Factory
387.08 Miha Artnak
o: ZEK advance
387.09 cubemen studio
o: magmabooks
387.10 J. Tuominen, Jukka
       Pylväs
o: Jenni&Jukka
387.11 Shivamat
387.12 daniel neye / trb.
387.13 ASH
o: The Leisure club
       Mogadishni
/:   Victor Ash
387.14 boris dworschak
o: Prickie
387.15 Draplin
       Gary Longfellow
       Draplin
/:   Aaron James Draplin

388.01 Draplin
388.02 123klan
/:   123klan©
388.03 Fase
       Allah Rabbit
388.04 Accident Grotesk!
388.05 Three Negative
388.06 Gints Apsits
o: Apsits stencil
       division
388.07 Carsten Raffel
/:   Christina Schultz /
       christinaschultz.de
388.08 Draplin
o: Grizzly Habitat
/:   Aaron James Draplin
388.09 Alëxone
388.10 Fase
:   Allah Rabbit
388.11 J. Tuominen, Jukka
       Pylväs
o: Jenni&Jukka
388.12 Naho Ogawa
o: P&R
388.13 Shivamat
388.14 Sanjai Bhana
o: Soma Traditional
       Medicine Clinic &
       Wellness Centre
388.15 Microbot
o: Urban Science

389.01 viagrafik
389.02 Sammy Stein
389.03 Sammy Stein
389.04 HelloBard.com
o: Stupid Devil
389.05 Mini Miniature Mouse
o: myself
389.06 Nando Costa
389.07 Dimomedia Lab
389.08 Attak
389.09 Povilas Utovka
o: CAC TV
389.10 Sammy Stein

390.01 Lapin
390.02 bleed
o: Bleed
390.03 Leon Vymenets
o: personal branding
390.04 Steven Harrington
/:   sh
390.05 Superpopstudio
o: Réseau IDée asbl /
       billy-globe.org
390.06 Carsten Raffel
390.07 Alëxone
o: GM crew
390.08 Positron
o: Yatta
390.09 YOK
390.10 YOK
390.11 Inocuodesign
390.12 Critterbox LLC
o: Gary Baseman
390.13 Lolo
390.14 Adhemas
o: Ricardo Almeida
390.15 Salon Vektoria
o: Transfertex
390.16 Blindresearch

391.01 Critterbox LLC
391.02 Büro Brendel
391.03 ruse76
391.04 seacreative
391.05 Lindedesign
391.06 Magnetofonica
o: Reynaldo Vazquez-Hmto
391.07 Boris Hoppek
o: bimbo sculptures
391.08 onrushdesign / front
o: Self Initiated
391.09 +ISM
391.10 Attak
391.11 june
o: june

391.12 Semisans
o: University of
       Southern Indiana
       Social Work Program
391.13 Alëxone
391.14 Mutabor Design
o: audi
391.15 Flying Förtress

392.01 Linoleum
392.02 Fakir
o: Fakir
392.03 Dr. Alderete
o: Heineken
392.04 Keep Left Studio
392.05 Graeme McMillan
o: Mcmillan Klinker
392.06 Tsuyoshi Hirooka
392.07 human empire

393.01 Ottograph
o: kmdq(painting with
       the guests)
393.02 austrianillustra-
       tion.com
o: buero8/wien
/:   tom mackinger
393.03 interspectacular
393.04 Ryohei Tanaka
393.05 Naho Ogawa
393.06 Gianni Rossi
o: Revolver film
393.07 Lapin
o: ENSERmqz
393.08 Stockbridge Interna-
       tional
o: Supporto Hardcoliko
393.09 actiondesigner
393.10 Blindresearch
393.11 Akiza
393.12 Alëxone
o: alexone.net
393.13 Onlyforthefuture
393.14 Onlyforthefuture
394.01 Christian Walden
o: Shake Your Tree
394.02 Christian Walden
o: Shake Your Tree
394.03 Nanospore, llc
394.04 Kallegraphics
o: Marius Martinussen
394.05 Thomas Nolfi

395.01 Joe A. Scerri
395.02 Three Negative
395.03 Ryohei Tanaka
395.04 Fellow Designers
o: Memfis Film

396.01 decoylab
o: EGO Magazine

397.01 ROM studio
o: Habita Hotel
397.02 Tohyto

398.01 Extraverage
       Productions

399.01 strange//attraktor:
o: The Von Heymann
       Family
399.02 The Skull Dezain
399.03 Alëxone
399.04 Adhemas
o: Oficina de Criação
399.05 Miki Amano
o: Poketo
399.06 Bionic Systems
o: GCS Catering, Germany
399.07 Extraverage Productions
399.08 viagrafik
o: player mag
399.09 Alëxone

400.01 Hjärta Smärta
400.02 Laborator
o: authors font
400.03 Frederique Daubal
o: koslik
400.04 Dan Abbott
400.05 Dan Abbott
400.06 Leon Vymenets

401.01 Tsuyoshi Hirooka
o: MTV Japan
/:   MTV Japan
401.02 ten_do_ten
o: Casey, Colleen and
       Edie Rei Lurie
401.03 ROM studio
o: Habita Hotel

402.01 Studio Sans Nom
o: Prate™ Computer
       Channel
402.02 Studio Sans Nom
o: Prate™ Computer
       Channel
402.03 Dan Sparkes
o: Kuildoosh
/:   Graham Dews
402.04 cisma
402.05 Dan Sparkes
o: Kuildoosh
/:   Graham Dews
402.06 viagrafik
o: pyramid editions

402.07 viagrafik
o: style express berlin
402.08 Tsuyoshi Hirooka

403.01 Koadzn
403.02 Jason Kochis
       Wes Abney
403.03 iaah
o: DC Comics
403.04 Mikkel Grafixico
       Westrup
o: graffitgalleriet.dk
403.05 Extraverage
       Productions
403.06 Laborator
o: authors font
403.07 Magnetofonica
o: Carlos Malavé
/:   Laura González Ron
403.08 KesselsKramer
o: ao
403.09 Laundry
o: gold frontz
403.10 Keep Left Studio
o: Universal Mind
403.11 Keep Left Studio
o: Universal Mind
403.12 Keep Left Studio
o: Universal Mind

404.01 Laundry
o: Joanna
404.02 Ninjacruise
404.03 Laundry
o: Girl Skateboards

405.01 Strukt Visual Network
/:   Donny Delgado
405.02 Alëxone
o: my old dirty french
       car
405.03 Ninjacruise
405.04 Hausgrafik
o: Gruntz Magazin
405.05 Laundry
o: The Rock Collection
405.06 Hula Hula
o: Jeremyville
405.07 Karen Jane
o: Shopaholics Anonymous
405.08 space3
o: freshcotton.com
405.09 Razauno
405.10 Mikko Rantanen
o: The Hand Magazine
405.11 archetype : interactive
o: cyprus cafe
405.12 Niels Shoe Meulman
o: Koopal

405.13 KesselsKramer
o: Capricious Magazine

406.01 Keep Left Studio
o: Becker Entertainment
406.02 Graeme McMillan
406.03 ZIP Design
406.04 DTM_INC
406.05 XYZ.CH

407.01 ten_do_ten
407.02 Dan Sparkes
o: Kuildoosh
/:   Graham Dews
407.03 The Skull Dezain
407.04 The Skull Dezain
407.05 The Skull Dezain
o: Refill magazine
407.06 Studio Maverick
o: pico
407.07 Studio Erosie

408.01 123klan
408.02 Regina
408.03 Salon Vektoria
408.04 Mikkel Grafixico
       Westrup
o: Glock193
408.05 Sellout Industries
408.06 Resin[sistem] design
408.07 viagrafik
o: pyramid editions
408.08 ehquestionmark
o: demon
408.09 Microbot
408.10 Dan Sparkes
o: Kuildoosh
/:   Graham Dews
408.11 Extraverage Productions
408.12 Laundry
o: The Rock Collection
408.13 Cherrybox Studios
/:   JESSICA KNAPP
408.14 ehquestionmark
o: bushra

409.01 Sellout Industries
409.02 Salon Vektoria
409.03 Dimaquina
o: Movida
/:   Ebenezer Bond
409.04 Razauno
409.05 Jun Watanabe
409.06 MvM / Maarten van
       Maanen
409.07 Tsuyoshi Hirooka
409.08 SHOK1
409.09 viagrafik
o: pyramid editions

409.10 DTM_INC
o: Headrush
409.11 Tsuyoshi Hirooka
409.12 Makak Factory

410.01 Tsuyoshi Hirooka
410.02 Laundry
o: Local Logos
410.03 viagrafik
o: pyramid editions
410.04 Labor für visuelles
       Wachstum™
o: Mywolrd™
410.05 Konstantinos
       Gargaletsos
o: BBC
/:   Point Blank Inc
410.06 Tsuyoshi Hirooka
410.07 Power Graphixx
410.08 onrushdesign / front
410.09 Lukatarina

411.01 Plastic Kid
o: Linus
411.02 spin
o: Ilena Makri
411.03 Sellout Industries
o: trouble inc
411.04 Blu Design
o: O galeria
411.05 Kallegraphics
411.06 paulroberts.tv
o: Pacific Island Motion
       Pictures
411.07 Laurent Fétis
411.08 Dan Sparkes
o: Kuildoosh
/:   Graham Dews
411.09 William Morrisey
411.10 No-Domain
411.11 Power Graphixx
411.12 Tsuyoshi Hirooka
411.13 zime SOL crew
o: streetart

412.01 Dan Sparkes
o: Kuildoosh
/:   Graham Dews
412.02 viagrafik
o: Pyramid editions
412.03 Dan Sparkes
o: Kuildoosh
/:   Graham Dews
412.04 Dan Sparkes
o: Kuildoosh
/:   Graham Dews
412.05 viagrafik
o: pyramid editions

412.06 Dan Sparkes
o: Kuildoosh
/:   Graham Dews
412.07 Dan Sparkes
o: Kuildoosh
/:   Graham Dews
412.08 austrianilllustra-
       tion.com
o: Fabienne Feltus
412.09 Power Graphixx
412.10 Extraverage
       Productions
412.11 Faith
412.12 Dan Sparkes
o: Kuildoosh
/:   Graham Dews
412.13 Omochi
o: Yokohama Date
       Wakuwaku
412.14 Mikkel Grafixico
       Westrup
o: Regret915
412.15 The Skull Dezain
412.16 cryogenicx.com

413.01 Dimomedia Lab
413.02 cubemen studio
o: humus
413.03 Resin[sistem] design
413.04 MaMadesign AB
413.05 Mattisimo
o: Jennifer Louie,
       jewelry maker
413.06 Stockbridge Interna-
       tional
o: Spa
413.07 Maak
413.08 Povilas Utovka
o: rütrüt
413.09 Tnop™ & ®bePOS!+IVE
o: Various Clients
/:   Segura Inc.,
       ®bePOSI+IVE design
413.10 derfaber
413.11 MH grafik
o: Simon Beyeler &
       Jola Furrer
413.12 Airside
o: 4 The Record

414.01 Klaus Wilhardt
o: Ulrik Jantzen
       Photography
414.02 Jenni Tuominen, J.
       Pylväs
414.03 Polygraph
o: MdN corporation
414.04 DTM_INC
o: Danny Geerlof

414.05 Friends With You
o: FWY
414.06 Station
o: Kosmik Voodoo
414.07 Engine
o: Audio+Visual
414.08 Mattisimo
o: Embassy Row
414.09 cubemen studio
414.10 Oc/Om/Oy/Ok
o: LDN

415.01 Nando Costa
o: Iconologic
415.02 Nando Costa
o: Iconologic
415.03 Out Of Order
415.04 Omochi
415.05 Tsuyoshi Hirooka
415.06 jl-prozess
o: flucht
415.07 +ISM
415.08 Polygraph
o: MdN corporation
415.09 MaMadesign AB
415.10 Formikula
o: Edition 52
415.11 Tnop™ & ®bePOS!+IVE
o: Various Clients
/:   Segura Inc.,
       ®bePOSI+IVE design
415.12 Omochi
o: Kuishinbo
415.13 resistro®
415.14 Carlos Bêla
415.15 MaMadesign AB
420.13 01 Kontrapunkt
o: giv din hånd

421.01 29 degres
o: Anonymus
421.02 Floor Wesseling Ix
       Opus Ada
o: vspa psychological
       conference group
421.13 03 projekttriangle
o: MAT / University of
       California Santa
       Barbara USA
421.15 04 base
o: Socialist Party of
       Europe (PES)

422.01 Simon & Goetz
o: World Model
       Association
422.02 Kontrapunkt
o: denmark.dk

422.03 David Maloney
o: Cornerstone Church
/:   Airhart & Co.
422.04 Kontrapunkt
o: The Danish Security
       Intelligence Service
422.05 Designunion
o: K-M-Sistas
422.06 3 deluxe
o: Rosenrot
422.07 Brighten the corners
       Studio for Design
       London & Stuttgart
o: Cilt, the National
       Centre for Languages
422.08 Studio Dumbar
o: Champalimaud
       Foundation, Portugal
422.09 Moniteurs
o: Creative Commons
422.10 sunrise studios
o: The Human
       Waterproject
422.11 HardCase
o: Federal Press and
       Information Office,
       Odeon Zwo
/:   Dirk Ostmann
422.12 ABC&Z
o: Porretta Terme
       (Bologna, Italy)
       Turistic Promotion
422.13 29 degres
o: Glaxo Smith Kline
/:   virus Ideenlabor
422.14 Klauser Weibel Design
o: Pfadi Kanton
       Solothurn
422.15 Atelier Mühlberg
o: Pastoralkreis
       Frauenfeld Gachnang
       Uesslingen

423.01 Kontrapunkt
o: forsvarsministeriet
423.02 Superlow
o: Gay Health Community
       Norway
423.03 cabina
o: Gobierno de la Ciudad
       de Buenos Aires
423.04 HardCase
o: Hanover City Council,
       Odeon Zwo
/:   Michael Kronacher
423.05 HardCase
o: Federal State of
       Hesse, AReA
/:   Antonio Pace

423.06 Brighten the corners
o: DfES, Department for
       Education and Skills
       (UK)
423.07 MWK - Zimmermann und
       Hähnel
o: Alexander-Von-
       Humboldt-Stiftung
423.08 Mark Sloan
o: National Kidney
       Foundation
423.09 zookeeper
o: LPO
423.10 Magnetofonica
o: VTV-Goverment TV
       Channel
/:   VTV
423.11 ABC&Z
o: Il Quarzo - Turistic
       Association
423.12 Dimaquina
o: Fernando Gabeira
423.13 Kimera
o: Producciones
       Educación Aplicada,
       DIF Hidalgo (México)
/:   Producciones
       Educación Aplicada,
       DIF Hidalgo (México)
423.14 Hula Hula
o: Magdalena BayKeepers

424.01 Magnetofonica
o: VTV
/:   Laura Sofía González
       Ron
424.02 Fupete Studio
o: Gruppoll
/:   Fabio Lattanzi
424.03 granit di Lioba
       Wackernell
o: Centro sociale la
       Chimica, Verona
424.04 Floor Wesseling Ix
       Opus Ada
o: happyChaos
424.05 the red is love
o: Maisumi*Agency
/:   Rosso
424.06 Emmi Salonen
424.07 Fase
o: accesoya!
424.08 Gints Apsits
o: UNCR
424.09 derek johnson
o: Shake
424.10 Maya Hayuk
424.11 Maya Hayuk

424.12 ABC&Z
o: Handicap Association
424.13 Judith Zaugg
o: Dr. S. Heiniger
424.14 Jeremyville

425.01 sunrise studios
o: Whale Care
425.02 Superpopstudio
o: Réseau IDée asbl /
       billy-globe.org
425.03 Floor Wesseling Ix
       Opus Ada
o: happyChaos
425.04 Shivamat
o: greenpeace
425.05 Mikel Mikel
o: Macmillan Cancer
       Support
/:   Wolff Olins
425.06 HandGun
o: Troubl Media
425.07 HandGun
o: Alone
425.08 Floor Wesseling Ix
       Opus Ada
o: vspa psychological
       conference group
425.09 Emil Hartvig
o: Evil Panda
425.10 human empire
425.11 Floor Wesseling Ix
       Opus Ada
o: cimedart philosophy
       magaine
425.12 anna-OM-line.com
425.13 Carsten Raffel
o: The World Dismay
       Company
425.14 Labor für visuelles
       Wachstum™
o: grellschwarz
425.15 Salon Vektoria

426.01 Superpopstudio
o: Réseau IDée asbl /
       Billy-globe.org
426.02 Grandpeople
o: Senter for Byøkologi
426.03 Jeremyville
426.04 human empire
426.05 the Legalizer
o: Danmarks Sociale
       Forum
426.06 310k
o: legalize campaign
426.07 Out Of Order
426.08 Pentagram
o: The Young Foundation

427.01 onlab
o: German Federal Agency
       for Civic Education
       and raumtaktik
427.02 44 flavours
o: Spanish Fly
/:   Patrick Fuchs
427.03 The KDU
427.04 Loïc Sattler
o: Commodite
427.05 Inocuodesign
o: Serie B Underground
       Magazine

428.01 Extraverage
       Productions
o: Youth For Europe
       Association
428.02 Niels Shoe Meulman
o: Watson & Lewis
428.03 viagrafik
428.04 viagrafik
o: pyramid editions
428.05 viagrafik
428.06 viagrafik
o: pyramid editions
428.07 Floor Wesseling Ix
       Opus Ada
o: ixopusada
/:   Aditude
428.08 june
o: designer for asia
428.09 Atelier Mühlberg
o: Schule Zürich Nord
428.11 Bringolf Irion
o: Sozialdepartement
       Stadt Zürich
428.12 cabina
o: Gobierno de la Ciudad
       de Buenos Aires
428.13 Parra
o: areyougeneric.org
428.14 Loïc Sattler
o: vazz (association)

429.01 Mytton Williams
o: The Countryside
       Agency
429.02 Semisans
o: Evansville Department
       of Urban Forestry
429.03 Superpopstudio
o: Réseau IDée asbl /
       billy-globe.org
429.04 29 degres
o: Agence Romande de
       Renseignement
/:   Piment communication

429.05 Rune Mortensen Design
       -Studio
o: The Norwegian Labor
       Party
429.06 AmorfoDesignlab™
o: Pastilla Digital™
429.07 Power Graphixx
o: POM2
429.08 Attak
o: Stuurgroep
       Dorpsbelang
       Combinatie
429.09 MWK - Zimmermann und
       Hähnel
o: World Humanity Fund
429.10 Atelier Mühlberg
o: Schule Zürich Nord
429.11 Pantiestudio
o: Empresarios Com-
       prometidos con la
       Ecología
429.12 cabina
o: Braga Menendez
429.13 Pixel Storm
o: Università della
       Svizzera Italiana
       (USI)
/:   HGK Luzern
429.14 ABC&Z
o: Comune di Milano
429.15 VIAO1
429.16 Atelier Mühlberg
o: Schule Zürich Nord

430.01 Nando Costa
430.02 JDK
o: Sanctuary
430.03 a+morph
o: Kristin Guttenberg
430.04 MvM
o: Rhijnhof
430.05 Studio Output
o: BBC Radio 1
430.06 Chris Rubino
o: Keep A Child Alive
430.07 BankerWessel
o: Folkpartiet (SE)
430.08 Kosta Lazarevski
o: Red Star
/:   Kosta Lazarevski
430.09 zookeeper
o: kfum spejderne
430.10 Kontrapunkt
o: nagoya univercity of
       arts and sciences
430.11 dainippon
o: Design for Asia

431.01 Floor Wesseling Ix
       Opus Ada
o: happyChaos
431.02 Alexander Fuchs
o: Kulturamt
       Berlin-Pankow
/:   Weißensee School of
       Art Berlin
431.03 Bodara
o: Migrationsmuseum,
       Zurich, Switzerland
431.04 MaMadesign AB
o: SSE Business Lab/
       Gonnabe
431.05 Floor Wesseling Ix
       Opus Ada
o: ixopusada
431.06 dainippon
o: Design Quarterly,
       Shoeisha
/:   Photo: Masanori Ikeda
431.07 dainippon

436.01 Futro
o: Olympic Center Pag

437.01 stylodesign
o: CyberByke
437.02 jum
o: ethos skateboards
437.03 Simon & Goetz
o: Möser Austria
437.04 Simon & Goetz
o: Ballgreen

438.01 Trafik
o: Sport communication
438.02 Büro Destruct
o: RedBull
438.03 Skin Design
o: Ask Sarajevo
438.04 zookeeper
o: Mission motos - Shaw

439.01 AKA
o: Ideenhaus
       for T-Mobile
       (Snowboardteam)
439.02 Velvet
o: Orangetime Expo
439.03 zookeeper
o: Luka
439.04 Draplin
o: Grenade Gloves
/:   Matt Kass
439.05 cabina
o: Sergio Resumil

439.06 JDK
o: Snowboarding Opens
439.07 zookeeper
o: redeye
439.08 GWG
o: Bodymakerpro
439.09 Toxic design
o: Volkers Extreme
/: Atombravo
439.10 Salon Vektoria
439.11 Yorgo Tloupas
o: Black Crows skis
439.12 viagrafik
o: Triplus clothing
439.13 29 degres
o: AFFS | FSSV

440.01 Christian Rothenhagen
o: threebros
440.02 3 deluxe
o: North Kiteboards
440.03 viagrafik
o: drake sports
440.04 The Vacuum Design
o: Freebord
440.05 Carsten Raffel
o: Shivamat
440.06 bleed
o: Qwatee
/: Element Skateboards
440.07 viagrafik
o: fatum
/: RiceHouse
440.08 I&EYE
o: MPG
/: Manila Dragons Rowing
    Team

441.01 Niels Shoe Meulman
o: Revert
441.02 J6Studios
o: Thomi Hawk
441.03 Kimera
441.04 3 deluxe
o: Fanatic
441.05 AmorfoDesignlab™
o: DMAT™
441.06 Parra
o: Nike Europe
441.07 Konstantinos
    Gargaletsos
o: The Times
441.08 J6Studios
o: Houston Area Knife
    Stickers
441.09 Systm
o: KSI
441.10 chemicalbox
o: tropical sunset

441.11 viagrafik
o: player mag

442.01 Ariel Pintos
o: Ken-Zen Dojo
    Venezuela
442.02 Michaël Pinto
442.03 Transittus
o: Universe Sports
442.04 Ketchup Arts
o: ollie magazine
442.05 Coutworks
o: Byakkotai Outerwear
442.06 Shivamat
442.07 Carsten Raffel
o: Shivamat
442.08 GUAK
/: PAU MISSER
442.09 Attak
o: Kleine Tour
    Steenbergen

443.01 anna-OM-line.com
o: Happy Sports
443.02 Digart Graphics
443.03 Studio Maverick
443.04 weissraum.de(sign)
o: Elevator Kiteboards
443.05 Floor Wesseling Ix
    Opus Ada
o: ixopusada
443.06 J6Studios
o: Alumni Skateboarding
443.07 Guadamur
o: Necia Polaca
443.08 Guadamur
o: Necia Polaca
443.09 Ohio Girl Design
o: Girl Skateboards
443.10 Ohio Girl Design
o: Girl Skateboards
443.11 Ohio Girl Design
o: Girl Skateboards
443.12 Kosta Lazarevski
o: girl's workout
    - aerobic studio
443.13 Christian Albriktsen
o: The 50-50 Company
443.14 Carsten Raffel
443.15 Carsten Raffel
443.16 Marcar/kindness
o: O'Neill Europe

444.01 enginesystem
o: Instant Winner
444.02 enginesystem
o: Instant Winner
    Skateboards

445.01 Bionic Systems
o: One Industries
    Motocross, USA
/: Bionic Systems /
    Honda is a registered
    trademark of Honda
    Motor Co.
445.02 Bionic Systems
o: One Industries
    Motocross, USA
/: Bionic Systems /
    Kawasaki is a regis-
    tered trademark of
    Kawasaki Motor Corp.,
    USA
445.03 Nish
o: FTC
445.04 ROM studio
o: La Silla
/: Powerleue
446.03 Simon & Goetz
o: Rotwild/ADP
    Engineering
/: player mag
446.13 Formgeber
o: Tremendous
/: Gordon College
    Athletics - Fighting
    Scots
446.14 Formgeber
o: Tremendous

447.01 Lunatiq
o: Salomon
447.02 Michaël Pinto
o: Decathlon
447.05 bleed
o: Skistar/Hemsedal
    Skicenter
/: Surf
447.06 Yo Freeman
o: 2005
447.08 the red is love
o: Easy Fishing
447.10 National Forest
o: Element Skateboards
447.11 National Forest
o: Element Skateboards
/: Hofstra University
447.12 National Forest
o: Element Skateboards
/: Lucky Dog Ultimate
447.13 National Forest
o: Element Skateboards

448.01 3 deluxe
o: Fanatic
448.02 Engine
o: Fuel

448.03 3 deluxe
o: Fanatic
448.04 C100
o: North Kiteboarding
448.05 leBeat
o: rheincoast surfboards

449.01 A-Side Studio
o: 5boro
/: A-Side Studio
449.02 44 flavours
o: young boys sevetal
/: patrick fuchs
449.03 Jenni Tuominen, Jukka
    Pylväs
o: Numero magazine

450.01 Fase
450.02 JDK
o: JAKE BURTON
/: Trouble
450.07 Floor Wesseling Ix
    Opus Ada
o: club2000
450.08 Draplin
o: Snowboarder Magazine
/: Primedia, Pat
    Bridges,
    Editor-in-Chief

451.01 Magma
o: Starshot
451.02 Emil Kozak
o: Skatebarcelona.com
/: Emil Kozak
451.03 National Forest
o: Element Skateboards
451.04 Raredrop
o: Sun yoga
451.05 viagrafik
o: player mag
451.06 TGB design
o: Jazzy Deportistas
451.07 Lukatarina
o: Tae-Kwon-Do Club
    Tiger
451.08 J6Studios
o: Ricochet Research and
    Development
451.09 J6Studios
o: International Knife
    Throwers Hall of Fame
451.10 Michael Genovese
o: GAM 3 Copenhagen DK.
451.11 VIA01
o: Starshot
451.12 leBeat
o: rheincoast surfboards

451.13 Emil Kozak
o: Lando Footwear
/: Emil Kozak
451.14 I&EYE
o: Paint Inn
451.15 I&EYE
o: 2DIE4 Sports
451.16 Ariel Pintos
o: Club de Kendo Chacao

452.01 Jenni Tuominen, Jukka
    Pylväs
o: Numero magazine
452.02 National Forest
o: Element Skateboards
452.03 National Forest
o: Element Skateboards
452.04 Accident Grotesk!
o: Vespa Tuning Center

453.01 3 deluxe
o: Fanatic
453.02 3 deluxe
o: North Kiteboards
453.03 3 deluxe
o: Fanatic
453.04 3 deluxe
o: Fanatic
453.05 3 deluxe
o: Fanatic
453.06 3 deluxe
o: North Kiteboards
453.07 3 deluxe
o: North Kiteboards
453.08 Magma
o: Starshot
453.09 National Forest
o: Element Skateboards
453.10 WGD
o: Snowboard graphics
    contest by Monson
    Snowboards

454.01 Emil Kozak
o: Instant Winner
454.02 Nish
o: Analog
454.03 JDK
o: Burton Snowboards
454.04 NeoDG
o: sukata jiu jitsu
/: neodg
454.05 3 deluxe
o: North Kiteboards
454.06 Flying Förtress
o: GreenHill Skateshop
454.07 Adam Cruickshank
o: Nike / Publicis Mojo
    Melbourne

454.08 struggle inc.
o:　　JEENYUS SNOWBOARDS
454.09 Guak
/:　　Pau Misser
454.10 Axel Peemöller

455.01 Büro Destruct
o:　　Rawlex
455.02 JDK
o:　　Burton Snowboards
455.03 viagrafik
o:　　fanatic snowboards
455.04 C100
o:　　Forum snowboarding
455.05 Flying Förtress
o:　　Hessenmob Skateboards
455.06 Flying Förtress
o:　　Diem Skateboard
　　　Trucks
455.07 inkgraphix
o:　　Scess Performance
　　　Dance Group
/:　　Patrice Potuznik
455.08 3 deluxe
o:　　Fanatic
455.09 Shinpei Yamamori
o:　　Be.BiKE
455.10 3 deluxe
o:　　Fanatic
455.11 Guak
o:　　Saturn
/:　　Pau Misser
455.12 Alexander Wise
o:　　Street Machine
455.13 Dan Sparkes
o:　　Ken Piyyr Skateboards
/:　　Graham Dews
455.14 Supermundane
o:　　Droors
455.15 Alexander Wise
o:　　Street Machine
455.16 Coutworks
o:　　Byakkotai Outerwear

456.01 bleed
o:　　Hard Rocx
456.02 Tnop™ & ®bePOS|+|VE
o:　　Nike USA
/:　　Arlo Inc.
456.03 Shinpei Yamamori
o:　　Be.BiKE
456.04 Draplin
o:　　Nike
456.05 Intercity
o:　　Carhartt
456.06 Kontrapunkt
o:　　dgi byen
456.07 JDK
o:　　Burton Snowboards

456.08 Kontrapunkt
o:　　adidas-salomon ag
456.09 A-Side Studio
o:　　Salomon
456.10 Dan Sparkes
o:　　Ken Piyyr Skateboards
/:　　Graham Dews

457.01 backyard 10
o:　　North Kiteboards
457.02 Shinpei Yamamori
o:　　Be.Bike
457.03 Keloide.net
o:　　Adikora kite surf
457.04 Sesame Studio
o:　　Board Culture
457.05 Yo Freeman
o:　　CTRL Clothing
457.06 JDK
o:　　Cris Copley
457.07 Yorgo Tloupas
o:　　Empire Snowboards
457.08 3 deluxe
o:　　Fanatic
457.09 viagrafik
o:　　fanatic snowboards

458.01 viagrafik
o:　　fanatic snowboards
458.02 A-Side Studio
o:　　FSC
458.03 Sesame Studio
o:　　Froth
458.04 Nish
o:　　FTC
458.05 Scott Duke
o:　　GP2 SERIES
/:　　The "GP2 SERIES" logo
　　　is a trademark of
　　　Formula One Promo-
　　　tions and Administra-
　　　tion Limited. Used
　　　with kind permission.
458.06 Mattisimo
o:　　Nike, Geoff Hollister
　　　Athletic Club
/:　　Nike
458.07 typotherapy+design
　　　inc.
o:　　rpm spinning and
　　　gravity studio
458.08 Yorgo Tloupas
o:　　Rossignol Snowboards
458.09 Yorgo Tloupas
o:　　street machine

459.01 Draplin
o:　　Snowboard Magazine
/:　　Mark Sullivan,
　　　Jeff Baker
459.02 bleed
o:　　Hard Rocx
459.03 Resin[sistem] design
o:　　Sailboard/kite club
459.04 Michaël Pinto
o:　　Decathlon

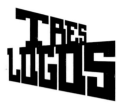

A Collection of Selected Logos

Edited by Robert Klanten, Nicolas Bourquin, Thorsten Geiger

Layout and design by Nicolas Bourquin and Thorsten Geiger
Cover design by Nicolas Bourquin
Index typeface: "T-STAR Mono Round" by Mika Mischler
Foundry: www.die-gestalten.de
Art direction by Robert Klanten

Preface by Robert Klanten and Nicolas Bourquin
Chapter texts and interviews by Roland Müller
Translations by Ian Pepper
Proofreading by Sonja Commentz

Production management by Martin Bretschneider
Editorial support Japan by Junko Hanzawa
Consultancy by Ralf Grauel
Printed by Offsetdruckerei Grammlich, Pliezhausen, Germany

Published by Die Gestalten Verlag, Berlin 2006

ISBN-10: 3-89955-158-3
ISBN-13: 978-3-89955-158-7

© dgv - Die Gestalten Verlag GmbH & Co. KG, Berlin 2006

Bibliographic information published by the Deutsche Nationalbibliothek.
The Deutsche Nationalbibliothek lists this publication in the Deutsche Nationalbiblio-
grafie; detailed bibliographic data is available on the Internet at http://dnb.d-nb.de

For more information please check: www.die-gestalten.de
Respect Copyright - encourage creativity!